# Research Methods
# in Palliative Care

# Research Methods in Palliative Care

## Julia M. Addington-Hall
Chair in End of Life Care, School of Nursing and
Midwifery, University of Southampton, UK

## Eduardo Bruera
Professor and Chair, Department of Palliative Care and
Rehabilitation Medicine, The University of Texas MD
Anderson Cancer Center, Houston, USA

## Irene J. Higginson
Professor of Palliative Care and Policy, Department of
Palliative Care, Policy and Rehabilitation, King's College
London, UK

## Sheila Payne
Help the Hospices Chair in Hospice Studies, International
Observatory on End of Life Care, Institute of Health
Research, Lancaster University, UK

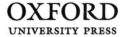

OXFORD
UNIVERSITY PRESS

# OXFORD

UNIVERSITY PRESS

Great Clarendon Street, Oxford OX2 6DP

Oxford University Press is a department of the University of Oxford.
It furthers the University's objective of excellence in research, scholarship,
and education by publishing worldwide in

Oxford New York

Auckland Cape Town Dar es Salaam Hong Kong Karachi
Kuala Lumpur Madrid Melbourne Mexico City Nairobi
New Delhi Shanghai Taipei Toronto

With offices in

Argentina Austria Brazil Chile Czech Republic France Greece
Guatemala Hungary Italy Japan Poland Portugal Singapore
South Korea Switzerland Thailand Turkey Ukraine Vietnam

Oxford is a registered trade mark of Oxford University Press
in the UK and in certain other countries

Published in the United States
by Oxford University Press Inc., New York

British Library Cataloguing in Publication Data

Data available

Library of Congress Cataloging in Publication Data

Data available

Typeset by Cepha Imaging Pvt. Ltd., Bangalore, India
Printed in Great Britain
on acid-free paper by
Biddles Ltd., King's Lynn, Norfolk.

ISBN 978-0-19-853025-1

10 9 8 7 6 5 4 3 2 1

Whilst every effort has been made to ensure that the contents of this book are as complete,
accurate and up-to-date as possible at the date of writing, Oxford University Press is not
able to give any guarantee or assurance that such is the case. Readers are urged to take
appropriately qualified medical advice in all cases. The information in this book is
intended to be useful to the general reader, but should not be used as a means of
self-diagnosis or for the prescription of medication.

# Contents

Section 5 **How to …**

# List of Contributors

**Julia M. Addington-Hall**
School of Nursing and Midwifery,
University of Southampton, UK

**Michael I. Bennett**
St Gemma's Hospice and
University of Leeds, UK

**Eduardo Bruera**
Department of Palliative Care
and Rehabilitation Medicine,
The University of Texas MD
Anderson Cancer Center,
Houston, USA

**Malcolm Campbell**
School of Nursing, Midwifery
and Social Work,
University of Manchester, UK

**Massimo Costantini**
Unit of Clinical Epidemiology,
National Cancer Institute,
Genova, Italy

**Michele Crossley**
Institute for Health Research
Liverpool John Moore's
University, UK

**Sue Davies**
School of Nursing and Midwifery,
University of Sheffield, UK

**Marjolein Gysels**
Department of Palliative Care, Policy
and Rehabilitation,
King's College London, UK

**Richard Harding**
Department of Palliative Care, Policy
and Rehabilitation,
King's College London, UK

**Irene J. Higginson**
Department of Palliative Care,
Policy and Rehabilitation,
King's College London, UK

**Christine Ingleton**
Centre for Health and Social Care
Research,
Sheffield Hallam University, UK

**Laura Kelly**
Surrey and Sussex Healthcare
NHS Trust, Surrey, UK

**Margaret O'Connor**
School of Nursing and Midwifery,
Monash University, Frankston,
Australia

**Sheila Payne**
International Observatory on
End of Life Care, Institute of Health
Research, Lancaster University, UK

**Yolanda Zuriarrain Reyna**
Department of Palliative Care and
Rehabilitation Medicine,
The University of Texas MD
Anderson Cancer Center,
Houston, USA

**Anita Sargeant**
School of Nursing and Midwifery,
University of Sheffield, UK

**Jane Seymour**
School of Nursing,
University of Nottingham, UK

**Frances Sheldon[1]**
School of Social Sciences,
University of Southampton, UK

**Patrick Stone**
St George's University of London
and NHS Trust, London

**Peter Speck**
Department of Palliative Care and
Policy, Kings College London;
School of Psychology, University
of Southampton, UK

**Chris Todd**
School of Nursing, Midwifery
and Social Work,
University of Manchester, UK

[1] Frances died during the writing of this book; her wisdom and expertise in palliative care are evident in the chapter she co-authored for it; she is greatly missed.

# Chapter 1

# Introduction

## Julia M. Addington-Hall

This is, as far as we can ascertain, the first research methods textbook to be focused specifically on palliative care. Given the wide range of other research methods textbooks available, the first task facing us is perhaps to justify the need for such a volume; surely the needs of both neophyte and experienced researchers in palliative care can be adequately met by existing texts. We have written this textbook because we think that palliative care presents particular challenges to researchers, both because of the ethical and practical difficulties which result from working with very ill patients and their families and because of the range of research questions considered to be within the domain of palliative care. New researchers, experienced researchers working in palliative care for the first time and skilled palliative care researchers encountering a question which cannot be answered by their existing research skills would all benefit, we suggest, from a text written specifically for them by researchers with real experience of palliative care research and of the challenges it presents; a text which also encompasses in one volume the range of research methods available to address the physical, psychosocial and spiritual problems of patients and their families.[1] This textbook therefore provides an introduction to the use in palliative care of clinical trials, of survey research, of epidemiological research methods and of qualitative research methods. In all cases, the chapters are written by researchers who are experienced both in the method itself and in applying it within palliative care. In addition, in the final section, a number of issues facing all palliative care researchers are addressed, including how to write a proposal, how to obtain research ethics approval and how to write a paper. Again, these chapters are permeated by an understanding of the challenges facing palliative care researchers and of the contexts in which they work.

Our aim is to contribute to an increase in both the quality and the quantity of palliative care research. Although the amount of palliative care research is increasing, as evidenced by increasing numbers of articles relevant to palliative care indexed in databases such as MEDLINE (a >2-fold increase between 1987 and 2005) and the growing number of palliative care journals, palliative care still has an underdeveloped research base; a meeting of leading supportive, palliative and end-of-life care academics from the UK, the USA and Canada recently concluded that the 'overall pool of investigators and number of research efforts remain proportionately small'.[2] There are still many unanswered questions: participants in this meeting, for example, acknowledged that each of the three countries would have their own priorities, but still identified 10 areas where they considered there to be an urgent need for research. These were:

> measuring symptoms and symptom clusters; study of the biological bases of complex symptom clusters; enhancing research in symptom interventions; family and informal care-giving; the impact of poverty; societal beliefs and approaches to death and end of life care; measuring quality of life within different cultural milieus; performance of the health care system; understanding and responding to transitions in care goals; use of technology to enhance care; and knowledge transfer.[2]

A different group of palliative care researchers might well have generated a different list of areas requiring research (and, indeed, a rather different list was produced in the UK as part of the process of developing evidence-based guidelines for supportive and palliative care[3]). They are unlikely to have too much difficulty in identifying priorities for research in palliative care, however; we currently lack the evidence we need to enable all patients with life-threatening illnesses to live as fully as possible for as long as possible, and to enable us to support their families appropriately both before and in bereavement. More high quality palliative care research is therefore needed. This text is designed to help researchers to design and deliver good research studies in this challenging but important research field.

## The challenges of palliative care research

The World Health Organization (WHO) currently defines palliative care as:

> … an approach that improves the quality of life of patients and their families facing the problem associated with life-threatening illness, through the prevention and relief of suffering by means of early identification and impeccable assessment and treatment of pain and other problems, physical, psychosocial and spiritual.[1]

Some of the challenges inherent in palliative care research can be identified from this definition. First, and fundamentally, palliative care is concerned with people with life-threatening illnesses. Although the WHO definition goes on to say that 'palliative care … is applicable early in the course of the illness',[1] and the principles and practice of palliative care are increasingly recognized as beneficial for people earlier in their disease trajectory, from the point of diagnosis,[4] the majority of people who receive palliative care are in the last months, weeks or days of life.[5,6] Palliative care is concerned with the prevention and relief of suffering because, for many, if not all, this period of their lives is associated with distressing physical symptoms and increased dependency on others as their bodies deteriorate, and with concomitant psychological, social and existential issues. Palliative care research is therefore by definition concerned with a sick patient group who are going to get sicker. This brings with it concerns about whether palliative care research can ever be ethical and, if it can, how to conduct ethically sensitive studies. These are rehearsed below and discussed in detail elsewhere in the text (Chapters 2, 3 and 10).

It also produces practical challenges. It can be difficult to recruit patients to studies because many are too ill to participate (or are thought to be so by the health professionals caring for them), are unable to give informed consent or die before they can be recruited. In addition, as will be discussed below, palliative care patients are a heterogeneous population, and only a minority may therefore 'fit' the study criteria. A recent well-designed and carefully executed large-scale palliative care trial found that only 31 per cent of the screened population was eligible for the study, a fairly typical figure in palliative care.[7] Patient attrition is a major issue in longitudinal studies: only 46 per cent of patients in this trial provided follow-up data at 8 weeks.[7] This, however, greatly exceeds the 32 per cent of patients who completed a clinical trial lasting only a few days in another setting.[8] Not only are recruitment and retention challenging, but the poor health status of many palliative care patients also impacts on data collection (whether quantitative or qualitative), not least because they often have limited concentration and tire easily. It also impacts on the researchers themselves, who are brought face to face with their own mortality as well as often having to deal with multiple losses as research participants die (Chapter 10).

Whilst the WHO definition makes clear that palliative care is concerned with life-threatening illness, it does not clarify this in any way. Palliative care services vary enormously across and between countries in the characteristics of the patients they see in terms of prognosis, diagnosis and the complexity of their problems. Whilst palliative care patients are united in living with a life-threatening illness, they are a very heterogeneous population. This presents challenges in designing good studies (Chapters 2 and 3). These are magnified by the difficulty of accurately judging prognosis, in most settings an (or even the) important determinant of whether patients with life-limiting illnesses are eligible for palliative care services and, by extension, for palliative care studies.

A further challenge for palliative care research is that it is investigating 'an approach that improves the quality of life of patients'.[1] It is therefore concerned not with what traditionally are seen as objective outcomes such as survival and physical indicators of disease regression, but with more subjective outcomes such as 'quality of life' and pain. The science of outcome measurement is relatively young, and the development of outcome measures is particularly challenging in palliative care (Chapter 7). The paucity of good outcome measures is seen as a particularly important obstacle to progress in palliative care research.[9]

Palliative care is concerned with improving the quality of life not only of patients but also of their families. The WHO definition expands on this by stating that 'palliative care ... offers a support system to help the family cope during the patient's illness and in their own bereavement'.[1] Palliative care research also, therefore, has to have the families of palliative care patients within its sight. This requires it not only to engage with the ethical and practical challenges inherent in working with very ill patients, but also to engage in the challenges involved in carrying out research with family members both before the patient's death and into bereavement. This begins to illustrate why palliative care research, like palliative care itself, needs to be multidisciplinary, drawing on a range of research methodologies and on researchers from different professional and academic backgrounds to meet its aims. It is not a narrowly focused field of research endeavour, where adequate research progress can be made by research drawing on any one school of research, whether that be, for example, research informed by the biomedical model, by qualitative research informed by the social sciences or by epidemiological research. Palliative care encompasses physical, psychological, social and spiritual (or existential) issues; it 'uses a team approach to address the needs of patients and their families'.[1] Palliative care research needs to do the same if it is to be able to make progress in addressing all of these issues: it needs to draw on the full range of available research methods, using the one that most appropriately answers the question in hand.

## Ethical issues

As already outlined, palliative care patients may experience physical, psychological, social and spiritual (or existential) distress. They will usually become increasingly dependent on others for help with activities of daily living, although the speed of this will vary with, for example, dependency being more long-lasting in conditions such as heart failure and chronic respiratory diseases than in cancer. Many, if not all, will experience a range of physical symptoms which may change rapidly and which will require prompt and effective intervention. They may have psychological or cognitive symptoms, they may experience spiritual distress and their illness may result in a number of family issues and practical problems. These can lead to palliative care patients being seen as being a particularly vulnerable group, needing special protection in relation to research. Vulnerability in terms of research ethics can be defined as the 'increased potential that one's interest cannot be protected'[10] (p. S26). To view palliative care patients as being vulnerable therefore requires them to be categorized as a group as being less able than other research participants to protect their own interests. There are good reasons to believe that some palliative care patients at least may fall into this category (see Chapters 3 and 10 for fuller discussion of these issues). For example, there is increasing recognition of the high incidence of cognitive impairment and reduced capacity amongst some populations of palliative care patients.[11] Where this reduces patients' ability to understand information about research studies and to make an informed choice about participation, it does make them vulnerable in research terms. Palliative care patients who are resident in in-patient units are also highly dependent on their health care providers; this can make them particularly susceptible to coercion (albeit unintentional), resulting in 'informed choices' which are not truly autonomous and again render them vulnerable. Patients living in the community may similarly be dependent on their health care providers and/or have developed close relationships with them and not want to disappoint them by not taking part in a study; they too may therefore be vulnerable. Indeed, Raudonis[12] has objected to enrolling palliative care patients in studies at all precisely because they are a 'captive audience', dependent on health professionals for their care.

The concept of vulnerability is useful in reminding researchers of the particular care they need to take to ensure that all research participants are able to make autonomous informed decisions about participation in palliative care studies. The question of whether all palliative care patients should be regarded as vulnerable simply because they have a life-threatening illness (and are dying) in the absence of more specific evidence about what they are vulnerable to is more contentious.[10,13] This is, however, the stance taken by most, if not all, Research Ethics Committees and Institutional Review Boards (see Chapter 17 for advice on how to work with ethical committees).

Linked to this is the question of whether palliative care research is ethical at all. The arguments for palliative care being a special case in which the normal safeguards for protecting participants are not adequate include that, as outlined above, palliative care patients are inherently vulnerable; that participants cannot because of their limited life expectancy be expected to benefit directly from the research;[14] that patients have limited time left and the cost to them of participating in research will always therefore outweigh the benefit; and that, as discussed above, as they are a captive audience they are unable to make voluntary choices about research participation.[15] There is now general agreement within palliative care at least that it is not a special case and that the usual methods for protecting research participants, for weighing the risks and benefits of participation for individuals and for ensuring that they are making autonomous, informed decisions to participate therefore apply.[15,16] It can be difficult to persuade Research Ethics Committees of this, however. Health professionals too may be concerned about the ethics of including palliative care patients in research, seeing research as an additional and unnecessary burden on already burdened patients. This overlooks the possibility that patients may receive benefits from participating in research. As Fine has argued:

> It is just as important to note that participation in research can have anti-comiogenic value, that is, bring an overriding sense of purpose and meaning to the patient and family. That is, instead of additive burdens, there is oftentimes perceived benefit, through 'helping', 'companionship', 'attention', and similar positively viewed attributions of being involved in a social enterprise[17] (p. S58).

Even very sick patients may wish to participate in research for altruistic reasons, to give something back to society, or even to make some sense of their situation.

There is beginning to be a small body of literature which has asked palliative care patients themselves their views on research participation. A qualitative research study of Australian hospice in-patients found that all wanted to participate in research.[18] Supporting Fine's argument, the most common reasons for this were altruism, enhancement of a sense of personal value, the assertion of continuing autonomy and the importance they attached to doctors seeking to improve palliative care via research. They rejected the idea that they were not capable of autonomous consent. A quantitative study in the USA found that nearly half of hospice patients were interested in participating in interview or survey research, or in therapeutic research.[19] Their informal caregivers were more interested in research, both for themselves and for the patient. Younger patients were more interested in research, but those aged over 75 were as interested as other people of the same age. A small UK study of hospice in-patients reported that two-thirds would be willing to participate in a trial; this reduced to half for the most invasive trial scenario (involving venepuncture and random drug allocation) and increased to three-quarters for a reflexology trial.[20] All three of these studies dealt with hypothetical situations rather than with patients' actual experiences of research participation, which may be different. However, a study from the USA of patients who had participated in research interviews indicated that they were positive about their experience.[21] These studies suggest that palliative care patients take a more positive attitude to research participation than health professionals and ethical review committees might expect. A note of caution is needed in that the patients represented here were, by definition, well enough to give consent and to participate in research; they do not, therefore, represent the views of all palliative care patients. These findings do, however, provide further evidence for the view that, whilst great care must be taken to adopt the highest possible ethical standards in palliative care research, there is no reason to consider all palliative care patients as inherently vulnerable and requiring special ethical protection.

Ethical issues in palliative care research are considered from the perspective of clinical trials in Chapters 2 and 3, and from the perspective of qualitative research in Chapter 10: issues specifically related to research ethics committees are considered in Chapter 17. Given the centrality of ethical issues to both palliative care and palliative care research, it will come as no surprise to the reader to find that they also occur throughout the book. It could, indeed, be argued that the whole book is concerned with the ethics of palliative care research in that it is primarily focused on enabling researchers to choose an appropriate research method, to design a high quality study and then to execute this successfully; as Cassarett *et al.* argue:

> ... a study is only ethically sound if its risks are reasonable in proportion to its potential benefits, and the knowledge to be gained. Thus, palliative care researchers ... must demonstrate that their research questions are important, their methods are appropriate to produce valid results, and that their findings are generalizable[16] (p. S5).

## Outline of the book

This book begins with a section focused on clinical trials. In Chapter 2, Bennett introduces the principles of designing clinical trials in palliative care. In Chapter 3, he is joined by Reyna and Bruera in considering the particular ethical and practical issues involved in designing and conducting clinical trials in palliative care.

The next section is concerned with survey research (Section 2). In Chapter 4, I introduce the principles underlying the design of scientific research surveys, with particular emphasis on sampling and on response rate, and on why these matter. Chapter 5 is concerned with methods of data collection in surveys, questionnaire design and the piloting of questionnaires.

The next three chapters introduce epidemiological research methods (Section 3). In the first, Chapter 6, Costantini and Higginson consider the use of experimental and quasi-experimental research designs in palliative care. Chapter 7 by Higginson and Harding is about outcome measurement, while in Chapter 8 Gysels and Higginson provide an introduction to systematic reviews, together with a summary of systematic review methods.

Section 4 is concerned with qualitative research methods. In the first chapter (Chapter 9), Payne provides a comprehensive overview of qualitative methods of data collection and analysis. In a companion chapter to Chapter 2, in Chapter 10 Sheldon and Sargeant consider ethical and practical issues in palliative care research from the perspective of qualitative research. Crossley then reflects in Chapter 11 how qualitative research should be evaluated. In Chapter 12, Ingleton and Davies provide a guide to evaluating palliative care services, with particular emphasis on mixed method research. Chapter 13 by Seymour discusses ethnography, in which researchers become involved in the daily lives of a small group of patients. The last chapter in this section, Chapter 14 by O'Connor, is focused on documentary analysis and policy, and introduces discourse analysis.

The final section of the book, Section 5, is rather different from the previous sections in that it does not introduce specific research methods; instead it aims to answer questions readers may have about 'how to' do particular things in research. In Chapter 15, Kelly and Stone address the question of 'how to develop a research question'. Once the question has been developed, the next stage in the research process is to write the research proposal and (often) to obtain funding; this is addressed by Todd in Chapter 16. In Chapter 17, Speck provides advice on how to obtain research ethics approval, and in Chapter 18 Campbell answers the question of 'how to use a statistician'. Finally, I consider what to do once the study is completed by addressing 'how to write a paper'.

## Conclusion

It is our hope that this textbook will provide a useful introduction to the range of research methods available to help us understand more about the experiences of people in the last months, weeks and days of life and of their families, and to develop and test effective interventions to improve their care. As the authors emphasize throughout the book, what is essential is that the right research methods are chosen to address the question of interest, and that the resulting study is then planned and delivered to the highest possible standard. Palliative care needs to be underpinned by a firm foundation of innovative, high quality and diverse research; we hope that this textbook will help make this a reality.

## References

1. World Health Organization (2005) http://www.who.int/cancer/palliative/definition/en/ Accessed 20 October 2006.
2. Hagen NA, Addington-Hall J, Sharpe M, Richardson A, Cleeland CS (2006) The Birmingham International Workshop on Supportive, Palliative, and End-of-Life Care Research. *Cancer* **107**: 874–81.
3. Gysels M, Higginson IJ (2000) *Improving Supportive and Palliative Care for Adults with Cancer: Research Evidence.* London: National Institute of Clinical Excellence.

4. **Ahmedzai, SH, Walsh TD** (2000) Palliative medicine and modern cancer care. *Seminars in Oncology* **27**: 1–6.

5. **Eve A, Smith M, Tebbitt P** (1997) Hospice and palliative care in the UK 1994–5, including a summary of trends 1990–5. *Palliative Medicine* **11**: 31–43.

6. **Lamont EB, Christakis NA** (2002) Physician factors in the timing of cancer patient referral to hospice palliative care. *Cancer* **94**: 2733–7.

7. **Abernethy AP, Currow DC, Hunt R, Williams H, Roder-Allan G, Rowett D, Shelby-James T, Esterman A, May F, Phillips PA** (2006) A pragmatic $2 \times 2 \times 2$ factorial cluster randomised controlled trial of educational outreach visiting and case conferencing in palliative care—methodology of the Palliative Care Trial. *Contemporary Clinical Trials* **27**: 83–100.

8. **Reymond L, Charles MA, Bowman J, Treston P** (2003) The effect of dexamethasone on the longevity of syringe driver subcutaneous sites in palliative care patients. *Medical Journal of Australia* **178**: 486–9.

9. **Kaasa S, De Conno F** (2001) Palliative care research. *European Journal of Cancer* **37** Suppl 8: S153–9.

10. **Agrawal M** (2003) Voluntariness in clinical research at the end of life. *Journal of Pain and Symptom Management* **25**: S25–32.

11. **Casarett DJ** (2003). Assessing decision-making capacity in the setting of palliative care research. *Journal of Pain and Symptom Management* **25**: S6–13.

12. **Raudonis BM** (1992) Ethical considerations in qualitative research with hospice patients. *Qualitative Health Research* **2**: 238–49.

13. **Koenig BA, Back AL, Crawley LM** (2003) Qualitative methods in end of life research: recommendations to enhance the protection of human subjects. *Journal of Pain and Symptom Management* **25**: S43–52.

14. **Janssens R, Gordijn B** (2000) Clinical trials in palliative care: an ethical evaluation. *Patient Education and Counselling* **41**: 55–62.

15. **Addington-Hall JM** (2005) Palliative care research in practice. *Canadian Journal of Nursing Research* **37**: 85–93.

16. **Casarett DJ, Knebel A, Helmers K** (2003) Ethical challenges in palliative care research. *Journal of Pain and Symptom Management* **25**: S3–5.

17. **Fine PG** (2003) Maximising benefits and minimising risks in palliative care research that involves patients near the end of life. *Journal of Pain and Symptom Management* **25**: S53–62.

18. **Terry W, Olson LG, Ravenscroft P, Wilss L, Boulton-Lewis G** (2006) Hospice patients' views on research in palliative care. *Internal Medicine Journal* **36**: 406–13.

19. **Williams CJ, Shuster JL, Clay OJ, Burgio KL** (2006) Interest in research participation among hospice patients, caregivers, and ambulatory senior citizens: practical barriers or ethical constraints? *Journal of Palliative Medicine* **9**: 968–74.

20. **Ross C, Cornbleet M** (2003) Attitudes of patients and staff to research in a specialist palliative care unit. *Palliative Medicine* **17**: 491–7.

21. **Emanuel EJ, Fairclough DL, Wolfe P, Emanuel LL** (2004) Talking with terminally ill patients and their caregivers about death, dying, and bereavement: is it stressful? Is it helpful? *Archives of Internal Medicine* **164**: 1999–2004.

# Section 1

# Clinical trials

Chapter 2

# Principles of designing clinical trials in palliative care

Michael I. Bennett

## Introduction

Clinical practice in palliative care is focused on improving the quality of life for people that are facing advanced and incurable disease. A key element of this process is intervening to control the symptoms of advanced disease, for example pain, fatigue, nausea, breathlessness and psychological distress. These clinical interventions or treatments may take many forms, including professional assessment and advice, medicines, surgical procedures and complementary therapies.

A reasonable question that patients and clinicians may ask is 'what is the benefit or harm that a particular treatment will bring about?' Sadly, for a range of treatments in health care, and particularly so in palliative care, we simply do not have the answers to these questions. This can sometimes leave everyday decision making in clinical practice as little more than a coin-tossing process; for example, do we use metoclopramide or cyclizine for this patient's nausea?

Clinical trials are essentially experiments to test and quantify the benefits and harms of a particular clinical treatment. In the absence of good quality evidence from clinical trials to guide decisions, less reliable means are often used.[1] This leads to significant variations in practice and runs the risk of exposing patients to useless treatments. Perhaps worse still is that we may cause unnecessary harm by denying patients treatments that may turn out to be effective if subjected to a clinical trial, or giving treatments that turn out to have reliably more side effects than benefits.

This chapter will focus on designing experimental studies that seek to examine the effects of clinical interventions.

## Clinical trial terminology

### Experimentation

Observation and other descriptive methodologies are useful techniques to identify whether a relationship or association exists between one variable and another. An experiment is simply a test that is conducted to explain the relationship between two or more variables, i.e. is the relationship one of cause and effect? For example, you may discover through repeated observation that when you give a certain drug to nauseated patients who have been admitted to your in-patient unit, their symptoms improve greatly. There is clearly a relationship between giving the drug and patients feeling better (an 'association'). What is not clear is whether giving the drug actually *causes* the improvement. Until this is tested within a clinical trial, other explanations may be equally valid. For example, the patient may improve because they feel safe and less anxious now they have been admitted to your unit; they may be taking a Chinese herbal remedy that they have not told you about; they have been removed from an emetic substance at their home, and so on.

## Hypothesis

A good research question in clinical research is usually presented in the form of a hypothesis or an assumption about something that is observed in clinical practice. Hypotheses can also be thought of as formal statements of predictions. To use the example above, the hypothesis might be that the drug causes the reduction in nausea (an equal hypothesis is that admission to the in-patient unit causes symptom improvement). In order for this assumption about cause and effect to be valid (discussed below), we can design an experiment or clinical trial to test whether patients given the drug do in fact become less nauseated.

Despite having a clear assumption or hypothesis about the outcome of the trial, it is essential that this is just an assumption and that the investigator (experimenter) does not have evidence or an overwhelming belief to the contrary. This state of not knowing is called 'equipoise' and is an essential component of ethical research practice. It is discussed in more detail in the following chapter (Chapter 3).

## Efficacy and effectiveness

Clinical trials can be subdivided into explanatory and pragmatic trials. An *explanatory trial* seeks to determine whether a treatment has efficacy, i.e. whether it works under ideal conditions. Data from these types of trials help the understanding of mechanisms or biological principles by which a treatment might work. Such trials normally investigate a single causal factor, very often (but not always) a drug.

*Pragmatic trials*, on the other hand, investigate effectiveness: whether the intervention works in typical clinical practice conditions for a patient with the condition. These trials often investigate more than one variable at a time.

For example, while an explanatory trial might compare a new drug with a placebo (an inactive substance), a pragmatic trial might compare the new drug with best current treatment and identify whether it works better in older versus younger patients, or in those with more advanced disease versus patients with less advanced disease, and so on. The investigator usually wishes to address both efficacy and effectiveness, and it is sometimes difficult to distinguish an efficacy trial clearly from an effectiveness trial. This distinction between theoretical and practical may, however, offer a useful perspective for making design choices in complex cases.

## Variables

A variable is any characteristic that can vary across people or situations that can be of different levels or type. Examples are age, sex, pain intensity, number of vomits in 24 h, length of stay in a hospice, and so on.

There are two main types of variable: dependent and independent. Dependent variables are those that will be measured to determine whether any experimental effect has occurred. In the example above, the subjective intensity of nausea or the number of vomits in 24 h may be useful dependent variables. A reduction in both would obviously be expected if the drug (or other intervention) was effective.

Dependent variables need to be measurable and appropriate. Clinical research in palliative care often deals with subjective measures such as patients' report of their symptom intensity. This can be difficult to record in ill patients, but an added challenge is that the measuring process also needs to be sensitive enough to detect small but important changes. A scale that only has 'a lot better' or 'a lot worse' as outcomes will not detect modest improvements in symptoms (Chapter 7). Dependent variables also need to be appropriate. For example, we may hope to improve a patient's quality of life (QoL) by giving them the anti-emetic drug. However, QoL may well be influenced by other things that are happening to the patient, for example changes in their place of care, a deterioration in their pain levels due to disease progression or unexpected events in the family affecting the patient's mood. Even if nausea improves, QoL as a whole may not. If we only measure QoL, a true effect of the drug may then be missed.

Independent variables are those that are studied to determine whether they are the cause of any effect or outcome. Commonly, the independent variable in a clinical trial will be the intervention itself—the dose of drug or the duration of therapy for example. Some independent variables can be controlled. The dose of drug or other characteristics of the intervention are examples of this. Others are fixed, such as gender and age.

## Confounding

The power of the clinical trial or experiment relies on its ability to examine the effect of the independent variable on the dependent variable and deduce whether a cause–effect relationship exists. To do this, the potential effects of other variables on the dependent variable need to be excluded. If these effects are not excluded, confounding (or bias) of the clinical trial can occur, which can render the results impossible to interpret.

There are several potentially confounding variables that are usually known at the start of the trial, such as age and gender. Others, however, can be subtle, such as place of care, style of clinician or the patient's own behaviour within the trial, and there will be several more completely unknown to the investigator, sometimes called 'chance' effects. The influence of known variables is usually managed by stratifying recruitment and allocation so that equal numbers of men and women are recruited or allocated, etc. The challenge comes when trying to deal with subtle or unknown variables. Techniques for addressing this aspect include randomization, blinding and use of placebos, and are discussed in more detail below.

## Validity

A critical element of all clinical trials is whether the results they give represent 'the truth', which is usually described as validity. Important aspects of a trial's validity are discussed in more detail below but commonly include whether the intervention was given consistently, that the effects of other variables were excluded and that outcomes were measured using sensitive instruments. An additional measure of whether the results of a trial represent the truth is that they can be repeated by different investigators or within another group of similar subjects. This is referred to as reliability. A clinical trial design can be reliable but not necessarily valid (the design merely ensures consistent results) and so it is important to consider all measures of validity when designing a clinical trial.

# Basics of clinical trial design

## Treatments, controls and placebos

The design of any clinical trial relies on establishing the effects of the independent variable. The simplest design is to compare the outcomes (changes in dependent variable) when the independent variable is present and when it is absent, using two groups in a clinical trial. These two situations are commonly called the intervention and the control arms, respectively.

Clinical trials that examine treatment effects on subjective symptoms are challenging because of the large number of influences on symptom expression.

Although a physical explanation for the symptom is often sought (e.g. a large cancer eroding through the femur causing pain), a range of psychological and social influences impact on the interpretation and expression of physical sensations by the patient. Clearly then, a patient who has high expectations that a given treatment will be effective is likely to respond positively. This is called a placebo effect—the change in a patient's illness attributable to the symbolic import of a treatment rather than a specific pharmacological or physiological property. An added complication is that the passage of time often changes symptom expression, either because of natural physical fluctuations or because other external influences also fluctuate.

Placebo effects can be quite impressive. In many placebo-controlled trials of analgesics, improvements in pain scores of around 30–40 per cent in the placebo group are not uncommon. A recent example involved a trial of gabapentin in cancer neuropathic pain.[2] In this study, both treatment and placebo achieved a reduction in pain intensity of 30 per cent. By day 10 of the study, 62 and 64 per cent of patients had experienced good pain control in the gabapentin and placebo groups, respectively.

The control arm is thus a critical element of the clinical trial. Explanatory trials will normally involve a placebo control because of the need to establish some intrinsic efficacy of the treatment over a non-treatment. The control arm of a pragmatic trial is more likely to be a comparative treatment, perhaps one that is regarded as the current best treatment or 'gold standard'. Some trial designs of course incorporate all three: study intervention, standard comparator and placebo. This allows the study intervention to be assessed alongside both controls. Another approach is to use an 'active placebo', a treatment that has some pharmacological or physiological effect, but not on the dependent variable under study. The purpose of this type of control is to maintain the patient's belief that they are taking an active treatment rather than inactive placebo and to prevent them distinguishing between the two arms. Common examples of active placebos used in some clinical trials of analgesics include benzodiazepines and anti-muscarinic drugs. Both types of drugs provide a mixture of sedation or dry mouth which may convince the patient of an active treatment. This helps to maintain the trial's validity in properly assessing the placebo response.

The use of placebos (active or inactive) within clinical trials in palliative care is controversial[3,4] (Chapter 4), despite limited evidence of effectiveness of many treatments currently used.[5]

## Parallel or crossover design

These design types refer to the arms of the clinical trial.[6] In parallel designs, patients are allocated to one of the arms and stay with this allocation throughout the trial. If patients are allocated one arm at the start of the trial but are then swapped to the other arm, the design is called crossover and each patient in the trial receives intervention and control. Other terms that are used for these designs are 'between subjects' and 'within subject', signifying that the intervention and control are being compared between different patients or within each patient, respectively. The crossover trial appears to be superior because it reduces the confounding effects of the patient themselves—each arm is tested on the same patient. However, as you might expect, there are advantages and disadvantages to each type.

The crossover design largely eliminates between-patient variation and, because of this, the validity and reliability of the trial are greater than for a parallel trial with the same number of patients. The corollorary of this of course is that for any given level of validity, fewer patients are required in a crossover design than in a parallel design.

There are problems with a crossover design, however, which can be magnified in a palliative care context. As patients are required to cross over treatments, the length of the trial is often longer than that of a similar trial with a parallel design. Increased length introduces two difficulties. First, the patient's condition or symptom may undergo natural fluctuations such that by the time of the second arm, symptoms are naturally better or worse, regardless of which arm they are currently allocated to. The patient may of course undergo other interventions such as radiotherapy for their pain, or have been given an additional treatment for their symptom by their normal clinician, albeit inadvertently. The second problem is that palliative care patients are, by definition, ill with advanced disease and their disease can accelerate without warning. This can result in the patient dropping out of the trial, either because they are too ill to continue or because they have unexpectedly died. In trials performed in palliative care, the number of drop-outs at the end of the study may be large enough to invalidate the results.

A further complication of crossover designs is called 'order' or 'carry-over' effects. These refer to the effects from the first study arm on the dependent variable persisting into, and influencing, the second arm. For example, carry-over effects may be mediated by persistence of drug or its metabolites (prolonged elimination of the drug from the patient's body), a long-lasting change in physiology caused by the treatment, or behavioural effects (the patient may have less stamina or be less willing to complete outcome measures accurately).

An interesting example of an order effect is illustrated in a clinical crossover trial that examined the effects of clinician posture on patients' ratings of compassion during a 'breaking bad news' consultation.[7] Patients clearly ranked clinicians who sat down as more compassionate than those who stood.

For some unexplained reason, however, they ranked the clinician in the second sequence as more compassionate than the first, regardless of the clinician's posture. This might be because the patients had had time to adapt to the bad news in the second sequence, and so thought of the clinician as more compassionate.

In contrast, parallel designs are shorter but require larger numbers of patients, although it is not simply twice the number required in a crossover design if two 'arms' are studied. This can result in fewer drop-outs and eliminates carry-over effects. Parallel designs are most useful for clinical situations in which the symptom may not be stable or the risk of drop-out is high. This is a very real problem, as illustrated in one recent study where only 12 of 38 palliative care patients who were entered into a short clinical trial lasting only a few days completed the trial.[8]

Crossover designs are best for studies in uncommon but relatively stable conditions or when single research centres are used, because fewer numbers are needed. A special type of crossover design called 'n-of-1' trial is sometimes used in this latter situation. This refers to a randomized crossover trial in one patient, and is most helpful for clearly determining whether an individual patient responds best to one drug or another, or one drug versus placebo.

## Randomization

### Rationale

The randomized controlled trial (RCT) is regarded as the most robust method for evaluating new treatments. It is normally attributed to Sir Austin Bradford-Hill.[9] Since then it has become the 'gold standard' for much investigation in the clinical sciences.

Randomization is a technique to ensure that as few differences as possible exist between different arms of a trial by giving every patient an equal chance of being allocated to each of the experimental conditions. For example, patients are randomly allocated to arm A or arm B, or to sequence A (drug first, placebo second) or sequence B (vice versa). One key feature of a randomized trial is that is tackles the central issue of confounding. Randomization ensures that known and unknown confounding variables are distributed equally, and allows greater confidence that any effects are due to the intervention. Successful randomization allows for valid statistical interpretation of 'raw' results, i.e. estimates that are unadjusted for other patient characteristics. However, successful randomization does not guarantee a perfect balance in risk factors between groups due to the play of chance, so adjusted analyses can also help in further interpretation of outcome results. An important aspect of randomization is that it does not eliminate confounding variables; it merely distributes such variables equally. This reduces the overall bias in the clinical trial.

In a clinical trial report, it is important to document that random allocation of treatment assignment was successfully achieved. The CONSORT statement suggests that the sequence generation, allocation concealment and implementation be reported.[10]

## Sequence generation

Simple randomization is the most basic method of random treatment assignment. This can be thought of as tossing a coin for each trial participant, A being allocated with 'heads', B with 'tails'. However, it is not usually performed using a real coin toss, as issues of concealment, validation and reproducibility arise (see below). Simple randomization is usually achieved using a sequence of random numbers from a statistical textbook, or a computer-generated sequence. Each patient recruited to the trial is allocated according to the next number in the sequence, e.g. AABABABBBA (A and B represent different arms or sequences).

In a large trial (at least 1000 subjects), simple randomization should give a balance in number of patients allocated to each of the groups in the trial, but for a small study the numbers allocated to each group may not be well balanced. In small trials, to maintain good balance, block randomization may be used. Blocks with equal numbers of As and Bs (A = intervention and B = control, for example) are used, with the order of treatments within the block being randomly permuted. A block of four has six different possible arrangements of two As and two Bs. A random number sequence is used to choose a particular block, which sets the allocation order for the first four subjects. Similarly, treatment group is allocated to the next four patients in the order specified by the next randomly selected block. The process is then repeated. Permuted block randomization ensures treatment group numbers are evenly balanced at the end of each block.

Stratified block randomization can further restrict chance imbalances to ensure the treatment groups are as alike as possible for selected prognostic variables or other patient factors. A set of permuted blocks is generated for each combination of prognostic factors. For example, in a trial of chemotherapy for breast cancer, suitable stratification factors might be menopausal status and oestrogen receptor status. A set of permuted blocks is generated for those women who are pre-menopausal and oestrogen receptor negative, another set for those who are pre-menopausal and oestrogen receptor positive, and so on. Stratification can add to the credibility of a trial, as it ensures treatment balance on these known prognostic factors, allowing easy interpretation of outcomes without adjustment.

Methods of allocation such as alternate allocation to treatment group, or those based on patient characteristics such as date of birth, order of entry into the clinic or day of clinic attendance, are not reliably random and are therefore inappropriate. Such allocation sequences are predictable, and not easily concealed, thus reducing the guarantee that allocation has indeed been random, and that no potential patients have been excluded because of prior knowledge of the intervention.

## Concealment of the allocation process

It is very important that those responsible for recruiting patients into a trial are unaware of the group to which a participant will be allocated, should they agree to be in the study. This avoids both conscious and unconscious selection of patients into the study. 'Allocation concealment' is the term used to describe this process, and underpins successful randomization strategies. For multicentre clinical trials, central randomization by telephone, interactive voice response system, fax or the Internet are ideal methods for allocation concealment. The clinician or data manager at the participating site assesses eligibility, gains consent and makes the decision to enrol a patient, then calls the randomization service to get the treatment allocation. Central randomization also enables trial coordinators to monitor randomization rates, and have a record of all allocated patients for potential follow-up.

For single-centre clinical trials, it is usually possible to identify a staff member not involved with the trial who can keep the randomization list or envelopes, preferably in a location away from the clinic or ward where patients are being assessed. For example, pharmacy staff may be able to undertake randomization. They should be instructed to keep the list private, and only to reveal a treatment allocation after receiving information demonstrating that the patient is eligible and has consented to the trial.

In situations where remote randomization may not be feasible or desirable, a set of opaque tamper-resistant envelopes may be provided to each participating site. The envelopes should look identical, and each should have the trial identification and a sequential number on it. Inside is the treatment allocation and usually a trial identifier for the patient (e.g. unique sequential number). After assessing eligibility and consent, as described above, the next envelope in sequence is opened.

## Implementation

The trial statistician (or others not directly involved in recruiting patients to the trial) commonly generates the randomization sequence. Methods that allow a permanent record of the sequence created are important to validate its randomness later if required. A clinical trial report should clarify who generated the sequence, the method used, and how concealment was achieved and monitored. There should be some demonstration that randomization was successful. This is usually achieved by providing a table in a report comparing the major baseline demographic and prognostic characteristics of the two treatment groups.

# Blinding

## Rationale

Blinding usually refers to keeping patients, investigators and those collecting and analysing clinical data unaware of the assigned treatment, so that they should not be influenced by that knowledge. This is important as the expectations of both patients and investigators can influence findings, particularly in palliative care where there is subjectivity in symptom assessment. Blinding is used to reduce this confounding.

The relevance of blinding will vary according to the clinical trial context. Blinding is much more important in trials assessing symptom management than trials assessing chemotherapy for example, where the response criteria are more objective such as survival or biochemical markers of disease. Clinical staff involved in a clinical trial should be blinded to treatment allocation to minimize possible bias in patient management and in assessing disease status. This bias might manifest in the decision to withdraw a patient from a study or to titrate the dose of medication, and could easily be influenced by knowledge of which treatment group the patient has been assigned to. Clinical trials that do not include blinding in general report larger effect sizes for treatments than blinded trials.

## Single or double blind

The term single blind means that either the patient (most commonly) or the investigator does not know the treatment allocation. In a double blind trial, neither party is aware of the treatment allocation. Blinding means more than just keeping the initial allocation hidden ('allocation concealment'). It also refers to maintaining the concealment throughout the clinical trial. Both patients and investigators may detect differences in the appearance of the treatment (size, colour, duration, administration, etc.), so these aspects should be identical for each treatment group.

Using placebos in a clinical trial will only allow proper assessment of the placebo effect if the patient and investigator are unable to detect differences between the placebo and the treatment. Sometimes, there are unavoidable differences in the appearance of two treatments, for example one drug tablet is blue and the other is red. One method of maintaining blinding in this context is to use a 'double dummy' approach. Here, an identical placebo for each treatment is given alongside the alternative drug—blue drug plus red placebo, or vice versa.

Blinding can be difficult to achieve or is sometimes impossible. This is particularly true when the intervention is not a drug: it is not possible to blind the patient to whether they are receiving counselling or not, for example, or nurses to the fact that the patient has been randomized to receive one wound dressing regime rather than another. Single blind trials (e.g. the investigator is not blind to the allocation) are sometimes unavoidable, as are open (non-blind) trials.[11]

## Blind assessment of outcome

In a double blind trial, it is implicit that the assessment of patient outcome is done in ignorance of the treatment received. Such blind assessment of outcome can often also be achieved in trials which are open (non-blinded). For example, a shuttle walking test for breathlessness before and after treatment can be assessed by someone not involved in running the trial.

Sometimes blind assessment of outcome may be more important than blinding the administration of the treatment, especially when the outcome measure involves subjectivity. An example is measuring the effects of blood transfusion in palliative care. Despite the best intentions, some treatments have unintended effects that are so specific that their occurrence will inevitably identify the treatment received to both the patient and the medical staff (e.g. nebulized local anaesthetics for cough resulting in tell-tale pharyngeal numbness). Blind assessment of outcome is especially useful when this is a risk.

# Determining sample size of a clinical trial

## Null hypothesis and errors

Having designed an ideal clinical trial that has appropriate controls against which to compare the treatment, and minimizes bias through randomization and blinding, we want to find out how many patients will need to be recruited to tell us whether the treatment is effective or not.

To answer this question, we need to review our hypothesis.

Let us return to the working hypothesis we discussed at the beginning of the chapter, that a certain drug reduces nausea in cancer patients, and imagine that we have designed a clinical trial to test this cause–effect relationship. When determining whether the drug works, it is convention to test the opposite hypothesis, called the 'null hypothesis', which would state that the drug has no effect at all in our patients. This is done because it is easier to show that a hypothesis is wrong than to show that it is correct. Therefore, if it can be shown that the null hypothesis is wrong, then we must accept the alternative, that the drug does actually work.

There are two types of error that affect the interpretation of clinical trials. The first is called 'type I error' in which a true null hypothesis is rejected, even though no difference between drug and control exists. This sometimes happens if the two groups are not equal in some aspect, or blinding or allocation are inadequate. It can lead to the acceptance of a treatment that does not work. A type II error is the opposite: a null hypothesis is accepted when the drug does actually work. This error also happens when there has been poor allocation, but is particularly true when the sample size is too small. In other words, the clinical trial is not sensitive enough to detect a treatment difference.

## Primary versus secondary outcomes

It is essential to specify the main outcome variable which will be used to decide the result of the trial. This is usually called the primary outcome or primary end-point. It is important that only one primary outcome is chosen; if that variable is statistically significant, then it would be reasonable to conclude that the treatment under investigation had 'worked' or was superior to its comparator. We usually need to specify the size of any effect that we might expect to see if the drug or treatment does actually work. For example, we might state that a new drug for nausea would reduce symptom scores by 50 per cent whereas a placebo control might only reduce scores by 20 per cent. Previous research can be used to help determine the likely size of any effect, perhaps from preliminary trials, observational case studies, and so on.

Often trials will want to investigate a number of additional variables, perhaps related to potential side effects. These too should be specified in advance, and are called secondary outcomes or secondary end-points. Although statistical analysis is usually performed on secondary outcomes, the interpretation is different from the result of analysing the primary outcome. The main analysis of a trial should first answer the original questions relating to the primary outcome. Sometimes researchers wish to investigate other hypotheses, but such results should be presented cautiously and with much less emphasis than the main findings. This particularly applies to subgroup analyses where we might seek out a group of patients in which the treatment is especially effective.

## Power calculations and significance levels

To minimize the chance of an incorrect conclusion to the trial, we need to determine what power our trial will have to prevent a type I or II error from occurring. The 'power' of a clinical trial is the probability that the null hypothesis will be correctly rejected and is commonly set at 80 per cent, or sometimes 90 per cent if it is especially important not to miss a real treatment effect.

Using our primary outcome or end-point, we can choose to design a trial that will show either superiority over a control arm, or equivalence. The latter design is used to show that a new treatment is just as effective as the gold standard treatment. At this stage of the clinical trial design, it is essential to consult a statistician (Chapter 18). They will calculate the number of patients needed to complete the study using information on a number of aspects, including primary outcome measure, the study design, effect size of clinical importance, desired power and the desired significance level.

The desired significance level is the probability ($P$-value) of obtaining a treatment effect in the study if the null hypothesis is actually true. It is accepted convention to use a level of 5 per cent or $P = 0.05$ as the cut-off ($P$ is a value that can be calculated from statistical tests on the data). This means that if the null hypothesis were true (no difference between arms exists), then there is less than a 5 per cent probability of observing a true effect by chance alone. If the effect seen has a $P$-value $<0.05$ (5 per cent), then we can conclude that it is very unlikely to have occurred because of chance alone, and we then accept the effectiveness of the treatment (i.e. we reject the null hypothesis). Of course, it still means that if 20 different researchers conducted identical trials, one of them would observe an effect by chance alone, even though the treatment may be useless. For this reason, significance levels are sometimes set lower at 1 per cent or $P = 0.01$. The lower the significance level, the less likely it is that a type I error will occur.

## Conclusion

RCTs have drawbacks. They are usually expensive to run, take a long time to conduct and are carried out on selected patient subsets. The high degree of selectivity may limit the ability of clinical trials to explain the effects of treatments once the treatments are used in more heterogeneous real world populations. Despite these drawbacks, randomized clinical trials with adequate levels of blinding and minimization of other sources of bias are able to provide the highest level of evidence to support or reject treatment effects. Other clinical trial designs exist that have not been covered in detail here. These include prospective cohort studies, which are observational rather than experimental, and are often used when randomization is impractical or unethical (Chapter 6). Evidence from randomized clinical trials can be pooled to examine a true effect size of a particular treatment, and there are several rules that govern whether such data can be pooled. The power of this meta-analytic approach lies in the fact that a larger aggregate sample size usually reduces the probability that observed treatment effects, or lack of, are due to chance alone, resulting in fewer type I and II errors (Chapter 8). Designing and conducting clinical trials of treatments in palliative care is difficult but remains an important process in building the scientific basis for this clinical specialty. Clinical trials are therefore a necessary component of a broader research process that seeks to improve the quality of life for palliative care patients. In the next chapter, some of the ethical and practical challenges involved in designing and conducting clinical trials in palliative care are addressed.

## References

1. Issacs D, Fitzgerald D (1999) Seven alternatives to evidence based medicine. *British Medical Journal* **319**: 1618.
2. Caraceni A, Zecca E, Bonezzi C, Arcuri E, Yaya Tur R, Maltoni M, Visentin M, Gorni G, Martini C, Tirelli W, Barbieri M, De Conno F (2004) Gabapentin for neuropathic cancer pain: a randomized controlled trial from the Gabapentin Cancer Pain Study Group. *Journal of Clinical Oncology* **22**: 2909–17.
3. Hardy J (1997) Placebo controlled trials in palliative care: the argument for. *Palliative Medicine* **11**: 415–8.
4. Kirkham SR, Abel J (1997) Placebo controlled trials in palliative care: the argument against. *Palliative Medicine* **11**: 489–492.
5. Bell RF, Wisloff T, Eccleston C, Kalso E (2006) Controlled clinical trials in cancer pain. How controlled should they be? A qualitative systematic review. *British Journal of Cancer* **94**: 1559–67.
6. Mazzocato C, Sweeney C, Bruera E (2001) Clinical research in palliative care: choice of trial design. *Palliative Medicine* **15**: 261–4.
7. Strasser F, Palmer JL, Willey J, Shen L, Shin K, Sivesind D, Beale E, Bruera E (2005) Impact of physician sitting versus standing during inpatient oncology consultations: patient's preference and perception of compassion and duration: a randomized controlled trial. *Journal of Pain and Symptom Management* **29**: 489–97.
8. Reymond L, Charles MA, Bowman J, Treston P (2003) The effect of dexamethasone on the longevity of syringe driver subcutaneous sites in palliative care patients. *Medical Journal of of Australia* **178**: 486–9.
9. Bradford-Hill A (1951) The clinical trial. *British Medical Bulletin* **7**: 278–82.
10. Moher D, Schulz KF, Altman DG (2001) The CONSORT statement: revised recommendations for improving the quality of reports of parallel group randomized trials. *Annals of Internal Medicine* **134**: 657–62.
11. Ahmedzai SH, Brookes D (1997) Transdermal fentanyl versus sustained-release oral morphine in cancer pain: preference, efficacy, and quality of life. The TTS-Fentanyl Comparative Trial Group. *Journal of Pain and Symptom Management* **13**: 254–61.

Chapter 3

# Ethical and practical issues in designing and conducting clinical trials in palliative care

Yolanda Zuriarrain Reyna, Michael I. Bennett and Eduardo Bruera

## Introduction

Clinical trials provide the strongest evidence for the effectiveness, efficiency and acceptability of clinical interventions.[1,2] As discussed in the previous chapter (Chapter 2), without evidence from clinical trials, clinicians lack an important source of information to guide their clinical practice. This is a particular issue in palliative care where clinical research has not evolved at the same pace as clinical and educational palliative care programmes.[3] As a consequence, there is limited evidence for many of the interventions used in palliative care. Most of the pharmacological interventions in common use have not been tested in robust, well-powered clinical trials. This is also true for most counselling techniques, for the use of complementary and alternative medicines, and for other palliative care practices such as the use of hydration, the use of oxygen therapy and practices related to nutrition. As a consequence, practice varies widely between centres (and indeed, between clinicians within centres), and the establishment of consensus regarding optimum treatments is difficult.

If palliative care patients are to receive the best possible care, it is important that clinical trials become more widespread in palliative care and that the evidence base for palliative care interventions increases as a consequence. The previous chapter has focused on the principles of designing clinical trials in palliative care. In this chapter, a number of ethical, administrative and methodological issues that need to be addressed in the process of conducting clinical trials in palliative care are reviewed, and solutions discussed.

## Ethical issues

### Basic ethical principles

Ethics plays a crucial role when integrating medical science, patient choice and cost in making appropriate decisions. There are four basic principles of ethics: beneficence, non-maleficence, respect for autonomy and justice.[4]

**Beneficence** is the obligation to further the welfare or well-being of others and also includes the obligation to prevent and remove harms and to weigh and balance risks and benefits of the action. Palliative care research is usually designed to improve the patients' or families' quality of life. It implies this principle of beneficence, to do the best for patients and families.

**Non-maleficence** is enmeshed with beneficence. It refers to avoiding the affliction of evil or harm and promoting good.

**Autonomy** refers to the potential of the individual to be self-determining, and includes recognizing a patient's capabilities and perspectives, including his or her right to hold views, to make choices and to take actions based on personal values and beliefs. Informed consent is based on this principle of autonomy. For patients to be able to exercise informed consent, they need to receive adequate, relevant and comprehensive information. Only patients who are mentally competent to make such a decision can give informed consent. This is a particular challenge in palliative care because cognitive failure, fatigue and depression are frequent. Confidentiality is also an element of the principle of autonomy. Individuals have the right to control the disclosure of medical information pertaining to them.[5]

**Justice** refers to how benefits and burdens are distributed among all members of society. Balancing individual patient needs with societal needs and cost is difficult for physicians. It is ethical and necessary to do it better in the future. Clinical trials may offer both a societal and personal benefit.

While ethical considerations are important in all research, randomized clinical trials in palliative care place additional ethical demands on the research design. As has already been argued (Chapter 2), controlled trials are necessary in palliative care, and there are some ethical guidelines for clinical research that are useful for palliative care research.[6,7] Ethical guidelines are not necessarily different for palliative care research, but there are special considerations in this patient population[8] (Chapter 1). These include patient vulnerability, treatment allocation and issues around gaining consent. These are discussed below.

### Patient vulnerability

Palliative care patients are a particularly vulnerable group, for whom there is often no second opportunity to improve care. Palliative care patients usually suffer from devastating physical and psychosocial symptoms.[9] Terminally ill patients are in an unstable situation and are usually receiving a combination of drugs.

The word vulnerability is often used in an inexact fashion. Levine defines vulnerability states as those in which individuals are relatively or absolutely incapable of protecting their own interests. He also added that when measured against the highest standards of capability, every person is relatively vulnerable.[10] Palliative care patients are vulnerable for a variety of reasons: they are often dependent on others to meet their physical care needs; they are at increased risk of adverse effects associated with experimental treatments; and their ability to make an informed choice about participation may be reduced temporarily, intermittently or permanently due to cognitive impairment. This vulnerability must be protected, but this does not mean that research participation must be prohibited. Vulnerable persons may be included in research if research bears direct relevance to their medical condition and carries the opportunity of medical benefit to those enrolled or the opportunity to advance knowledge for the class of patients to which they belong and, recognizing the risk of enhanced vulnerability, dedicated safeguards are in place.[9]

## Treatment allocation and use of placebo

The idea of allocating vulnerable patients to less than optimal care is therefore contentious. One issue is the use of placebos. The latest revision of the Declaration of Helsinki strongly supports the use of active controls instead of placebos in clinical trials, except in cases where there are not any proven prophylactic, diagnostic or therapeutic methods.[11–13] In palliative care, these Helsinki rules appear to be less of a threat to the use of placebos in clinical trials since there are so few proven therapies, thereby justifying the use of placebos. The complication is that anecdotal therapies, whose efficacies have not been disproved, have become normalized in modern palliative care.[14] Due to severe patient distress, some argue that withholding an established although unimproved treatment would be unethical.[15] The decision is between what is theoretically correct in terms of trial design if the intention is to conduct an explanatory trial (Chapter 2) and what is seen as acceptable within palliative care. This contentious issue has not been resolved.

The vulnerability of palliative care patients has also focused attention on whether conducting the clinical trial is justified ethically at all. For a trial to be ethically justifiable, there must be real uncertainty as to whether the new treatment is superior to no treatment, or to existing treatments. This is *theoretical equipoise*.[16] Freedman proposes a different understanding of equipoise termed *clinical equipoise*, which exists when there is an honest, professional disagreement among expert clinicians about the preferred treatment.[17] Some authors have argued that this means the treatments in a trial must be precisely balanced (theoretical equipoise), i.e. no empirical grounding for a preference for one treatment over another in a trial can exist.[18] Even when theoretical equipoise exists, it is often difficult to convince others that there is equipoise between trial conditions. This is because the new service, which requires evaluation, is often perceived to be more desirable by professionals, patients and their families.

Equipoise is important in the context of randomized controlled trials (RCTs) because if it is present it means that participants will not suffer relative harm from random assignment to a particular treatment arm: if there is reason to prefer one arm over another, patients assigned to the other arm are at a disadvantage. If equipoise is present, it should not be possible consistently to predict the results of a study in advance, and over a number of RCTs those proving or failing to prove a hypothesis will be approximately equal in number.[19]

Studies have confirmed that investigators often do not know in advance what they will discover, reflecting adherence to equipoise in the design and conduct of randomized trials.[20,21] However, there is a concern that clinical trials sponsored by the pharmaceutical industry result in biased findings.[22] In 2000, Djulvegovic *et al.* examined the quality of 136 published RCTs on multiple myeloma to evaluate whether the uncertainty principle or equipoise was upheld comparing studies favouring experimental treatments over standard ones according to the source of funding.[19] Equipoise was seen in studies funded by non-profit-making organizations, with 53 per cent proving a hypothesis versus 47 per cent failing to prove it ($P = 0.60$). However, in trials supported solely or in part by commercial organizations, new treatments were significantly favoured over standard treatments, with figures of 74 versus 26 per cent ($P = 0.004$). The violation of equipoise in commercially funded studies may occur because treatments that are more efficacious than standard therapy are being tested, so patients are being enrolled into trials with inferior comparative therapies. This violation of equipoise could also be explained by the decision of a sponsor to prevent the publication of negative studies.[22] Determination of equipoise should be a quality control measure in randomized trials, and no trial should be approved without explicit consideration of the uncertainty principle.[23] This is of particular importance in palliative care, where ethical concerns are heightened because of the vulnerability of the patient group.

In a 2004 article, Fries and Krishnan[24] consider that equipoise should be replaced by 'positive expected value'. This allows for placebo-controlled RCTs with predictable results. This is because the ability to design clinical trials for success, and therefore to be able to predict outcomes in advance, implies the ability to cull weak drugs early in the approval process and improve the efficiency of drug development. This in turn reduces the cost of pharmaceuticals,[25] and identifies those drugs that are most likely to be clinically useful and of positive value.[24] The acceptability of this to research participants, and to those tasked with judging the ethical implications of research, has yet to be determined, as has the question of whether it raises particular issues for palliative care research.

## Consent

A major issue for palliative care research is how to obtain informed consent from patients. Patients engaged in research must understand their options after receiving the relevant information, and must be able both to use that information to reach a decision and to communicate that decision clearly.[26]

Obtaining informed consent is a particularly delicate issue, since patients often misunderstand the process of randomization[27] and can find it especially difficult to make such decisions at such a worrying time, especially if doctors do not take the issue very seriously.[28] In addition, there is the problem of how to describe the trial, since not all patients and families will have had the full and frank discussion with their doctors required for open acknowledgement of the patient's condition and prognosis.[29,30] Overcoming these difficulties is possible, but each trial needs to develop carefully an appropriate protocol and procedure to solve the problems the specific trial brings up.

The following issues are relevant.[9] First, language should be particularly simple and the consent form should be concise. This is due to the physical and mental fatigue as well as the psychosocial distress that are often present in both patient and family. Secondly, the patient and/or relative should be given adequate time to read the consent form carefully and discuss it with other family or staff members. Thirdly, mental status should be assessed in patients who are given a consent form (see below). Next, all members of the palliative care team need to be aware and supportive of the research project. It can be distressing for the patient or relative to learn that a member of the team whom they particularly trust is unaware or unsupportive of a given research project. Finally, patients need to know that they can withdraw from a study at any time.

Informed consent in terminally ill patients is problematic because the stability and duration of consent are uncertain, and may be influenced by events emerging in the course of the study. Patients in the palliative care setting are at particular risk of developing a confusional state. More than 80 per cent of patients develop severe cognitive failure before death.[31] Contributing factors include age, polypharmacy, institutional setting, the common occurrence of dehydration, infection and hypoxia, and direct damage to the central nervous system induced by the underlying chronic disorder. Often cognitive impairment may not be obvious to health professionals or family members, as people can mask the worrisome signs of loss of mental function.[32] Cognitive deficits raise significant concern about some patients' ability to understand a study completely. In addition, the inclusion of patients with poor cognition in clinical trials results in poor science because they frequently drop out of a study due to complications or non-compliance.[32] So, in general, these patients should be identified and excluded from clinical trials.

One major exception to this proposal is clinical research into the assessment and management of delirium, because of the high prevalence and devastating consequences of this syndrome on patients, families and staff,[33] and also in studies of palliative sedation. There are two potential methods of obtaining consent for research that requires the recruitment of patients that lack capacity.

### Proxy consent

Consent can be obtained by proxy in patients in whom cognitive failure has already occurred. Under these circumstances, the informed consent of patient's representative will usually be required, although practice varies between countries (in England, Wales and Northern Ireland, there is, for example, no legislation supporting proxy consent[34]). Authorized representatives may be legally mandated individuals or family members recognized by the professional staff as sharing responsibility for family care. In the USA, there is still a lack of clear regulatory protection.[35]

Guidelines and proposed regulations in the USA recommend that a close friend or family member serve as a proxy. The general consensus is that proxies should make decisions regarding research participation in a similar manner to those decisions regarding clinical care. The proxy's decision should reflect a substituted judgement, i.e. what the person would decide if they could decide for themselves.[36,37]

### Advanced consent

Proxy consent may not be adequate in the case of research that presents risks and potential discomforts without reasonable prospect of benefit to the subject's health. A common proposal by which another person can enrol a patient is a research advance directive.[32] Prior to incapacity, the potential subject indicates the kinds of research they would or would not participate in. Research advance directives may have a useful role in palliative care research[36] because they may be a useful way to ensure that proxies use substituted judgements in research; research shows that in general, there is poor agreement between patient and proxy.[38] They may also assist proxies who are reluctant to decide: 60 per cent of proxy decision makers declined to allow their relative to participate in the study because of the reluctance to decide for the patient. There is some evidence that the use of research advance directives is feasible, especially in end-of-life research. For example, Breitbart *et al.* used advanced consent to recruit subjects for a study to test the efficacy and safety of potential treatments for delirium in hospitalized AIDS patients.[39] The investigators obtained informed consent from all subjects admitted to hospital who were not delirious. Subjects were then enrolled if they became delirious. Here the model is not an advance directive. Instead the immediacy and specificity of the study make the decision an advanced consent. Another recent study used a similar advanced consent to support a randomized control trial of two antimuscarinic drugs in the management of noisy respirations associated with retained secretions ('death rattle').[40]

## Practical issues

### Integration of service with the research

There are large areas of clinical practice in palliative care that are based on clinical experience rather than high-quality evidence.[41] Research is essential in order to be confident that the practice is best practice. There is a need to change the culture of palliative care so that research is seen as an integral and essential part of the discipline, and also to be eclectic in the approach to research and the choice of methodologies that are employed[42] (Chapter 1). There is a need to encourage specialist trainees to take time out to do research. Some ethical and practical issues are shown in Figure 3.1.

Adequate research can only take place in areas where excellent care is provided. It is important for researchers with an interest in palliative care to have access to clinical facilities with an adequate concentration of patients in order to interact closely with clinicians.

### Design considerations

Multicentre studies work best

Patients and families are generally willing to cooperate with research if they understand the purpose and potential benefits expected from the study. Obtaining sufficient patient numbers is itself a particular difficulty in palliative care research. Multicentre studies (four or five palliative care units) are better because in some cases it is not easy for small hospitals or palliative care centres to design a study, but they can participate in patient recruitment, and

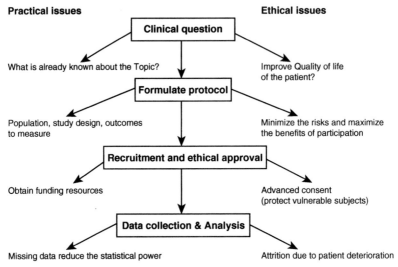

**Fig. 3.1** Practical and ethical questions to apply in a randomized controlled trial.

contribute to the significance of the study designed. In this way, the designed study can be done in a shorter time.

## A short-term study is better than a long study

In palliative care, the patient has limited life expectancy and any delay may seem considerable or, worse still, be equivalent to receiving no intervention at all. Patients often die before they can enter the study or data can be collected.

## A simple design with a limited number of outcomes is best

This may not be easy to achieve because larger numbers of measurements than those normally performed in clinical practice will be necessary to control for confounding variables (e.g. confusion in a patient receiving an analgesic).

## Frequent follow-ups are needed

This is because the patients change very rapidly. Deciding on the timing of measurements is crucial for the success of a trial. Yet in palliative care, timing is problematic as it is dictated by the unpredictable course of the illness, and often there is only a short time between eligibility and death. All of these problems add to overall attrition. In order to optimize results and minimize attrition, it is best to follow-up patients by visiting them in their homes or by telephone, rather than expecting them to return to the hospital or palliative care unit.

## Conducting the trial

The low number of successful trials probably bears witness to the particular difficulties associated with conducting RCTs in palliative care.[43]

**Data collection** represents a major difficulty in palliative care research. Patients, and also caregivers, may have difficulty completing standardized measures, and there is often substantial loss of data.[44,45] Researchers often have no choice but to rely on assessment by proxy and retrospective accounts if a sufficient data set is to be collected. However, the views of informal caregivers and health professionals do not necessarily reflect those of patients.[46]

Ideally, the same person should not be responsible for collecting the data and for conducting the study: careful data collection and skilled data analysis are both vital for good clinical research in this complex area, and combining both roles can threaten the quality of the study, not least because these roles require rather different skills, in addition to the workload implications. Funding limitations mean that this is not always possible; it may also not be desirable at an early stage of a clinical researcher's career when they need to learn by experience the realities of clinical research in palliative care.

**Regular monitoring of recruitment** is necessary to identify early any accrual problems due, for example, to the study being based in an inappropriate clinical setting, excessive criteria for exclusion, other competitive research studies, and so on. It will also identify whether large numbers of those approached are refusing to participate and enable the reasons for this to be identified. These may be related to, for example, the study being excessively complex, to the consent form being poorly worded or to the researcher being inexperienced and needing more coaching in how to approach people. Regular monitoring will also enable the amount of missing data to be identified, which may be due to the number of outcome measures used, to specific characteristics of the ones chosen or to questionnaire design. Early identifications of these problems will allow for changes in the protocol before too much time has passed.

## Analysing and reporting the trial

Missing data are a particularly important problem in clinical trials. Clinical trials need to enrol a sufficiently large sample to be sure that differences between the intervention and control groups can be detected. If the study is too small, it may fail to detect a difference, not because the intervention has no effect, but because the study has insufficient statistical power (type II error) (Chapter 2). Enrolling subjects is not by itself enough; they also need to provide adequate data. Missing data impact on researchers' ability to interpret research findings and, if enough are missing, can make meaningful data analysis impossible.

Because of the frailty of patients in palliative care services, there is often considerable loss of data through failure to complete measures. In the last week of life, even a simple three-item measure designed to elicit patient concerns may achieve less than a one-third response rate.[47] Missing data can present significant challenges to clinical researchers at the data analysis stage.

It is of great importance to approach a statistician very early in the process of designing the study (Chapter 18). The statistician will be instrumental in helping appropriately define the main aims of the clinical trial, the most appropriate analysis for the main outcome and all secondary outcomes, and the sample size required for the clinical trial. The statistician will also help to define the way of dealing with covariates, missing data, multiple comparisons and other problems that might emerge while conducting the trial.

As discussed in Chapter 2, the results of analyses planned in advance and based on pre-specified hypotheses are much more reliable than the results of analyses conducted after the study has been completed. One of the most common errors in palliative care research is to attempt to contact the statistician after the study has been designed or, even worse, when the study has already been conducted. At this point, there might be fatal errors in both the design and data collection that cannot be corrected by the statistician's intervention (Chapter 18).

Ideally, all clinical trials should be reported in scientific meetings and later published as original contributions. In palliative care, it is now quite possible both to present the data in good scientific meetings and to publish in a number of excellent peer-reviewed journals. This is a major improvement as compared with the state of palliative care development 10 years ago.

It is particularly important to publish the results of negative studies (those that did not disprove the null hypothesis) because preferential publications of positive studies may provide false impressions about the efficacy of a given therapeutic innovation.[48] It is also important to submit brief papers reporting on studies in which patient accrual was not possible so as to inform colleagues about why these studies were not completed.

Cooperative studies between different institutions pose a particular challenge for data analysis. It is not possible to conduct subgroup analysis for each of the centres due to lack of statistical power. Therefore, all the data are analysed as a pool. It is important for all participating centres to agree on the process for outcome measurement and data gathering. Even more important, it is crucial for all centres to reach the number of patients they agreed to include in the study, otherwise the whole collaborative study will not have enough power to conduct the statistical analysis and the whole study will collapse. The interdependent nature of collaborative studies is not always understood by centres that offer to participate and estimate a potential number of patients in an excessively optimistic way.

# Administrative issues

## Funding

Uncertain career structures and a relative lack of funding opportunities present challenges to the conduct of high quality clinical research in palliative care. This reflects the historic lack of funds and investment. Funding to support clinical trials is needed if the evidence base in palliative care is to grow, particularly as without dedicated funding clinicians will always find that clinical practice takes priority over research. In order to increase the amount of funding available, it is important that individuals who understand and can promote the importance of funding research in this area attain positions of influence within the different grant-giving agencies. It is also important that independent grant-giving agencies for clinical research in palliative care are developed and nurtured. In order to obtain funding, it is, of course, essential that grant applications are of the highest possible quality and able to compete with other areas of clinical research.

## Career opportunities in palliative care research

One of the major limitations of research in palliative care is the lack of designated granting agencies or even private organizations promoting career awards or funding grants. In the USA, the development of a body of knowledge in geriatrics and cancer was greatly supported by the establishment of the National Institute of Aging and the National Cancer Institute, respectively. There are established fundraising and research-supporting organizations for cancer, heart disease, rheumatic disease, AIDS and a number of other health care problems. Unfortunately, the lack of designated institutions leads to uncertainty in the long-term career planning of young investigators. With the exception of Canada, in most other countries palliative care investigators are required to submit to review panels with minimal or no expertise in palliative care. As a result, the level of expertise of the reviewers in palliative care issues is limited. Proposals are more likely to receive borderline scores and have great difficulty being funded.

Most Faculties of Medicine in North America and the overwhelming majority of those in the rest of the world have no palliative care departments in place. As a result, Faculty members willing to pursue a career in palliative research require appointment to other academic departments. The academic evaluation on an annual basis and the consideration for promotion and tenure will be made overwhelmingly by supervisors with limited understanding of the content and methodology of the individual's research projects.

The establishment of palliative care academic departments would do much to address the question of career pathways for clinical researchers in palliative care. The example of the UK, however, where such departments exist but where career pathways and funding are still an issue in clinical research, suggests that establishing these departments should be seen as an essential and important first step in addressing the question of career pathways, but not the final answer. Increased funding for research is also needed. It would therefore also help if existing private and public granting agencies established palliative care review panels and if powerful advocates for palliative care research infiltrated other panels (a process that has already begun). These measures would greatly improve career stability and would probably increase the attractiveness of palliative care research among young investigators.

## Cooperative research

Because of the lack of resources, it would be ideal to coordinate the effort of the different centres with an interest in developing clinical palliative care research as cooperative national or international groups or as research centres. For example, the European Association for Palliative Care Research Network in one of its initial studies, a cross-sectional survey of palliative care in Europe, has demonstrated the potential of palliative care research networks to work in a coherent and collaborative fashion.

The disadvantage of using some of the already established cancer research networks for palliative care research is that many centres that provide excellent palliative care are not represented within those organizations.

The future for palliative care research lies with networks, be they local, regional, national or international networks, of excellent clinical programmes receiving adequate funding to support their contribution to research studies.

## References

1. Jones B, Jarvis P, Lewis JA, Ebbutt AF (1996) Trials to assess equivalence: the importance of rigorous methods. *British Medical Journal* **313**: 36–9.
2. Gray JAM (1997) *Evidence-based Healthcare*. London: Churchill Livingstone.
3. Seymour J, Clark D, Hughes P, Bath B, Beech N, Corner J, Douglas HR, Halliday D, Haviland J, Marples R, Normand C, Skilbeck J, Webb T (2002) Clinical nurse specialists in palliative care. Part 3. Issues for the Macmillan Nurse role. *Palliative Medicine* **16**: 386–94.
4. Beauchamp TL, Childress JF (1983) *Principles of Biomedical Ethics*, 2nd edn. New York: Oxford University Press.

5. Anderson GR, Glesnes-Anderson VA (1987) *Health Care Ethics*. Rockville, MD: Aspen, pp. 25–26.

6. Bradford-Hill A (1963) Medical ethics and controlled trials. *British Medical Journal* i: 1043–9.

7. Beecher HK (1996) Ethics and clinical research. *New England Journal of Medicine* 274: 1354–60.

8. Casarett D, Karlawish JHT (2000) Are special ethical guidelines needed for palliative care research? *Journal of Pain and Symptom Management* 20: 130–9.

9. Bruera E (1994) Ethical issues in palliative care research. *Journal of Palliative Care* 10: 7–9.

10. Levine RJ (1988) *Ethics and Regulation of Clinical Research*. New Haven, CT: Yale University Press, pp. 187–90.

11. Temple R, Ellensberg SS (2000) Placebo-controlled trials and active-control trials in the evaluation of new treatments. *Annals of Internal Medicine* 133: 455–70.

12. Emanuel EJ, Miller FG (2001) The ethics of placebo-controlled trials—a middle ground. *New England Journal of Medicine* 345: 915–919.

13. Enserink M (2000) Helsinki's new clinical rules: fewer placebos, more disclosure. *Science* 290: 418–9.

14. Vase L, Riley JL, Price DD (2002) A comparison of placebo effects in analgesic trials versus studies of placebo analgesia. *Pain* 99: 443–52.

15. Fine PG (2003) Maximizing benefits and minimizing risks in palliative care research that involves patients near the end of life. *Journal of Pain and Symptom Management* 25: S53–62.

16. MacDonald N, Weijer C (2004) Ethical issues in palliative care research. In: Doyle D, Hanks GW, Cherny N, Calman K, (ed.) *Oxford Textbook of Palliative Medicine*, Vol. 3. Oxford: Oxford University Press, pp. 76–83.

17. Freedman B (1987) Equipoise and ethics of clinical research. *New England Journal of Medicine* 317: 141–5.

18. Shaw LW, Chalmers TC (1970) Ethics in cooperative clinical trails. *Annals of the New York Academy of Sciences* 169: 487–95.

19. Djulbegovic B, Lacevic M, Cantor A, Fields K, Bennett C, Adams JR (2000) The uncertain principle and industry-sponsored research. *Lancet* 356: 635–8.

20. Machin D, Steinning S, Parmar M (1997) Thirty years of Medical Research Council randomized trials in solid tumours. *Clinical Oncology* 9: 100–14.

21. Colditz GA, Miller JN, Moster F (1989) How study design affects outcomes in comparison of therapy, I: Medical. *Statistics in Medicine* 8: 441–54.

22. Dieppe P, Chard J, Tallon D, Egger M (1999) Funding clinical research. *Lancet* 353: 1626.

23. Lilford RJ, Jackson J (1995) Equipoise and the ethics of randomization. *Journal of the Royal Society of Medicine* 88: 552–9.

24. Fries J, Krishnan E (2004) Equipoise, design bias, and randomized controlled trials: the elusive ethics of new drug development. *Arthritis Research and Therapy* 6: R250–5.

25. Toroyan T, Roberts Oakley A (2000) Randomisation and resource allocation: a missed opportunity for evaluating health care and social interventions. *Journal of Medical Ethics* 26: 319–22.

26. Appelbaum PS, Grisso T (1988) Assessing patient's capacities to consent to treatment. *New England Journal of Medicine* **319**: 1635–88.

27. Featherstone K, Donovan JL (1998) Random allocation or allocation at random? Patients' perspectives of participation in a randomized controlled trial. *British Medical Journal* **317**: 1177–80.

28. Edwards JL, Gilford RJ, Hewison J (1998) The ethics of randomised controlled trials from the perspectives of patients, the public, and healthcare professionals. *British Medical Journal* **317**: 1208–12.

29. Todd C, Still A (1984) Communication between general practitioners and patients dying at home. *Social Science and Medicine* **18**: 667–72.

30. Todd C, Still A (1993) General practitioners' strategies and tactics of communication with the terminally ill. *Family Practice* **10**: 268–76.

31. Bruera E, Miller L, McCallion J, Macmillan K, Krefting L, Hanson J (1992) Cognitive failure (CF) in patients with terminal cancer: a prospective study. *Journal of Pain and Symptom Management* **7**: 192–5.

32. Bruera E, Spachynsky K, MacEachem T, Hanson J (1993) Cognitive failure in cancer patients who agree to participate in clinical trials. *Lancet* **341**: 247.

33. Bruera E, Fainsinger R, Miller MJ, Kuehn N (1992) The assessment of pain intensity in patients with cognitive failure: a preliminary report. *Journal of Pain and Symptom Management* **7**: 267–70.

34. General Medical Council (2002) Research: the roles and responsibilities of doctors. http://www.gmc-uk.org/guidance/library/research.asp#Adults%20who%20lack%20capacity Accessed on 10 October 2006

35. Scott YH, Appelbaum PS, Dilip VJ, Olin JT (2004) Proxy and surrogate consent in geriatric neuro-psychiatric research: update and recommendations. *American Journal of Psychiatry* **161**: 797–806.

36. Karlawish JHT (2003) Conducting research that involves subjects at the end of life who are unable to give consent. *Journal of Pain and Symptom Management* **25**: S14–24.

37. Karlawish JHT, Casarett D, Klocinksi J, Sankar P (2001) How do AD patients and their caregivers decide whether to enrol in a clinical trial? *Neurology* **56**: 789–92.

38. Muncie HL Jr, Magaziner J, Hebel R, Warren JW (1997) Proxies' decisions about clinical research participation for their charges. *Journal of the American Geriatric Society* **45**: 929–33.

39. Breitbart W, Marotta R, Platt MM, Weisman H, Derevenco M, Grau C, Corbera K, Raymond S, Lund S, Jacobson P (1996). A double-blind trial of haloperidol, chlorpromazine, and lorazepam in the treatment of delirium in hospitalized AIDS patients. *American Journal of Psychiatry* **153**: 231–7.

40. Rees E, Hardy J (2003) Novel consent process for research in dying patients unable to give consent. *British Medical Journal* **327**: 198.

41. Hanks G, Kaasa S, Robbins M (2004) Research in palliative care: getting started. In: Doyle D, Hanks GW, Cherny N, Calman K, (ed.) *Oxford Textbook of Palliative Medicine*, Vol. 5.2. Oxford: Oxford University Press, pp. 128–38.

42. Coyle N, Adelardt J, Foley KM, Portenoy RK (1990) Character of terminal illness in the advanced cancer patient: pain and other symptoms during the last 4 weeks of life. *Journal of Pain and Symptom Management* **5**: 83–93.

43. Grande G, Todd C (2000) Why are trials in palliative care so difficult? *Palliative Medicine* **14**: 69–74.

44. Rinck GC, van den Bos GAM, Kleijnen J, de Haes HJCJM, Schade E, Veenhof CHN (1997) Methodological issues in effectiveness research on palliative cancer care: a systematic review. *Journal of Clinical Oncology* **15**: 1697–707.

45. McWhinney IR, Bass MJ, Donner A (1994) Evaluation of palliative care services: problems and pitfalls. *British Medical Journal* **309**: 1340–2.

46. Slevin ML, Plant H, Lynch D, Drinkwater J, Gregory WM (1988) Who should measure quality of life, the doctor or the patient? *British Journal of Cancer* **57**: 109–12.

47. Rathbone GV, Horsley S, Goacher J (1994) A self-evaluated assessment suitable for seriously ill hospice patients. *Palliative Medicine* **8**: 29–34.

48. Dickersin K (1997). How important is publication bias? A synthesis of available data. *AIDS Education and Prevention* **9**: 15–21.

# Section 2

# **Survey research**

Chapter 4

# Survey design

Julia M. Addington-Hall

## Introduction

Perhaps more than any other research method presented in this volume, surveys are part of the language and fabric of contemporary life. The findings from the latest 'survey' feature regularly in the media, covering a wide range of issues from, for example, the electorate's views of the Government's current policy initiative to perhaps surprising reports of the frequency of alien abductions amongst teenage inhabitants of Notting Hill. Rarely do the reporters of these surveys or, presumably, the readers apparently differentiate between surveys on the basis of their origin, their sample, their design, and so on; a survey is a survey and all can be equally trusted or distrusted. This situation causes much angst and gnashing of teeth amongst researchers with an understanding of survey research methodology; asking a group of people some questions can result in reliable, robust information or in utter rubbish, depending on the methods used. This chapter will introduce the principles underlying the design of scientific research surveys, with particular emphasis on sampling and on response rate, and on why these matter. It provides essential introductory information for those considering conducting a research survey, but will also interest anyone wanting to make sense of the plethora of survey results presented daily in the media.

## What is survey research?

All surveys, of whatever quality or type, probably have in common the fact that they ask people questions, and then present or analyse the responses quantitatively, using statistics. Survey research consists of a set of scientific procedures addressing the three key components of surveys: the selection of those to whom the questions will be asked (sampling); the design of the questions (questionnaire design); and the choice of the best data collection method. Each of these components has been, and continues to be, the subject of considerable research. This is because in scientific survey research, the object of the exercise is not simply to describe the views of the people who complete the questionnaire, but rather to draw valid, reliable and unbiased conclusions about the population from which these people were drawn.

In order to do this, survey research has a number of distinguishing features.[1] It usually involves collecting data about a defined population, normally by drawing a sample from this population. The sample is drawn in a way that is fixed and objective, and is usually based on statistical probability theory. Quantitative data are collected, with questions being asked (or other measurements applied) in a standardized way to each person, in order to obtain comparable results across the whole sample; results are summarized and analysed statistically. Inferences are then drawn from the sample to the whole population. Surveys may be used to describe the attributes, attitudes and opinions, knowledge and beliefs, or behaviour of a population at a given time point. For example, a palliative care organization in the UK funded a national survey of hospice staff and volunteers to ascertain their opinions about changes facing palliative care in the UK and their attitudes to, for example, euthanasia.[2] They are also used to study associations between variables; in this example, views on a number of contemporary issues were found to be associated with professional group. Surveys are not able to establish 'cause and effect' relationships between variables; longitudinal surveys, which follow the same population over time, are better able to analyse these relationships than cross-sectional surveys, however.

Perhaps because of the familiarity we all have with survey findings, it is easy to overlook the human skills and other resources required to complete a robust and reliable survey successfully: it is not an easy option, requiring little more than writing a few questions and administering them to a readily available pool of putative research participants. At each stage of the research process, care needs to be taken to minimize sources of bias in order to ensure that the final inferences drawn from the sample about the population are as valid and reliable as possible. This requires careful planning, attention to detail and, for anything other than very simple surveys, access to appropriate specialist advice. The first stage in this process, sampling, is considered next.

## Sampling

As already discussed, the central purpose of a survey is to be able to draw reliable, valid and unbiased inferences about the population of interest, not just about the people who participated in the survey (the sample). The sample therefore needs to be representative of the population. The sampling frame is fundamental to ensuring this, as is the use of probability sampling procedures.

Before discussing these, however, it is necessary to define what is meant by two key terms in the following text.

- Units: individual patients, patients, members of public, hospices, hospitals, etc.
- Population: the complete set of units from which a sample is selected and to which the sample-based results may apply.

## The sampling frame

The sampling frame is a list of all the units in the population who are eligible to be sampled. It is fundamental to the success of surveys, and defects can seriously affect the representativeness of the sample; it is therefore worth spending time ensuring that the quality of the sampling frame is as good as possible. A key question to ask is how comprehensive it is: does it include the complete population and, if not, who is excluded? This is important because a sample can only be representative of the sampling frame, and an incomplete sampling frame is therefore an important threat to the representativeness of the survey; it introduces coverage error to the study.

The comprehensiveness of the sampling frame will be determined in part by its construction. Any sampling frame based upon telephone directories, for example, will exclude the small minority without a telephone (usually older and socially deprived members of the population) and, increasingly, those who only have a mobile telephone (conversely, younger and more affluent members). Sampling from e-mail addresses introduces similar biases. In palliative and supportive care, constructing a sampling frame of women with breast cancer from records of patient and support organizations will exclude older women and those from more socially deprived backgrounds, as well as others who prefer not to use these services. Using the records of hospice-based bereavement services as a sampling frame for a population of bereaved people will exclude the majority of those bereaved by causes other than cancer, and probably under-represent men; it would, however, be an entirely appropriate sampling frame where the population of interest is users of these services.

Current interpretation of data protection legislation in the UK, and of similar privacy laws elsewhere, is causing new challenges in constructing complete sampling frames, particularly in contexts such as palliative and supportive care where the population of interest would, as in the examples above, usually have been those using particular services or those with a specific diagnosis, and sampling frames would consequently have been constructed from medical or other records. Individuals now normally need to give their consent to their personal information being forwarded to researchers, who can no longer access this information from medical or administrative records directly.

This changes the characteristics of the population being surveyed to include only those who 'opt in' to research, who will differ in important—and often unknown—ways from the total population. If almost everyone in fact 'opts in', this may not matter. If, however, this is not the case, then the researcher needs to consider carefully whether to proceed with a survey design, given that their ability to make valid, reliable and unbiased inferences from the sample to the population has fallen at the first hurdle: the construction of the sampling frame. If they proceed, they need both to be aware, and to make later users of their data aware, of the ways in which their sampling frame deviates from the population of interest. This, of course, applies to any researcher using a flawed sampling frame; the amount and type of coverage error need to be considered and discussed.

Errors can occur in sampling frames for more prosaic reasons than changes in data protection legislation. It is not unknown, for example, for clerical or administrative errors to occur at some stage of its construction. In a recent survey, for example, a national organization responsible for maintaining registers of all deaths in England used all deaths of people aged over 65 years in specified time periods as the sampling frame, despite being instructed to use only deaths from causes other than cancer, changing the population about which inferences could be drawn.[3] Obviously, such errors need to be avoided; attention to detail is a useful if not essential characteristic of a survey researcher. Any report or paper about a survey should make it clear who was included in the sampling frame (and thus had a chance to be sampled for the survey) and the characteristics of those who were excluded, where known. This will enable the reader to judge whether, in this respect, the survey was indeed representative of the population of interest and whether in reality it might more correctly be seen as representative of a rather different population.

In addition to questioning the comprehensiveness of the sampling frame, it is also important to consider whether it is possible to calculate the probability of selection of each person sampled from the sampling frame. As will be discussed in the next section, an essential characteristic of probability sampling procedures is that each member of the target population has a calculable and non-zero probability of being sampled. This necessitates them being on the sampling frame in the first place, and that the probability of them being selected can be calculated. The most straightforward situation is where every sampling unit occurs only once on the sampling frame. Many sampling frames in palliative care are essentially of this nature, although care must be taken to remove duplicate entries which might arise from, for example, individuals attending more than one palliative care service, having contacted a number of different support services or, indeed, working for several different health care organizations. If the researcher is unaware of duplicate entries and allows them to remain in the sample, then the individuals concerned will have a greater chance of being sampled than others in the sampling frame. What is important here is that the enhanced probability of them being sampled is unknown to the researcher, and the resulting data cannot be adjusted to take account of this; bias will therefore have been introduced into the inferences drawn about the population from the sample.

In some situations, individuals may occur more than once in the sampling frame, but this is known to the researcher who is therefore able to calculate the probability of selection for each individual in the sample and adjust the data accordingly. An example of this might be where a sampling frame is constructed of patients attending an oncology out-patient clinic by entering details of all patients attending the clinic over a specified period. Patients who attend most frequently would be entered most frequently on the sampling frame, and therefore have an increased chance of being sampled compared with those who attend only once. The frequency of visits for all sampled patients could be ascertained from medical records or by asking the patient, and used by a statistician to adjust the data derived from the survey to take account of the different chances of selection.

## Probability sampling procedures

The use of a probability sampling procedure is fundamental to the ability to draw inferences from the sample to the population; unless each individual in the sampling frame has a known and non-zero probability of selection, there is no statistical basis for saying that the sample is representative of the population.

### Simple random sampling

The basic probability sampling procedure is simple random sampling. We are all familiar with this as the process used to draw the winning ticket for prize raffles: all eligible tickets are placed in a hat, shaken, and the required number selected at random. In research, it is more usual for each unit on the sampling frame to be numbered sequentially, with each unit appearing only once and therefore having an equal chance of selection. Say there are 100 units in the sample and 20 are needed for the sample. The next stage is then to consult random number tables (in many statistics textbooks) or to use random number generators (available on many statistical packages or on the Internet[4]) to produce at random 20 numbers between 1 and 100; these then form the sample.

## Systematic random sampling

In reality, in most cases it quickly becomes cumbersome to number each unit in a sampling frame individually unless the list is computerized or very short. An alternative which is frequently used is therefore systematic random sampling. This is based on the same principles as simple random sampling but is more practical for anything but very small samples. This requires calculation of the 'sampling fraction': the proportion of the sampling frame that will be sampled. If, for example, a sample of 200 cancer deaths is required but there were 800 in an area, the sampling fraction would be 1:4. The next stage is to go through the sampling frame and select every fourth unit. However, in order to meet the requirements for random sampling, it is necessary first to select the starting point randomly between one and four (again using random numbers). In addition, it is important to check that the sampling frame is not organized in such a way that one random start would result in a sample that is systematically different from that resulting from another start and, if so, to re-organize it. To give an unlikely example, if hospices across the UK had all been asked to supply the names of four staff members, one doctor, one senior nurse, one care assistant and one administrator and they all presented their lists in this order, systematic random sampling would result in a sample of all doctors or all nurses, and so on, depending on the random start point.

## Stratified random sampling

Random sampling may result by chance in a sample that differs slightly from the population of interest. The 'fit' between the sample and the population can be improved by reducing the normal sampling variation by structuring the sampling procedure using a process called 'stratification'. This is only possible where relevant information is available in the sampling frame; depending on the study, this might, for example, be gender, age or professional group. It involves dividing the sampling frame into strata (layers) on the basis of the chosen defining characteristic, and then sampling from each stratum in turn using the usual random sampling procedures. This will result in a sample which matches the population more exactly on this characteristic than might otherwise have been the case; for example, in a survey of the attitudes of hospital nurses to caring for dying patients, it is reasonable to suppose that age may be an important characteristic. If simple random sampling is used, by chance the sample may differ from the population in this respect. However, if the sampling frame is re-organized by the nurses' age (in decades) and systematic random sampling is then used within each stratum, the sample will have the same proportion of those in each decade as the sampling frame (and thus, provided this is not subject to coverage error, the population).

It may be, however, that age is not primarily the characteristic of interest. Instead, there may be particular interest in how the attitudes of male nurses differ from those of women. Let us say that men make up only 1 in 10 of this workforce, and that it is estimated that a sample size of 100 is needed in each group to allow group comparisons (we will return to the subject of sample size below). A total sample size of 1000 would be needed to ensure a sample of 100 men. If, however, it was estimated that in fact 200 was the minimum group size needed, the total sample size would increase to 2000—an overall increase of 1000 just to obtain an additional 100 men. Fortunately, there is an alternative sampling strategy which overcomes this problem.

## Disproportionate stratified sampling

This allows a different sampling fraction in each stratum of the sampling frame; in the example above, it might, for example, be appropriate to sample all of the men to ensure a large enough sample group for subgroup analysis, but only one in four of the women. This can be a much more cost-effective way of ensuring a sufficiently large sample size of less common population groups. It is important to note that to combine subgroup samples to obtain overall estimates, it is necessary to weight subgroup samples to take account of the disproportionate sampling fractions (see Fowler[5] for a clear explanation).

## Multistage sampling

There are many situations where it is not practicable to construct an adequate sampling frame for the population of interest. Consider, for example, if in the example above the population of concern were all nurses working in acute hospitals in the UK. Just thinking about the amount of work involved in constructing a sampling frame that is not subject to considerable coverage error is enough to persuade any sensible researcher to decide on another research question immediately; leaving aside (although, of course, in reality one cannot) the issue of obtaining research ethics approval and gaining local research governance permissions, the researcher would need to identify every single acute hospital in the UK, negotiate access to the current staff list with addresses in each one, actually obtain these, check these for duplicates and organize them all in one massive sampling frame—before beginning to sample. Again, survey researchers have, of course, found ways around these problems which, while maintaining the principles of probability sampling, provide more practical approaches to sampling in situations where a sampling frame cannot initially be identified because of the size and/or breadth of the population of interest; the need for high quality sampling frames and the concomitant reduction in coverage errors if inferences are to be drawn from the sample to the population has fuelled the development of these methods by social survey methodologists, who have also been motivated by the need for methods which enhance the cost-effectiveness of data collection, as will be discussed below.

Where it is not possible to find a direct source for a sampling frame, it is necessary to identify some higher grouping which unites the units of interest. For example, hospital nurses all work in hospitals. Instead of directly sampling hospital nurses across the country, hospitals—the group into which hospital nurses cluster—can be initially sampled instead, using the same procedures of probability sampling specified above. Lists can then be obtained of all the nurses working in the sampled hospitals. At this stage, it may be decided to include all the nurses, or a sample may be taken; it is perfectly possible, for example, to apply the disproportionate sampling strategy discussed above at this stage of a multistage sampling design. More complex designs are also possible. For example, in order to obtain a nationally representative sample of deaths in England in such a way that was cost-effective for fieldwork, Cartwright and Seale first sampled regional health authorities, stratified by location in the north or south of England, then health districts and finally deaths.[6] The advice of a sampling expert is needed with such designs, not least because of the complexities of weighting data appropriately to take account of the design when drawing inferences about the population from the sample. This is because of the impact of the design on sampling error, to which we now turn.

## Sampling error

Imagine that in a survey of cancer patients, 50 per cent reported that they had pain in the last week. If all cancer patients in the population of interest completed the survey (in which case it was actually a census, not a survey), then it is possible to be confident that 50 per cent is indeed the 'true' rate of pain in this population, and to plan services accordingly. It is more likely, however, that a sample of cancer patients were randomly selected to participate in the survey, and that they are therefore one of many possible samples from the total population. In this case, their response will differ by chance to a greater or lesser extent from those of the population value, and it is not therefore certain that 50 per cent is the 'true' rate of pain. This variation from the true population value is known as 'sampling error'.[5] Sampling error decreases as sample size increases.[5]

Sampling error is an important problem for survey researchers who are, after all, not primarily interested in the scores of their research participants for their own sakes, but for what they tell them about the wider population from which they were drawn. Fortunately, probability theory indicates that if an infinite number of samples is drawn from the population of cancer patients (to use the above example), the sample estimates of the proportion in pain will form a bell-shaped normal distribution around the true population value. This enables the sampling error to be estimated and, for example, confidence intervals to be presented alongside the overall percentage[5] (p. 30). As this is based on probability theory, it only applies when probability sampling procedures have been used to draw the sample. Calculating sampling error is most straightforward for simple random samples, and standard tables of confidence ranges for sampling variability are available;[5] expert advice and the use of specialist survey data analysis software is recommended for more complex designs because of the risk of underestimating sampling error.

## Sampling size

An important question facing any researcher planning a survey is how large does the sample need to be. Getting this right matters: make the number too high and the survey may become unfeasible because the resources it requires exceed those available; make it too small and the sampling error may be so large that no useful inferences can be drawn about the population, and no comparisons made between subgroups. If resources were unlimited (which, of course they never are), then it might be a good strategy to go for the largest sample size possible (if we ignore the question of whether it is ethical to ask respondents to complete questionnaires unnecessarily); sampling error reduces as sample size increases. This effect is, however, as Fowler observes,[5] particularly pronounced at smaller numbers, with the same increase in sample size reducing sampling error more at low numbers (e.g. 50) than at higher numbers (>500). So, size matters, but gains from a further increase in sample size reduce as size increases. What then is the optimum sample size?

Statisticians will usually ask researchers seeking advice on sample size to identify key questions on the questionnaire and to decide how precise they require their estimates of the population value to be. For example, using the example above, is it adequate to know that there is a 95 per cent probability that the 'true' incidence of pain in the cancer population given a reported incidence of 50 per cent lies between, say, 40 and 60 per cent, or is this too imprecise and therefore more appropriate figures are 48 and 52 per cent? Given this information, the statistician can calculate the desired sample size (which would be considerably larger for the more precise estimate). This relies on there being reasonably reliable existing data to use in the sample size calculations. It also, as Fowler argues,[5] overlooks the fact that most surveys are designed to make many estimates, not just one, and that the desired precision may vary between estimates. He also observes that it is usually difficult to define the desired level of precision in advance. Moreover, he argues that the decision about sample size cannot depend solely on the need to reduce sampling error, because decisions to increase sample size may take resources away from optimum questionnaire design and data collection, and introduce other sources of bias (Chapter 4).

Fowler argues instead for the importance of deciding in advance what the key analyses to be undertaken are and the careful construction of an analysis plan, and then ensuring that the sample size is sufficiently large in each subgroup to enable all the desired subgroup analyses to be undertaken. He writes from the position of an experienced social survey researcher, and this is therefore advice to be followed (and the advice to construct an analysis plan is indeed good practice in any research study). It is likely, however, that funding bodies, in the UK at least, will continue to require conventional sample size estimates, based upon the identification of key questions and decisions about the degree of precision required in estimates. As with complex design issues, sample size is another area of survey research where expert advice is needed in all but the most simple cases (Chapter 18).

Before leaving this section, it is worth noting two misunderstandings about sample sizes in surveys which Fowler draws attention to.[5] The first is the notion that there is a 'typical' or 'appropriate' sample size which can be taken off the shelf and applied in all situations. As should now be clear, this is not the case; because it depends on the purpose and design of the individual survey, sample size has to be decided afresh for each survey.

The second misunderstanding is the idea that the adequacy of the sample depends on the proportion of the total population included in the sample. Unless more than 1 in 10 of the total population are sampled, in which case sampling error estimates are reduced, this is not the case; the ability of a sample to represent a population depends on the quality of the sampling frame and the use of probability sampling methods, not on the proportion of the population included.[5] Indeed, a sample which includes a higher proportion of the population may actually represent it less well if a consequence of the increased sample size has been that the researchers have paid less attention to other aspects of the survey and thus introduced other sources of error (Chapter 4). This illustrates how decisions about the ideal sample size cannot be made solely on the basis of achieving the lowest possible sampling error, important as this is. One important factor to consider is the impact of the size of the sample on the ability of the research team to maximize the response rate. The importance of a good survey response rate is considered next.

## Response rate

The response rate is the number of people interviewed (or completing a question-naire) divided by the number of people in the sampling frame. This is the basic statistic by which the success—or otherwise—of a survey is judged. The reason why such weight is placed upon the response rate is that if non-respondents differ from respondents in ways that are germane to the objectives of the survey, then non-response error is introduced into the survey;[7] the ability to draw inferences accurately from the sample to the population is impaired because the proportion of the sample from whom data are obtained differs systematically from the whole sample, and therefore from the population. If non-response was entirely at random, then it would not be such a concern: it would reduce the final sample size and increase sample error but would not introduce bias into the survey in the way that systematic differences between respondents and non-respondents do.

If the response rate is very high, perhaps 98 per cent, then even if the non-respondents differ systematically from respondents in ways related to the survey's aims this is unlikely to have much impact on estimates derived from the survey. If, however, the response rate is much lower, then it is likely that the respondents will be very different from the non-respondents, and the ability to make accurate inferences from the sample to the population would be severely compromised. When response rates are low, respondents are essentially self-selected and are not representative of the population. The survey may still have worth as, for example, a tool for generating hypotheses by exploring associations between variables, but non-response error means that it is unreliable as a source of estimates of wider population parameters.

What is an adequate response rate? Clearly, the response rate needs to be as high as possible, and Fowler[8] has argued that if it seems likely (perhaps on the basis of pilot data) that the response rate will fall below 70 per cent, researchers would get better estimates if they reduced sample sizes and concentrated efforts on increasing the response rate (ways to do this are discussed in Chapter 5). Mangione[9] categorized response rates as follows: 85 per cent or above 'excellent', 70–84 per cent 'very good', 60–69 per cent 'acceptable', 50–59 per cent 'barely acceptable' and under 50 per cent 'unacceptable'. This focuses attention on the need to obtain a high response rate because of the likelihood of non-response error with lower rates, and can be a useful aid when critically reading survey research findings. Palliative care surveys can achieve good response rates in surveys with health professionals,[10–12] with population sam-ples[6] and with patients and carers.[13,14] This is not, however, always the case, despite apparently appropriate design.[3,15–17] This is not surprising, given the particular challenges and sensitivities of recruiting severely ill patients and bereaved people into research studies. Nevertheless, as indicated above, caution does need to be used in interpreting the findings from surveys with low response rates, which is currently not always the case.[16,17] Every effort needs to be made to ensure that planned surveys achieve good response rates, and further methodological research is needed to find appropriate ways of increasing response rates in surveys with patients and bereaved relatives.

Response rates are not always calculated in the straightforward way indicated at the beginning of this section. This is due in part to the complexity of some multistage survey designs; to the difficulty in deciding, for example, when a response is a response (when, for example, should a partly completed questionnaire count as a response and when as a refusal?); and, perhaps, to the importance placed on achieving a good response rate leading some researchers to choose methods which maximize their response rates (by, for example, including only respondents and refusals and excluding those they were unable to contact). Groves and Lyberg[18] have argued that: '(t)here are so many ways of calculating response rates that comparisons across surveys are fraught with misinterpretations'.

In order to reduce confusion, the American Association of Public Opinion Research[19] have produced helpful and detailed standard definitions: these offer six different types of response rate as well as four versions of cooperation rates, used when only respondents successfully contacted by researchers are included, thus excluding that section of the sampling frame whom they could not contact. There are also formulae for three different refusal rates and three contact rates. It is unlikely that such a wide range of definitions will be necessary outside of complex social and public surveys, but their existence indicates both the complexities that can lie behind the apparently simple 'response rate' and the great importance placed upon it by survey researchers. What is essential in any survey is to know what happened to each unit in the sample (its 'disposition') and to have a clearly defined response rate; it may also be appropriate to include a cooperation rate, depending on survey design. A common failing is to publish information which does not allow the reader either to know what happened to the whole sample or to understand how the response rate was calculated.

The social survey research literature indicates that non-responders are likely to differ systematically from responders. Compared with responders, those who refuse to participate in surveys are more likely to be older people, to have lower incomes, to be less educated, to be single rather than married people, to be members of minority ethnic groups, to be from households with high mobility and to live in urban areas.[20] Similarly, compared with responders, those who researchers are unable to contact are more likely to be young people, older people, men, to have higher incomes and/or to be in employment, to live in single-person households, to live in households with high mobility and to live in urban areas.[20] It is important in any survey to seek to understand the ways in which the non-responders differed from the responders, with particular attention to characteristics related to the aims of the survey, as this enables an assessment to be made of the degree of bias introduced into the survey by the response rate. For example, in a national survey of the last 3 months of life of people aged over 65 years in England, it was important to know how those for whom information was available from bereaved relatives differed from those for whom it was not in terms of age at death and cause of death. This showed little difference between responders and non-responders, suggesting that little bias had been introduced.[3] However, as is often the case, information was not available on other important variables such as service use in the last 3 months of life, degree of symptom control, adequacy of family support, and so on; we do not know precisely what biases were introduced into the survey but, as the response rate was <50 per cent, we can expect there to be systematic differences between the responders and non-responders and the level of non-response error to therefore be significant. Thus, whilst it is important to document all known differences between responders and non-responders (and to expect authors of papers reporting survey findings to do so), it is also important to be aware that information is unlikely to be available on all the ways the two groups differ that are germane to the study aims, and that much of the impact of non-response error will therefore be unknown. This emphasizes the importance of reducing non-response error by achieving as good a response rate as possible. Ways of doing this are addressed in the next chapter.

## Non-probability sampling procedures

Before leaving this chapter, however, methods of sampling which do not use probability sampling procedures will be briefly considered. These methods are widely used outside of scientific survey research, for example by market research or by opinion polling organizations. The limitation of these methods is that the use of probability sampling procedures is essential if statistical estimates are to be made of population parameters from sample data, and the fact that these procedures are not used means that it is not possible to make reliable inferences about the population using these methods. Nevertheless, they do have their uses on occasions in research, provided that their strengths and limitations are understood.

One such method is quota sampling, where rather than drawing a random sample of the population of interest the surveyors identify the key characteristics of that population and then seek people who match those characteristics. For example, if the population of interest is women aged under 50 years and available statistics indicate that 60 per cent own their own home, and that 50 per cent have children under the age of 10, then fieldworkers would be sent out to find, say, 100 women aged under 50 years: 30 of whom have their own home and have children under 10 years; 30 of whom have their own home but do not have children; 20 of whom do not have their own home but do have children under 10 years, and 20 who have neither. Compared with identifying a sampling frame, drawing a sample and conducting fieldwork in such a way that a high response rate is achieved, this can be a rapid and cost-effective method. It does not, however, result in a truly representative sample because all members of the population have not had a calculable and non-zero chance of being sampled. If, for example, fieldworkers approached women in a local shopping street during the week, then the sample is likely to have excluded women who work, those who are too ill to shop, those who prefer to shop on the Internet, those who are skilled at evading fieldworkers with clipboards, and so on. If they used random digit dialling [in which telephone numbers from a specified exchange(s) are dialled at random] until they filled their quotas, again the women they succeeded in recruiting are likely to have differed systematically from other women aged under 50. Whilst this method has its uses, it does not result in a statistically representative sample, and the strong likelihood of systematic (but often unknown) differences between the sample and the population of interest needs to be kept in mind when considering the value of data obtained in this way.

An alternative approach is 'snowballing'. This is particularly useful in reaching members of hard-to-reach populations. These include groups whose members tend not to respond to requests to participate in surveys (such as young people and/or those living in transient urban communities), communities subject to social stigma, discrimination and/or prejudice (including members of ethnic minority groups, or employees fearing disciplinary action if they reveal workplace practices) and people engaged in illegal activities (including users of illegal substances or pornography). In some of these cases, developing a robust sampling frame is not an issue, but the reliability of a probability-based sample would be threatened by high non-response error due to a poor response rate. In others, developing an adequate sampling frame would be a near impossibility. In these cases, asking one member of the community of interest to recommend others and 'snowballing' a sample in this way may well be the only practical way forward. As with quota sampling, it is important to remember that the resulting sample will not be truly representative of the population of interest and to limit the conclusions drawn from the data accordingly. It may well, however, be better than no sample at all.

## Conclusion

This chapter has provided an introduction to the principles underlying scientific survey research, and has focused particularly on the issues of sampling and on the importance of achieving a good response rate. It has introduced the fundamental notion that the purpose of a survey generally is to be able to say something reliably about the population from which the sample has been drawn, rather than the sample being of interest in its own right. Following the correct sampling procedure is essential to achieve this, with the sampling frame and the use of probability sampling procedures being basic building blocks of sampling procedure. A number of different probability-based sampling procedures are discussed, and the need to consult experts in sampling statistics where appropriate is emphasized. The concept of sampling error is then introduced and the impact of sample size on this is introduced. The importance of achieving a good response rate to avoid non-response error is then emphasized. Finally, two non-probability-based methods of sampling are considered. The next chapter addresses methods of survey administration, questionnaire design and piloting.

## References

1. McColl E (2002) Design and use of questionnaires: a review of best practice applicable to surveys of health service staff and patients. *The Research Findings Register.* Summary number 778. http://www.ReFeR.nhs.uk/ViewRecord.asp?ID=778 Accessed 24 September 2006.

2. Addington-Hall JM, Karlsen S (2005) A national survey of health professionals and volunteers working in voluntary hospice services in the UK: I. Attitudes to current issues affecting hospices and palliative care. *Palliative Medicine* 19: 40–8.

3. Addington-Hall JM, Burt J, Shipman C, Ream E, Beynon T, Richardson A (2006) *Evaluation of the Department of Health Funded Education and Support Programme for District and Community Nurses in the Principles and Practice of Palliative Care: The Impact on Older People Dying from Non-malignant Disease.* London: Department of Health.

4. www.randomizer.org

5. Fowler FJ Jr (2002) *Survey Research Methods*, 3rd edn. Newbury Park, CA: Sage Publications.

6. Cartwright A, Seale CF (1990) *The Natural History of a Survey: An Account of the Methodological Issues Encountered in a Study of Life Before Death.* London: Kings Fund.

7. Groves RM (1989) *Survey Errors and Survey Costs.* Hoboken, NJ: Wiley Interscience.

8. Fowler FJ Jr (2002) *Survey Research Methods*, 2nd edn. Newbury Park, CA: Sage Publications.

9. Mangione TW (1995) *Mail Surveys—Improving the Quality*. Applied Social Research Methods Series, Volume 40. Thousand Oaks, CA: Sage Publications.

10. Sullivan AM, Lakoma MD, Billings JA, Peters AS, Block SD (2006) PCEP Core Faculty. Creating enduring change: demonstrating the long-term impact of a faculty development program in palliative care. *Journal of General Internal Medicine* 21: 907–14.

11. Field D, Reid D, Payne S, Relf M (2004) Survey of UK hospice and specialist palliative care adult bereavement services. *International Journal of Palliative Nursing* 10: 569–76.

12. Addington-Hall JM, Karlsen S (2005) A national survey of health professionals and volunteers working in voluntary hospices in the UK. II. Staff and volunteers' experiences of working in hospices. *Palliative Medicine* 19: 49–57.

13. Heyland DK, Groll D, Rocker G, Dodek P, Gafni A, Trnmer J, *et al.* (2005) Canadian Researchers at the End of Life Network (CARENET). End-of-life care in acute care hospitals in Canada: a quality finish? *Journal of Palliative Care* 21: 142–50.

14. Morita T, Akechi T, Ikenaga M, Kizawa Y, Kohara H, Mukaiyama T, Nakaho T, Nakashima N, Shima T, Matsubara T, Fujimori M, Uchitomi Y (2004) Communication about the ending of anticancer treatment and transition to palliative care. *Annals of Oncology* 15: 1551–7.

15. Morita T, Miyashita M, Shibagaki M, Hirai K, Ashiya T, Ishihara T, Matsubara T, Miyoshi I, Nakaho T, Nakashima N, Onishi H, Ozawa T, Suenaga K, Tajima T, Akechi T, Uchitomi Y (2006) Knowledge and beliefs about end-of-life care and the effects of specialized palliative care: a population-based survey in Japan. *Journal of Pain and Symptom Management* 31: 306–16.

16. Farber NJ, Simpson P, Salam T, Collier VU, Weiner J, Boyer EG (2006) Physicians' decisions to withhold and withdraw life-sustaining treatment. *Archives of Internal Medicine* 166: 560–4.

17. Hussainy SY, Beattie J, Nation RL, Dooley MJ, Fleming J, Wein S, Pisasale M, Scott WJ, Marriott JL (2006) Palliative care for patients with cancer: what are the educational needs of community pharmacists? *Supportive Care in Cancer* 14: 177–84.

18. Groves RM, Lyberg LE (1988) An overview of non-response issues in telephone surveys. In: Groves RM, (ed.) *Telephone Survey Methodology*. New York: John Wiley and Sons.

19. The American Association for Public Opinion Research (2000) *Standard Definitions: Final Dispositions of Case Codes and Outcome Rates for Surveys*. Lenexa, KS: AAPOR.

20. Lynn P, Buck N, Burton J, Jackie A, Laurie H (2005) *A Review of Methodological Research Pertinent to Longitudinal Survey Design and Data Collection*. Working Papers of the Institute for Social and Economic Research, paper 2005-29. Colchester: University of Essex.

Chapter 5

# Survey research: methods of data collection, questionnaire design and piloting

Julia M. Addington-Hall

## Introduction

The previous chapter has discussed the principles underlying the design of scientific research surveys where the interest is primarily in the population from which the sample is drawn, rather than in the sample itself. It focused on one of the three key components of surveys, namely the selection of those to whom questions are asked, and introduced a range of sampling methods designed to ensure that the resulting sample is representative of the population. The importance of achieving a high response rate was also discussed. In this chapter, the remaining two fundamental survey components are addressed. These are the choice of the best data collection method to meet the aims of the survey, given budgetary and other constraints, and the design and testing of the questionnaire. By the end of the chapter, the reader should be equipped with the basic information they need to design and execute a survey which enables them to draw valid, reliable and unbiased conclusions about the population of interest.

## Methods of data collection

In surveys, questions are asked in a standardized way to each person in order to obtain comparable results across the whole sample; results are then summarized and analysed statistically. The questions may be asked by a trained interviewer following a structured schedule, either in personal interview or over the telephone. Alternatively, the questions may be contained in a self-complete questionnaire which may be posted to the respondent, given to them to complete or, increasingly, e-mailed to them or accessed over the Internet. An important decision in any survey is the choice of the appropriate data collection method (or methods, as a number of studies now combine modalities in order to increase the response rate). No one method consistently outperforms the others, with each having strengths and weaknesses depending on the context and the study resources. The final decision about the data collection method will be based on, for example, the topic of the study, the characteristics of the study population, the volume and complexity of the data to be collected, the information available on the sampling frame, the size of the sample, and the financial and staffing resources available.

## Personal interviews

In many populations, personal interviews are likely to result in the best response rate, particularly when experienced and/or well trained interviewers are used. They are able to explain the study and answer any queries about it, and can provide additional motivation to participate to those respondents who welcome the opportunity to talk to an interested listener but would not enjoy completing a questionnaire. Rapport can be built up, increasing the likelihood, for example, that respondents will persist with lengthy questionnaires. Personal interviews are also valuable for complex questionnaires with a number of sections which apply to some respondents and not to others (the growing use of computer-assisted personal interviewing makes it increasingly easy for interviewers to use very complex questionnaires). Interviewers are also able to probe when respondents give inconsistent or inadequate answers and can therefore improve the quality of the data. Additional information can be collected: for example, the interviewer may be asked to make observations about the respondent's living arrangements or their apparent health status, or they may be asked to record precisely what medication the respondent is taking, listing details from the medication itself. They are also able to assess the apparent impact of the interview on the respondent and encourage them to seek appropriate support if necessary.

Personal interviews do have disadvantages, however. They require trained, well supported interviewers who are both available at the right time and in the right geographical area for the survey. They are usually, therefore, more expensive than other methods of data collection. For surveys in palliative and bereavement care, the interviewers need not only to be trained in survey research but also to be able to work with these populations; clinical staff may find it difficult to adjust to the structured method of questioning and thus be a risk to the quality of data collection, whilst non-clinical interviewers may lack the qualities necessary to be acceptable to these populations and/or to do so without an adverse impact on themselves. In any survey, there is a clear need to consider the interviewers' personal safety, and this can make it either a less appropriate method for areas of high crime or, if it is felt necessary for the interviewer to have an escort, a more expensive method. The usual advantage of personal interviews in terms of response rate may not apply in areas where a high proportion of the population is accessed via entry phones (for instance, in inner city areas). In terms of the data themselves, interviews may not be the best method when highly sensitive information is to be collected, as will be discussed below.

## Telephone interviewing

This method is used increasingly often because telephone interviews have many of the benefits of personal interviews in terms of a skilled individual administering the survey, with the added benefits of both a safe working environment for the interviewer and reduced costs. There is no need for the interviewers to be located near the respondents, fewer are generally needed because there is no travel time involved, and it is easier for their work to be supervised and for quality control to be ensured. A telephone survey is likely to result in a higher response rate than postal surveys, and to be more successful than interviews in, for example, inner city populations. It is becoming harder, however, to get a good response rate using this method as a result of growing intolerance of telephone salespeople, and the increasing use of answering machines to screen calls. People who do not have telephones, or for whom an accurate phone number cannot be obtained, will be excluded, potentially introducing bias into the survey. It may also be a less suitable method for populations where high levels of hearing loss are expected, such as the 'oldest old'; nevertheless, depending on local circumstances, they may prefer to be telephoned than to answer the door to a stranger. The questionnaire needs to be simpler for a telephone survey than for a personal survey, particularly with respect to question wording and response categories as respondents have to be able to hold all the information in their memory, without the help of visual aids, etc. It is also not possible to use self-complete questionnaires within the interview. Together with the fact that the interviewer has no control or knowledge of who can hear the respondent's answers, this may make this mode of data collection less suitable for personal or sensitive questions than other methods.

## Postal questionnaires

These surveys are less expensive than telephone or personal interview surveys, and require fewer staff and facilities. They can be used to survey populations who are widely dispersed, and those who for whatever reason are otherwise hard to reach. In terms of the questionnaire itself, the respondent is able to go and look up information, potentially increasing the accuracy of their response, and they are able to read and re-read questions rather than relying on their memory of what the interviewer said, enabling more complex response categories to be used. This may be the best method to collect personal or sensitive information. On the less positive side, however, the success of the survey is dependent on the accuracy of the address list, a particular problem in inner city areas and with younger populations where frequent changes of address are common (and with bereaved spouses, who often move after the loss of their partner). There is also no interviewer to explain the purpose of the study and to encourage respondents to consider participation. Respondents also need good literacy skills to participate. Response rates are therefore lower than for other modes of administration. In the absence of an interviewer, questionnaire design has to be particularly good, with a clear route through the questionnaire and precise, easy to understand instructions for the respondent. Levels of missing data are higher than in telephone or personal interviews. There is also no control over who actually completes the questionnaire. The cost savings involved when conducting a postal survey are therefore likely to be obtained at the cost of both reductions in the reliability and validity of the data itself and the introduction of biases into the sample.

## E-mailed or Internet surveys

The Internet and e-mail are said to offer 'the possibility of nearly instantaneous transmission of surveys at little or no cost'[1] (p. 9). E-mail and Internet surveys are probably cheaper than postal surveys, but this is dependent on the number of responses and on the surveyors having prior experience of web survey programming, as problems with this can remove any savings. They are thought to be a particularly rapid form of survey, but the evidence for this is mixed.[1] Studies which have compared response rates to e-mailed surveys with those to postal surveys have found the response rates to the latter to be higher.[1] The biggest problem with this method at present, however, is that coverage of the population by e-mail and the Internet is limited (although growing): this may be an appropriate method to reach particular populations (such as university employees) but would result in a biased sample in other circumstances (e.g. a survey of palliative care patients).

## Mixed-method surveys

The best way to increase the response rate whilst keeping survey costs down may be to combine data collection methods. For example, the questionnaire might initially be e-mailed out to the sample.[2] As discussed above, this has the advantage of being cost-effective and fast. It also, however, will result in a lower response rate than a postal survey. The next stage might therefore be to post the questionnaire to all non-responders, thus benefiting from the advantages of this modality whilst at the same time reducing costs compared with a postal-only survey because some people will have replied to the initial e-mail approach. Another approach might be to post the questionnaire initially, then to telephone the non-responders, and then send interviewers into the field to interview those who did not respond to the telephone survey. Combining modalities in this way can be very helpful in obtaining the highest possible response rate as it can reach respondents who would not be reachable by one method alone. It does presume, however, that the responses given to the survey questions have not been influenced by the method of administration. This is not necessarily so, and it is important that the question of whether the chosen methods do give equivalent data is researched and not taken for granted.[3–5]

## Conducting personal and telephone interview surveys

This section considers steps that can be taken in both personal and telephone interview surveys to increase the response rate, the role of the interviewer and other issues relevant to quality control in this context. There are two stages in achieving an interview, whether in person or by telephone. First, the sampled individual has to be contacted, and secondly they need to agree to cooperate. One reason why studies fail to achieve a good response rate is simply that too little effort is put into contacting the sample; this is often because the importance of achieving a high response rate is not understood.[6] The minimum number of contacts needs to be agreed in advance to ensure all interviewers work to the same standard. For almost all populations (with, perhaps, the exception of older people), these will need to be concentrated on evenings and weekends, and will therefore require interviewers able to work at these times. Fowler, an experienced survey researcher, recommends a minimum of six visits in urban areas, and at least 10 telephone calls for telephone surveys.[6] In some circumstances, it will be right to continue to try and make contact (at different times and on different days) until the end of fieldwork.[8] If resources will not allow such intensive fieldwork, a different method of data collection should be considered. Once contact has been made, the role of the interviewer is to enable the putative respondent to make an informed choice about participation in the survey. Their task is often made easier if a letter introducing the survey has been sent in advance. They need to be able to present the purposes of the survey effectively and accurately, and make clear to the respondent why their participation is being requested and why it is important. As Fowler suggests, it is relatively straightforward to secure the cooperation of many respondents as they agree to be interviewed quite readily; it is much more difficult to encourage someone who is predisposed to refuse without finding out what the survey is about to listen to information about the survey so that they are able to make an informed choice, or to persuade someone initially reluctant to participate to do so.[6] Interviewers need to be both well trained and well supported in order to be able to perform well in this respect; recruiting survey participants is a skilled task which, because of its effect on response rate, impacts directly on the survey's scientific credibility. Once they have secured agreement to an interview, the role of the interviewer is both to:

> train and motivate respondents to do a good job of being a respondent (and) to ask questions, record answers, and probe incomplete answers to ensure that answers meet the question objectives[6] (p. 118).

Again, these are skilled tasks and the interviewer needs to be well trained. They need to be able to tell the respondent what is expected of them, to explain about confidentiality, to answer any questions about the survey and, in particular, to be able to emphasize the importance of accurate responses. If the respondent is left unsure about the uses to which the findings will be put, is not assured of the confidentiality of their responses or does not appreciate that the most important thing they can do is to give accurate responses, they may not engage fully in answering the questions, they may withhold information or give misleading answers, all of which would threaten the validity of the study findings.[6] The interviewer then needs to go through the interview, asking each question exactly as written, in the order written, and using only such prompts and explanations as provided, and recording answers accurately, fully and legibly in pre-determined ways. If interviewers are inconsistent, then error will be introduced into the survey and the precision of survey estimates will be reduced; bias may also be introduced if interviewers interact with some groups of respondents differently than with others, or express their own views, thus encouraging respondents to choose some options rather than others. Once again, it is clear that survey interviewing, whether face to face or by telephone, is a skilled task.

Interviewers do not, of course, become skilled without appropriate training both in generic survey research interviewing skills and in the particular survey. The training needs to include an explanation both of why a good response matters and why the interview must be administered in a standardized way; the latter may be particularly important if the interviewer has a clinical background and is used to a different form of interviewing. The interviewers need to understand the purpose of the survey, including its research questions, who is sponsoring it and what is likely to happen to the findings. They need to understand the approach to confidentiality which is being adopted in the survey, and the general purpose of the questions. They then need to become very familiar with the interview itself, from the brief they are to follow when explaining it to the sample, through the instructions at the beginning of the interview itself, the format and structure of the interview, the question wording, the acceptable prompts and how to close the interview. They need to rehearse how to record the answers, whether on a computer or on paper. A training package may therefore need to include lectures, role play and computer-based tutorials.[6] In addition, a comprehensive interviewers' handbook should be prepared, providing all this information in written form. It is also important that some early interviews are either observed or recorded and then discussed, to enable the interviewer to refine their skills further. All this clearly takes time: in the Regional Study of Care for the Dying (the RSCD), a survey of the last year of life in the UK from the perspective of bereaved relatives, interviewers with previous experience of survey research attended a 2 day briefing and then submitted a tape-recorded interview, whilst those with no previous experience attended a 5 day briefing and submitted two tapes.[7]

Supervision needs to be provided throughout the period of fieldwork to ensure data quality. This is easiest for telephone interviews, where it is comparatively easy to listen into interviews periodically to ensure that interviewers are still asking questions exactly as written. Interviewers working in the field can be asked to tape interviews from time to time to enable these quality assurance checks to be made. Response rates should be monitored for all interviewers, regardless of the mode of data collection, as this will reveal those who are finding it difficult to make contact or to convert initial reluctance into an interview (without, of course, exerting undue pressure). Some may require further training, but others may not be suitable for the task and should be replaced if at all possible; the response rate is too important to the credibility of the survey to be put at risk by incompetent interviewers.[6]

Supervision will also go some way towards identifying interviewer falsification, defined as 'the intentional departure from the designed interviewer guidelines or instructions, unreported by the interviewer, which could result in contamination of the data'.[8] This has long been recognized as an issue in survey research and was, indeed, an issue for the forerunner of the RSCD.[9] It may involve the interviewer making up all or part of an interview, saying that the outcomes of their attempt to contact an individual was something other than it was, deliberately miscoding the answer to a question to avoid having to ask follow-up questions, or otherwise deliberately changing the data or misrepresenting the data collection process.[8] It is particularly likely to occur when the interviewer receives an incentive for the number of interviews they complete rather than being paid for the time they work, when they have a lot of interviews to complete in a short period, when subjects are difficult to approach, when the interviews are particularly long and complex, and when the interviewer has pressures in their own lives.[8] It is possible in palliative and supportive care that conducting emotionally difficult interviews without sufficient support may also help tip the balance for an interviewer to the point where the making up an interview seems a better option than collecting the data honestly.

Guidelines on how to avoid interviewer falsification have been issued.[8] These emphasize the importance of recognizing that interviewing is a skilled, often stressful job, of paying interviewers well, of periodically observing work and of verifying work; interviewers need to know this will happen for this to be an effective deterrent. For example, in the RSCD, the interviewers were not given the deceased's date or cause of death and, instead, asked for these in the interview. As soon as the interview schedule was returned to the Research Office, these were checked against information derived from the death certificate; fortunately, no fabricated interviews were detected. An alternative would have been to re-contact a percentage of respondents. When fabricated interviews are detected, it is necessary to discard all interviews completed by that individual.[9] The essential role played by interviewers in personal and telephone surveys is easy to overlook but, if they do not do their job well, the sample will not be representative of the population, sampling error will be introduced and bias may be introduced into sample estimates. It is therefore important that interviewers are well trained and supported, particularly in palliative and supportive care where they often have to contend with the emotional consequences of the subject matter as well as the exacting demands of survey research.

## Conducting postal surveys

As reviewed above, sending questionnaires by post has considerable advantages in terms of the costs and resources required, but usually results in lower response rates than would be achieved if an interviewer were employed, in either personal or telephone interviews. The key challenge in a postal survey is therefore designing it in such a way as to maximize the response rate. This is such an important issue for survey researchers that there is a considerable body of evidence to guide practice in this area.

Edwards *et al.* published in 2002 the findings of a systematic review into ways of improving the response rate to postal questionnaires.[10] They reviewed 292 papers, and found that the odds of completed or partially completed questionnaires being returned was more than doubled when a monetary incentive was used. Their recent meta-analysis of the role of monetary incentives in increasing responses to postal questionnaires has supported this.[11] The relationship between the amount of the money offered and response is not straightforward, however. In the systematic review,[10] a US$1 incentive doubled the likelihood of response but the marginal benefit decreased with each additional dollar, so that the odds of responding to a US$15 incentive was only two and a half times the odds of responding to no incentive at all. The meta-analysis similarly found a complex relationship between increases in the incentive and increases in response rate,[11] with decreasing returns between US$0.5 and US$5 and no statistically significant benefit above this. This may be because respondents become increasingly doubtful about the likelihood of receiving the incentive as the amount increases. This may help to explain why the likelihood of response was also almost doubled when incentives were not conditional on response. Some caution is needed in applying these results to the design of postal questionnaires in palliative care as a systematic review which looked specifically at predictors of increased response rate in a patient, rather than a general, population found no effects of incentives;[12] this may, however, have been because of a paucity of studies.

There was a slightly increased chance of response in the systematic review when non-monetary incentives were used, but significant variation between studies suggests that different incentives are more beneficial than others and that some populations respond better than others to these.[10] For example, the chance to enter a prize draw for a personal digital assistant (PDA) did not significantly increase the response rate for consultant obstetricians and gynaecologists;[13] this might well have been more motivating for research students unable to fund one from their own resources. Entering into a draw for a £100 gift voucher did not increase the response rate for a health survey of the UK general practice population.[14] A more effective non-monetary incentive seems to be the inclusion of a pen or pencil with the questionnaire: a UK study in a health setting demonstrated a significant improvement in response rate when a pen was included in the initial mailing,[15] whilst others have reported a significant increase when a pencil was included with the mailing to non-responders.[16] Short questionnaires were more effective than longer ones.[10] The systematic review in a patient population also found that shorter questionnaires improved response rates.[12] A study of US physicians suggests that for this population 1000 words is the threshold above which response declines.[17] Whilst as a general rule short questionnaires are best, in some circumstances response rates are actually higher for longer questionnaires;[18] this may because the longer questionnaire better enabled the respondent to represent their experience and was therefore more satisfying for them to complete. In terms of the appearance of the questionnaire, coloured ink increased the response rate, as did personalized questionnaires and letters.[10] The results of use of coloured paper versus white paper approached significance, as did whether the questionnaire was folded into a booklet rather than simply being stapled, suggesting that these might be useful strategies for increasing the response rate in some circumstances. The use of a brown envelope rather than a white one made little difference to the response rate, however. The odds of questionnaires being returned was more than doubled when recorded delivery was used to send the questionnaire rather than the standard post.[10] It was also increased when stamped return envelopes were used to return the questionnaire rather than business reply or franked envelopes, and when the questionnaires were sent out using first class rather than second class post. Using a stamp on the envelope did not make a difference, nor did using a commemorative stamp rather than an ordinary one.

In terms of contact with the sample, response rates were increased when participants were contacted before the questionnaires were sent out;[10] it did not seem to make a difference to the response rate if this was by telephone or letter (it might, however, make a considerable difference to the ethics of a palliative care study). The value of a pre-warning letter in health research is confirmed by the finding that it increased the response rate by half in a survey of sedentary patients from whom a low response rate was expected.[19] In the systematic review, response rates were also increased if there was follow-up contact, and if a copy of the questionnaire was included in the follow-up contacts.[10] In a patient population, using reminder letters and telephone contact were found to have the most significant effects on response rate.[12] If respondents were given an explicit option to opt out of the survey, response rates were decreased.[10] It made no difference to the response rate if the appeal to the respondent emphasized the benefit to the respondent of participating, if it emphasized the benefit to the sponsor or if it emphasized the benefit to society. Questionnaires were more likely to be returned if they originated from universities than if they originated from other sources, such as commercial organizations. Questionnaires which were of interest to the participants were more than twice as likely to be returned as less interesting questionnaires,[10] and response rates were also higher for questionnaires designed to be user-friendly as opposed to standard questionnaires.[10,20] The inclusion of sensitive (but not demographic) questions reduced the response rate, whilst including only factual questions as opposed to factual and attitudinal questions increased it.

Questionnaire design and administration is, as this review of the evidence illustrates, something which survey researchers take very seriously because of the threat posed to surveys by a poor response rate. Very little of this research has been conducted specifically in palliative care or even with seriously ill people, and the strategies discussed here to improve response rates in postal questionnaire surveys need further evaluation with these populations. It is not clear, for example, that the use of monetary incentives would be as effective as in the general population even if it were deemed appropriate from an ethical viewpoint; it could well be seen as putting undue pressure on a vulnerable population. The evidence for the use of non-conditional monetary incentives in a general population is, however, convincing and should be considered by all researchers designing a survey with, for example, health professionals or members of the general population. There is growing evidence for the benefits of including a pen or pencil, and this should also be considered, particularly with follow-up mailings where it may be cost-effective if it reduces the need for subsequent mailings.[16] The research evidence has now established beyond doubt that there is little point in conducting a survey into a topic that is unlikely to interest the sample or that cannot be presented in such a way that it will interest them. It has also been demonstrated that a shorter questionnaire is nearly always better than a longer one; including questions which are interesting but not essential to the survey's aim puts the response rate and therefore the scientific validity of the survey at risk. Sensitive questions should be avoided if possible. Questionnaires should be user-friendly; this means at the very least using language appropriate for the targeted population and presenting the questions in an easy to follow and attractive manner, and probably necessitates active user involvement in questionnaire design. The questionnaire and accompanying letter should be personalized. Coloured ink (and possibly coloured paper) should be used, provided of course that these do not reduce the legibility of the questionnaire. A pre-warning letter should always be sent, and this should come from an academic rather than commercial organization. Reminders are essential, and these should be accompanied by the questionnaire; at least two reminders are usually needed. To increase the response rate further, the envelope provided to return the questionnaire in should have a stamp on it. Following these guidelines will not guarantee a good response rate but they should help achieve one.

This section has begun to consider issues related to the design of the questionnaire in so far as these impact on the response rate obtained in postal surveys. In the next section, the design and testing of survey instruments is considered in more depth.

## The design of survey instruments

### Deciding what to measure

The first stage in designing a questionnaire or interview schedule is deciding exactly what is to be measured in the survey. It is very tempting to include questions which are interesting to the researchers but which are not essential to meeting the study's goal; the relationship between survey length and response rate highlighted above illustrates one of the dangers inherent in doing this. It also diverts resources away from the survey's aims and can have a detrimental effect on the study's time scales. It is also, however, very easy to omit questions which later prove to have been needed in important analyses. Fowler argues that a clear statement, perhaps in one paragraph, of what the survey is intended to achieve is an important first step in avoiding both unnecessary and missed questions.[6] The next stage is to list what needs to be measured if the survey is to achieve its aims, grouped into related categories or areas. Next, how the survey data are going to be analysed needs to be considered and an analysis plan developed. This should include consideration of what are the dependent variables in the planned analyses, the variables that the survey is intended to describe or predict; what are the independent variables, the variables which are needed to understand distributions and relationships; and finally what variables may be needed as control or intervening variables to explain associations in the data and to check out competing hypotheses.[6] For instance, if one of the purposes of the survey was to investigate predictors of days off work amongst carers of palliative care patients, the dependent variable would be a question about days off work, the independent variables might include the questions about the carer's physical and psychological health, the patient's dependency levels, levels of support from health and social services, and so on. Control variables might include age and gender, to see whether and how relationships were explained by these. A good knowledge of the existing literature on the impact of caring in palliative care would be needed to decide on appropriate independent variables together with, perhaps, findings from pilot work and the opinions of users and health professionals. Time spent on working out precisely what should be measured in the survey is well spent as it increases the scientific validity of the survey as well as saving time at later stages of the survey process.

## Survey instrument design

Once the content of the survey instrument has been decided, the actual questions can be designed. It will come as no surprise to readers of this and the preceding chapter that this is not a simple process. As Fowler states

> Designing a question for a survey instrument is designing a measure, not a conversational inquiry. In general, an answer given to a survey question is of no intrinsic interest. The answer is valuable to the extent that it can be shown to have a predictable relationship to facts or subjective states. Good questions maximise the relationship between the answers recorded and what the researcher is trying to measure[6] (p. 76).

Good survey questions are reliable and valid. Being reliable means that they provide consistent answers in comparable situations; two people in the same situation with, for example, the same amount of pain will answer the question in the same way, and the same individual will answer the question in the same way if asked it again shortly after the first administration. Being valid means that the measure measures what it is intended to measure.

## Does the question mean the same to everyone?

As discussed above, reliability is increased by standardized interviewing in which the questions are asked in the same way to each person. This relies, however, on the question meaning the same to every respondent, regardless of education or cultural background; it is essential that all respondents have the same understanding of what is to be reported. This is difficult to achieve and a major source of error in surveys. Many words used in health surveys appear at first glance to be straightforward, but on careful examination can be seen to have a number of interpretations: even a simple question such as 'how many times have you seen a doctor recently' relies on respondents having a shared understanding of what a doctor is (should they include hospital doctors only or GPs too; should they include their complementary therapists who are called 'Dr X'?) and of what 'seeing a doctor' involves (does this mean a booked consultation, a 'significant' conversation, contact by telephone as well as face to face, literally 'seeing' the doctor in the corridor?).[6] Such shared understandings are clearly unlikely. They therefore need to be provided by the question writer. This can be done by including a definition before the question and/or asking a series of questions from which the survey team can extract the information they want. In this example, the question might be reworded as follows: 'We are interested in any contact you have had with a medical doctor over the past month. This contact may have been in hospital, in your home, on the telephone or in the family doctor's surgery. First, I want to ask you about any contact you have had with hospital doctors. In the last month, how many times have you had contact with a hospital doctor?' This is still not a very good question as 'contact' is left undefined, but the use of definitions and of multiple questions has improved it compared with the initial question.

All key terms need to be defined in the survey instrument, and this then needs to be carefully tested to check that all respondents do share a common understanding of these terms (survey instrument testing is discussed below). This is particularly important when the survey instrument is being designed by health professionals or others with specialized knowledge of the subject matter; it is not uncommon to find palliative care questionnaires, for example, asking patients about their dyspnoea or enuresis, terms unlikely to be understood by the general population. It is also common for survey instruments written by a team of academics, all with PhDs, to use inappropriately complex language. Use of specialized or complicated language will lead to different members of the sample understanding questions in different ways and will, therefore, introduce error into the survey.

Other threats to a common understanding of questions include questions which ask about two things at once, which result in unreliable answers from respondents who would give different answers to each half of the question. Questions which are overly long or complicated will place too great a burden on the ability of some individuals to comprehend or remember the question (particularly in personal and telephone interviews) and will again threaten reliability. Questions which lead respondents to an acceptable answer, questions which contain negatives and double negatives, and imprecise questions should also be avoided.

### Does the question ask about a sensitive or threatening topic?

Particular care needs to be taken in constructing questions about sensitive or threatening topics.[21] Researchers are not always aware of what these are, particularly perhaps health professionals who are used to talking openly about bodily functions and other issues that the majority of the population consider private and/or embarrassing. Survey researchers can also be so used to asking questions about income that they forget how threatening many people consider this topic. Fowler suggests that if an answer to a question would be seen by society, or by a section of society, as undesirable, then the question itself should be seen as sensitive or threatening.[21] It will usually be necessary to pilot the survey instrument with the target population in order to identify these questions. Given the impact of sensitive questions on postal questionnaire response rates, it is important to be certain that these questions are central to the aims of the survey and, if not, to exclude them.

One of the problems with sensitive questions is social desirability effects on respondents' answers; respondents will usually want to reply to interviewers in a way that reflects well on themselves, they will also want to give answers which support their own self-image and the image they wish to project of themselves.[21] This may lead respondents to give an inaccurate answer. Postal questionnaire surveys avoid social desirability effects as an interviewer is not involved, but the benefits of this may be off-set by the impact of sensitive questions on response rates. In personal and telephone interviews, it is essential to have skilled non-judgemental interviewers who are comfortable with the subject matter and who are able to explain clearly to respondents why accurate answers matter. The accuracy of responses to sensitive questions within personal interviews can be improved by containing these questions in a self-complete questionnaire which the respondent completes alone and then places in a sealed envelope before handing the envelope back to the interviewer.

Response validity can also be improved by the use of open rather than closed questions to measure the frequency of undesirable behaviour, as otherwise the respondent is given information on what the 'acceptable' range is, leading to under-reporting. It can also help to construct long, rather than short, questions to give respondents time to consider their response, to ask whether the respondent has ever engaged in the undesirable behaviour before asking about current behaviour, and to write introductions to questions which make it clear that all possible answers are acceptable.

In addition to social desirability effects, sensitive and threatening questions can adversely affect the accuracy of responses because some responses could have adverse effects for respondents;[21] a doctor may, for example, understandably fear indicating that they have been involved in an act of euthanasia if this is outside the legal framework in their country of practice. This highlights the importance of confidentiality within survey research. It is good practice in all surveys, and essential in surveys dealing with sensitive or threatening material, to follow steps proposed by Fowler to protect confidentiality in surveys[21] (p. 30): minimize the use of names and other identifiers (hospital numbers should never, for example, be used as survey IDs); make sure that the survey IDs cannot be linked with identifiers by, for example, ensuring that the 'key' that links them is not stored on the same computer or in the same filing cabinet as the survey IDs or the identifiers and by destroying the identifiers as soon as possible; keep completed survey instruments in a locked filing cabinet; restrict access to survey instruments to those working on them; and see to their proper disposal.[23] In highly sensitive surveys, it may be appropriate for the survey to be anonymous, with no identifier used on the survey instrument at all, not even a survey ID; this is compatible with sending reminders if respondents are supplied with a postcard to return to a separate address when they return the questionnaire.

## Do respondents have the information they need to answer the question?

Once it is clear that respondents are able to understand the questions and, importantly, hold a common understanding of what they are being asked, the next important issue is whether they have the information needed to answer the question. Surveys are good at asking people about their first-hand experiences, their behaviours, beliefs, opinions and attributes; they are not designed to be used to collect second-hand information. Respondents may therefore fully understand a question but not be able to answer it because it asks for information which lies outside their experience. This is a particular issue when individuals are asked to act as proxy respondents for others. In most survey settings, the use of proxies would therefore be avoided or restricted to very limited information. In palliative care, there is often no alternative to the use of bereaved relatives as proxies for patients if information is to be obtained on the quality of care received at the end of life;[22] this makes it important that the strengths and weaknesses of the information obtained in this way are fully explored.[23] In addition to problems caused by lack of knowledge when acting as proxies, respondents may on occasion be unable to answer questions about their own health because information has not been shared with them by health professionals; patients may, for example, have an understanding of their health condition but not know the precise medical diagnosis.[21] Careful piloting is needed to identify these problems.

Respondents may once have known the information they need to answer a question but have difficulty recalling it. More recent and more salient information is remembered best so, if the needed information is unlikely to be of importance to the respondent, recall can be enhanced by asking about very recent events; the time period can be longer for more salient information. Recall can also be improved by designing the preamble to the question in such a way that it encourages the respondent to recreate the experience in their mind, and by asking a longer question as this gives the respondent time to recall their experience.

Respondents may recall the event but have difficulty deciding whether it fits in the time period of interest to the research. If it is important to the research for events to be placed in the right period, respondents can be encouraged to recall what was happening at the boundary of the period of interest and by use of a calendar. They can also be helped to decide when a significant event occurred by encouraging them to think about its timing in relation to other events such as birthdays and Christmas. Alternatively, if it is vital to know about events over a period, an initial interview can be held at which respondents can be informed that there is interest in what happens to them between then and a subsequent interview; this can increase the accuracy of recall at subsequent interviews.

## What constitutes an acceptable answer?

Respondents need clear instructions about what is an acceptable answer; they need to know, for example, whether their task is give a narrative answer, as in an open question, or to choose from amongst a limited number of acceptable options, as in a closed question. The form of the answer needs to fit the reality being described; asking respondents their views on a complex issue such as euthanasia with a simple agree/disagree format would, for example, prove frustrating to those with strongly held views as well as being unanswerable by those who neither agree nor disagree with it. It might, however, be an appropriate response format for a question about whether the respondent takes sugar in tea.

The response options for factual questions need to be as comprehensive as possible. It is good practice to include an 'other' category, however, as all possible answers will not be anticipated. It is important that response categories are mutually exclusive. For example, when measuring the frequency of events by offering a series of number ranges, each category must exclude the next: 1–5, 6–10, 11–15, and so on, not 1–5, 5–10, 10–15. If the latter is used, some respondents for whom 10 is the right answer will choose the second category whilst others will chose the third, introducing error.

When measuring people's beliefs, attitudes and opinions, the response task is different from that for factual questions as the respondent is not being asked to retrieve accurate information from memory, but to make a judgement. Respondents are often asked to give a rating along a continuum; for example, to describe care from a family doctor as 'excellent, good, fair or poor' or to rate pain on a scale from 0 to 10 'if 0 is no pain and 10 is the worse possible pain'. These are ordinal scales. A rating scale with two or three categories is easiest for respondents, but more valid information is provided by a larger number of categories as the responses will be spread across a larger number of categories. There is evidence that no more than 10 should be used, and that most respondents can only meaningfully use 5–7 categories.[21] Adjectival and numerical rating scales both have their uses: use of the former increases validity because the points on the scale are clearly defined so that all respondents are using the same terms, whilst use of the latter enables 10 points to be used which has advantages in some studies.[21] The adjectives used on adjectival scales have to be chosen carefully as they can change how respondents use the options; it is particularly important, for example, that the adjectives used are perceived by respondents in a linear fashion and that they measure only one dimension.

A different design is the use of the 'agree/disagree' rating format. This is often used when asking respondents their opinions on contemporary issues. A 5-point scale is usually used as it is important to include a middle value for those who neither agree nor disagree with the statement. An additional option should be included for those who do not know enough about the issue to have an opinion.[24]

## Is the survey instrument itself fit for purpose?

Once the questions have been designed, the questionnaire (or interview schedule) itself needs to be designed. This needs to be formatted in such a way as to make the task of reading the questions, following the questions and answering them as easy as possible. Some of the principles underlying the design of survey instruments are discussed above. If designed for use in a personal or telephone interview survey, it should contain a complete 'script' for the interviewer, with clear instructions about, for example, what sections should be asked to whom, how to record answers to each questions, what prompts are acceptable and how both to introduce and to terminate the interview. As already discussed, questionnaires designed to be self-completed need to be considerably simpler, with either no or very few skips, and with clear instructions about how to answer questions. In both cases, a good introduction needs to be provided, outlining why the survey is being done and why it is important, explaining confidentiality, and then making it clear to the respondent what their task is.

Whether or not the resulting survey instrument is fit for purpose cannot be ascertained by researchers alone; it is important to test the survey instrument with the target population to be sure that it is indeed measuring what it is intended to measure and it is doing so in a reliable way. The next section addresses these issues.

## Testing survey instruments

### Conducting pre-tests

The only way to identify problems with the design of survey instruments before data collection begins is to conduct a pre-test of the instrument. There are a number of ways of doing this.

A method frequently used by survey researchers in both personal and telephone interview surveys is the field pre-test.[21] This aims to identify and fix overt problems experienced by the interviewer and the respondent. Interviewers are trained in the same way as they would be in a full survey and then they administer the survey instrument to members of the target population; they are debriefed about what did and did not work. This method usually places reliance on experienced and sensitive interviewers who are able to identify problems, although members of the research team may accompany interviewers and observe the survey instrument in action for themselves. Once the interviews are complete, the amount of item non-response and the distribution of responses is usually examined. Presser et al.[25] caution against placing too much reliance on this approach, arguing that it relies on the problems with questions being big enough to be observable from the respondent's behaviour, and on respondents being aware that they are having problems with the question. It can therefore, for example, miss instances where the respondent completely misunderstands a question but gives no indication of this. Other methods include expert analysis, in which a researcher (who may or may not have been involved in constructing the question) reviews the questionnaire to gain an understanding of the response task and to note potential problems. This can be very useful in identifying structural or logical problems with the questionnaire. In terms of detecting problems with questions, however, its weakness is that it shows what might go wrong with the questions, not what does go wrong. It is also unlikely to identify problems caused by the researchers' understanding of terms or use of language differing from those of the sample. Focus group discussions, in which respondents are given the opportunity to react to different aspects of the proposed questionnaire, can be more useful in identifying these problems.[21] Behaviour coding also has a role here; this involves observation of the interactions between the interviewer and respondent whilst the survey instrument is completed and is good at identifying problematic questions from, for example, the fact that respondents asked for clarification, took longer to answer the question, or that the interviewer did not ask the question as written.[21] These methods differ in the types of problems they can identify. Multiple testing methods therefore need to be used in order to be sure that all respondents share the same understanding of the meaning of questions, and are able and willing to answer them accurately.[25]

## Using cognitive interviewing techniques

These techniques are drawn from psychology and the cognitive sciences and aim to probe how respondents answer survey questions.[25–27] They aim to uncover the thought processes involved in interpreting and answering a question; these are then analysed to identify problems with the question. They can also be useful in identifying structural and logical problems in the survey instrument.[27] There is general agreement about the value of cognitive interviews in survey research.[25] This is supported by the findings from a study which used cognitive testing in the development of a survey instrument to produce data on patient perspectives on in-patient hospital care;[28] despite the fact that many of the questions had been used in other in-patient surveys, more than 70 per cent of the items tested were revised or deleted as a result of the cognitive interviews. Given the growing evidence for the value of these techniques, it is surprising that there is little evidence of their use in palliative care research.[23] All researchers planning a survey should consider using these techniques to increase the validity of their survey questions. Cognitive interviews are one to one interviews, usually between a researcher and an individual from the target population. They are normally conducted in person, although they may now be done on the telephone.[26] Because they are labour-intensive and result in rich data, the sample sizes used in cognitive interview studies are generally small, with samples of 12 not being uncommon, although larger samples are preferable.[27] There are two main techniques: 'think aloud' and verbal probing. In the first, respondents are explicitly asked to 'think aloud' as they answer the survey questions, thus revealing how they go about answering the question. The advantage of this method compared with verbal probing is that because it is open-ended the respondent is able to come up with unanticipated issues, and there is less potential for interviewer bias. The difficulty with it is that it is an artificial task so that respondents need to be trained how to do it; it may place a burden on them and they may be resistant to it.[27] It may also interfere with the respondent's usual cognitive processes.[26] In contrast, with verbal probing the interviewer asks the survey question and the respondent answers it as usual. The interviewer then asks for specific information relevant to the question and to the specific answer given; they 'probe' into the basis for the respondent's answer. This avoids the necessity for training the respondent as the task is not fundamentally different from that involved in answering survey questions. Probing may be concurrent, one question at a time, or retrospective, at the end of the questionnaire. The latter technique can be used to test self-complete questionnaires where it is important to explore the respondent's ability to complete the questionnaire unaided. There is currently no consensus about the best method to use.[25]

## Conclusion

This chapter has considered the relative advantages and disadvantages of collecting survey data via personal interviews, telephone interviews, postal surveys, and e-mailed and Internet surveys. It has highlighted the added value which may result from combining methods in order to enhance response rates, whilst at the same time cautioning against presuming that data collected by different methods can necessarily be provided. The principles of conducting personal and telephone surveys have been reviewed, with particular emphasis on the role of the interviewer. The evidence base underlying the design of effective postal surveys has been analysed. The design of survey instruments was then considered, along with methods to test the resulting questionnaire. All three key components of survey design have been addressed in this or the preceding chapter: the selection of those to whom questions are asked; the choice of the best collection method to meet the aims of the survey; and the design and testing of the questionnaire. Working knowledge of these components, together with an understanding of the underlying principles, will enable readers to design palliative care surveys which produce results which are representative of their target population, and are reliable and valid.

# References

1. Schonlau M, Fricker RD Jr, Elliott MN (2002) *Conducting Research Surveys via E-mail and the Web.* Santa Monica, CA: Rand Corporation.

2. Dillman DA (2000) *Mail and Internet Surveys: The Tailored Design Method.* New York: John Wiley.

3. Addington-Hall JM, Walker L, Jones C, Karlsen S, McCarthy M (1998) A randomised controlled trial of postal versus interviewer administration of a questionnaire measuring satisfaction with and use of services received in the year before death. *Journal of Epidemiology and Community Health* 52: 802–7.

4. Hepner KA, Brown JA, Hays RD (2005) Comparison of mail and telephone in assessing patient experiences in receiving care from medical group practices. *Evaluation and the Health Professions* 28: 377–89.

5. Hawthorne G (2003) The effect of different methods of collecting data: mail, telephone and filter data collection issues in utility measurement. *Quality of Life Research* 12: 1081–8.

6. Fowler FJ Jr (2002) *Survey Research Methods*, 3rd edn. Newbury Park, CA: Sage Publications.

7. Addington-Hall JM, McCarthy M (1995) The Regional Study of Care for the Dying: methods and sample characteristics. *Palliative Medicine* 9: 27–35.

8. American Association of Public Opinion Research. Interviewer Falsification in Survey Research: Current Best Methods for Prevention, Detection and Repair of its Effects. 2003. www.aapor.org/pdfs/falsification.pdf Accessed 2 October 2006.

9. Cartwright A, Seale CF (1990) *The Natural History of a Survey: An Account of the Methodological Issues Encountered in a Study of Life Before Death.* London: Kings Fund.

10. Edwards P, Roberts I, Clarke M, DiGuiseppi C, Pratap S, Wentz R, Kwan I (2002) Increasing response rates to postal questionnaires: systematic review. *British Medical Journal* 324: 1183–91.

11. Edwards P, Cooper R, Roberts I, Frost C (2005) Meta-analysis of randomised trials of monetary incentives and response to mailed questionnaires. *Journal of Epidemiology and Community Health* 59: 987–99.

12. Nakash RA, Hutton JL, Jorstad-Stein EC, Gates S, Lamb SE (2006) Maximising response to postal questionnaires—a systematic review of randomised trials in health research. *BMC Medical Research Methodology* 6: 5.

13. Moses SH, Clark TJ (2004) Effect of prize draw incentive on the response rate to a postal survey of obstetricians and gynaecologists: a randomised controlled trial. *BMC Health Services Research* 4: 14.

14. Roberts LM, Wilson S, Roalfe A, Bridge P (2004) A randomised controlled trial to determine the effect on response of including a lottery incentive in health surveys. *BMC Health Services Research* 4: 30.

15. Sharp L, Cochran C, Cotton SC, Gray NM, Gallagher ME, TOMBOLA group (2006) Enclosing a pen with a postal questionnaire can significantly increase the response rate. *Journal of Clinical Epidemiology* 59: 747–54.

16. White E, Carney PA, Kolar AS (2005). Increasing response to mailed questionnaires by including a pencil/pen. *American Journal of Epidemiology* 162: 261–6.

17. Jepson C, Asch DA, Hershey JC, Ubel PA (2005) In a mailed physician survey, questionnaire length had a threshold effect on response rate. *Journal of Clinical Epidemiology* **58**: 103–5.

18. Mond JM, Rodgers B, Hay PJ, Owen C, Beumont PJ (2004) Mode of delivery, but not questionnaire length, affected response in an epidemiological study of eating-disordered behaviour. **57**: 1167–71.

19. Harrison RA, Cock D (2004) Increasing response to a postal survey of sedentary patients—a randomised controlled trial. *BMC Health Services Research* **4**: 31.

20. Fredrickson DD, Jones TL, Molgaard CA, Carman CG, Schukman J, Dismuke E, Ablah E (2005) Optimal design features for surveying low-income populations. *Journal of Health Care for the Poor and Underserved* **16**: 677–90.

21. Fowler FJ Jr (1995) *Improving Survey Questions: Design and Evaluation.* Thousand Oaks, CA: Sage.

22. McPherson C, Addington-Hall JM (2003) Judging the quality of care at the end of life: can proxies provide reliable information? *Social Science and Medicine* **56**: 95–109.

23. McPherson CJ, Addington-Hall JM (2004) Evaluating palliative care: bereaved family members' evaluations of patients' pain, anxiety and depression. *Journal of Pain and Symptom Management* **28**: 104–14.

24. Addington-Hall JM, Karlsen S (2005) A national survey of health professionals and volunteers working in voluntary hospice services in the UK: I. Attitudes to current issues affecting hospices and palliative care. *Palliative Medicine* **19**: 40–8.

25. Presser S, Couper MP, Lessler JT, Martin E, Martin J, Rothgeb JM, Singer E (2004) Methods for testing and evaluating survey questions. *Public Opinion Quarterly* **68**:109–130

26. Beatty P, Callegaro M, Whitaker K, Miller K, Calvillo A. Cognitive interviewing at the National Center for Health Statistics. www.cdc.gov/nchs/ppt/duc2002/cognitive-interviewing.ppt375,1,Cognitive Interviewing at the National Center for Health Statistics. Accessed 7 July 2006.

27. Willis GB (2005) *Cognitive Interviewing.* Thousand Oaks, CA: Sage Publications.

28. Levine RE, Fowler FJ Jr, Brown JA (2005) Role of cognitive testing in the development of the CAHPS Hospital Survey. *Health Services Research* **40**: 2037–56.

# Section 3

# Epidemiological research methods

Chapter 6

# Experimental and quasi-experimental designs

Massimo Costantini and Irene J. Higginson

## Introduction

This chapter uses classical epidemiological methods to describe the most common non-experimental study designs used in palliative care research. Most of this chapter is focused on methodological issues in testing hypotheses of association between two or more variables, using observational and quasi-experimental designs. Randomized studies are not discussed in detail, not because we think they are of little value in palliative care research, but because these are considered in detail elsewhere (Chapters 2 and 3).

Although different, all study designs have in common the aim to obtain the highest possible degree of internal validity from their results. When a study aims to estimate the association between variables, and/or to estimate a measure of effect, validity refers to the correct quantification of the association. A misrepresentation of effect is a bias. In other words, internal validity is the degree to which the results of a study are likely to be true and free of bias. Bias occurs for all study designs, experimental and non-experimental, at any stage of investigation, from study design to publication of the results.[1] This is relevant in the light of the increasingly recognized value of integrating different types of study in the process of construction of evidence, and in the effort to make the decision-making process, at any level, and not only in palliative care, more evidence based.[2]

Finally, choosing the most appropriate study design to answer a specific research question assumes that the researcher knows in detail the main aim of the study. This may seem self-evident, but it is often overlooked, as much of the controversy over the interpretation of the results of clinical research arises from disagreements or ambiguities over the questions posed by the research. The perfect design does not exist, but it is possible to find a good design to answer a well-defined specific question (Chapter 15).

This chapter cannot give all answers (in terms of detailed design descriptions), but seeks to help researchers and clinicians interpret and consider different options (in terms of study designs) for their questions.

**Table 6.1** Types of epidemiological designs

| Type of study | Artificial manipulation of the study factor | Randomization |
|---|---|---|
| Observational | No | No |
| Quasi-experimental | Yes | No |
| Experimental | Yes | Yes |

# Types of study design

The epidemiological approach is based on the structuring of research design. Kleinbaum et al.[3] classifies epidemiological research into three mutually exclusive types of studies: experimental, quasi-experimental and observational (Table 6.1). If there is artificial manipulation of the study factor, the study is experimental or quasi-experimental rather than observational. Random allocation (randomization) of the study factor (i.e. a treatment, an intervention) between groups of patients discriminates experimental from quasi-experimental studies (Table 6.1). These study designs are considered in detail in the remainder of this chapter.

# Observational studies

Observational studies are commonly further subdivided into two subtypes: descriptive and analytic studies.[3]

## Descriptive studies

Descriptive studies estimate the frequency of a disease, symptoms or problems in a population and in different subgroups. They are usually conducted when little is known about a problem, or little is known about the occurrence of a known problem. Studies describing the prevalence (i.e. the proportion with) of pain[4] or of severe communication problems[5] in different settings of patients, or temporal trends in home deaths,[6,7] are classical descriptive studies. A descriptive study has the advantage of being practical and feasible to plan and conduct, and in most cases can be analysed without a strong knowledge of statistics. These studies are very important for generating hypotheses that can be explored using other study designs.

Case reports or case series are probably the most descriptive studies of all. In a case report, a single unit (a patient or a small group of patients, or a setting such as a service or hospital) is described in detail to reveal something original, for example the positive clinical response to a drug never previously used for that problem. In 1998, Zylicz *et al.* described the anti-pruritic activity of paroxetine in five patients experiencing severe pruritus.[8] The paper described for each patient, clinical characteristics, therapy, response and adverse effects. Five years later, the same group published the results of a randomized controlled trial (RCT) indicating that paroxetine is effective in the treatment of severe pruritus.[9]

## Analytic studies

Analytic studies examine an association between a dependent variable and one or more independent variables. Possible causative factors are examined. The independent variable may be not only a characteristic of the patient or of the disease, but also a therapy or an intervention. The dependent variable is the outcome of interest, such as pain control, satisfaction or one or more dimensions of quality of life.

An analytic study is planned when enough is known about the problem and a specific *a priori* hypothesis can be evaluated. In analytic studies, we are interested in studying possible causal associations (or relationships) between variables. However, and very importantly, association does not necessarily imply a causal relationship. Variables may be associated in cross-sectional data sets, but it is not clear which change came first. Further variables may be associated with each other, but also with another variable, which was in fact the cause of the change, but has not been measured in the study. Caution is therefore needed when interpreting associations.

Analytic studies may be cross-sectional, longitudinal or case–control designs. Case–control studies compare groups of cases (subjects with the outcome of interest, e.g. disease) and one or more groups of controls (subjects without the outcome) with respect to a current or previous independent variable. This study design is rarely used in palliative care research because of the difficulty in identifying representative samples of persons with and without 'the outcome', e.g. 'disease'. Although it would be virtually impossible to select people according to whether they had a disease or not (since all people in palliative care have many diseases), it is conceivable that a case–control study could be conducted examining patients who did and did not have other outcomes, for example adequate pain control or their wish for place of death, met.

### Cross-sectional studies

In a cross-sectional study, a defined population is examined at one point in time or over a short period of time. With a cross-sectional design, you can limit the analyses to a descriptive level, but in most cases the relationship between a problem (or other health-related characteristics) and other variables of interest is evaluated. For example, in 1999, a survey was carried out in all the public hospitals of an Italian region in order to quantify the prevalence of (proportion with) pain among all adult patients hospitalized for at least 24 h (descriptive aim of the study).[4] However, the aim of the study was to describe the potential determinants of pain by demographic and clinical characteristics of the patients, and by types of units and hospitals (analytic aim of the study). As cross-sectional studies are very popular, discussing their limitation is essential. The most important limitation, often reported as length-biased sampling, is that all cross-sectional studies usually over-represent subjects with long duration and under-represent cases with short duration.

An example is useful to understand how this bias can affect the results of a cross-sectional study. Imagine that, as medical director of a hospice, you are worried because your team is slow in detecting and promptly treating pain during the first days after patients' admission to the hospice. To make evident the problem, you plan a small prevalence survey to study the point prevalence of pain (i.e. the proportion with pain at one point in time). On one afternoon, a medical student is asked to go around the ward interviewing patients and, using a standard questionnaire, to ask if they have pain. While this will give a snapshot of who has pain on one afternoon, it will not give a true picture of all patients admitted to the unit. Patients staying longer will be over-represented and those staying for shorter periods will be under-represented. Thus, it is likely that this approach will underestimate the prevalence of pain, because patients staying for a shorter period in your service (and, if you are right, with a higher probability of suffering from pain) are less likely to be included in the survey. In this instance, a more useful design would be to follow patients as they are admitted, so that all admissions are captured.

In cross-sectional studies, every association should be interpreted cautiously, as the cause and effect question affects all cross-sectional studies. Further, any temporal sequence between cause and effect is usually hard to establish. As a consequence, these study designs should be used to plan other analytic approaches that are more valid in estimating causal relationships between variables.

One particular variation of cross-sectional design which is worthy of note is the ecological study. In an ecological study, groups of individuals, rather than single individuals, are studied. The groups may be people living in a geographical area, people receiving care from one particular family doctor (or group practice), on one ward or even in one hospital. Independent and dependent variables related to the group are then contrasted. For example, in both London and then later in Genova (Italy), ecological studies analysed the relationship between community levels of deprivation and the proportion of people who died at home in that area.[10,11] In both studies, there was an inverse relationship between deprivation and dying at home, which was remarkably similar. However, these associations are found at the level of the group. This does not necessarily mean that the association will hold true for each individual living in those areas. To make such an assumption erroneously would be to fall for what is known as the ecological fallacy.

## Cohort studies

The cohort study is a design in which two or more groups of subjects are followed from exposure to outcome.[12] In its simplest form, it compares the experience of the group exposed to a study factor (exposed) with the other group not exposed to the factor (unexposed). The occurrence of the outcome is recorded for all subjects. If the exposed subjects have a higher or lower frequency of the outcome than the unexposed subjects, then an association between exposure and outcome is evident.

The main characteristic of a cohort study is that the population (both exposed and unexposed) is followed forward in time from exposure to outcome. The most common type of cohort study is prospective, when the data are collected prospectively from the beginning. However, they can be retrospective or historical (if the investigator goes back in time and retrospectively identifies exposed and unexposed using, for example, clinical records collected prospectively), or ambidirectional (when the data are collected both retrospectively and prospectively).

In cohort studies, information about the study factor, the factors that allow subjects to be classified into exposed and unexposed groups, is known at the beginning of the follow-up period. To be at risk of developing the outcome, the population must be free from the outcome at the beginning of the follow-up period (when 'it enters the cohort'). This study design allows us to estimate the incidence of the outcome of interest (i.e. new cases with the outcome in a population occurring within a defined period of time) and, by comparing incidence among exposed and non-exposed, to quantify the association between the study factor and the outcome.

Cohort studies can vary enormously in their size and complexity. This study design has many appealing features for palliative care research. More specifically, cohort studies are the best way to study the natural history of a disease, a disorder or a problem, and the temporal sequence between cause and outcome is usually clear. A better understanding of the natural history of many diseases and of their determinants is crucial for identifying possible effective interventions and for planning experimental studies. In palliative care, this approach could help to understand better the range of specific problems encountered by non-cancer patients during their advanced and terminal phase of disease.[13] Cohort studies also allow us to avoid the cause–effect dilemma, as the exposure to the independent variable precedes the outcome. They allow us to study many outcomes potentially arising from a single exposure, as well as allowing us to study infrequent exposure. They are not affected by the risk of length-biased sampling, as in cross-sectional designs. They also allow us to estimate incidence and the calculation of relative risk.

On the other hand, cohort studies have some limitations to take carefully into account, especially when they are used to evaluate an association between health interventions, such as the provision of new services and the outcome. Some selection bias is unavoidable in cohort studies, as in all non-randomized studies. To test an intervention, ideally the exposed and unexposed subjects should be the same in all aspects except for the exposure under study. The risk of selection bias must be taken into account in the development stage of the study (choosing an appropriate study design that allows minimization of the risk of bias), and explored, and if possible corrected, during the analysis of results.

In palliative care research, studies have compared the proportion of home deaths among a population of cancer patients followed by palliative home care services with a control population (usually composed of patients not followed at home). Most of these studies conclude that the higher proportion of home deaths among the first group as compared with the control group is a consequence of the effectiveness of the palliative home care services in reducing home deaths. Many of these studies tried to reduce the effect of a potential selection bias by matching cases and controls for some patient characteristics,[14,15] or by estimating the association after adjusting for a number of variables. In both cases, what the researcher cannot do is to reduce the selection bias by variables that are not known, or not measurable (such as the different attitudes of the two groups to being followed at home, and consequently to dying at home). This does not mean that these are invalid studies, but that the validity of the results should be discussed taking into account the possibility of misinterpretation of the results due to a selection bias.

Finally, an incomplete assessment resulting in a reduction of the study population available for analyses can result in a selection bias. Studies assessing the prevalence of symptoms among patients with HIV/AIDS in a palliative care service found more severe symptoms among those patients who were unable to self-complete questionnaires.[16] Incomplete assessment becomes very difficult to analyse when the compliance is different in the experimental group and in the control group. This means that selection bias may occur independently from the compliance obtained by the study. Even very little loss in assessment, if unequally distributed between the two groups, can produce a large distortion in the estimate of the association.

Note, however, that this type of selection bias can occur in observational, quasi-experimental and experimental studies. In fact it can (and frequently does) occur in many palliative care studies, because of the nature of the very ill population, who are unable to complete questionnaires. For example, imagine that you want to estimate the effectiveness of a new experimental service in controlling breathlessness by comparing it with standard services (Fig. 6.1). New patients admitted in both the services are evaluated for breathlessness by the nurses of the two services at baseline and after a month. Let us consider two different scenarios. In the first scenario you get a low compliance at the assessment (60 per cent overall), but this is equally distributed in the two groups. In the second scenario you get a higher overall compliance (85 per cent) but with a different proportion of assessments in the two groups (for example 100 per cent in the experimental service and only 70 per cent in the conventional service) (Fig. 6.1). Although the compliance is higher in the second scenario, the risk of selection bias is also much higher in this situation than in the first scenario. In the first scenario, you might reasonably assume (but you will never be sure!) that the factor which has reduced the completion of assessment took effect in the same way in both the groups, making your estimate of effect potentially free from selection bias. Note that selection bias invariably happens when different standards of assessment are planned for the two groups, or when the assessment is left to the professional of the services. In this case, you must expect that the professionals involved in the study, being more motivated, achieved a higher proportion of assessment (and probably of different quality). What you will not know easily, in scenario two, is whether the assessments were completed more frequently because patients had less

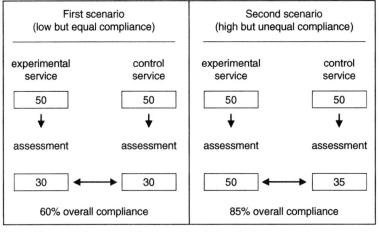

**Fig. 6.1** Cohort studies with different levels of compliance.

breathlessness or other problems, because they were more motivated due to the fact that they received the intervention, or whether the staff's higher motivation meant that more very ill people completed questionnaires. Each option would distort the result in different ways.

## Quasi-experimental studies

A quasi-experimental study is a study in which an intervention is deliberately introduced to observe its effects (the artificial manipulation of the study factor) without using randomization to create the comparisons from which the effects are inferred.[3,17] In other words, we study the efficacy (or the effectiveness) of an intervention, or, more specifically, its power to produce the effect under study. According to the classification used in this chapter, in a quasi-experimental study the intervention can be planned by the investigators (who implement the intervention themselves in a group of subjects or in a specific area), or can be planned by others not directly involved in the study.[3]

Assignment to the study factor under investigation (e.g. an intervention) is by means of self-selection (the individual or the unit chooses the intervention themselves), or by means of administrative selection, by which physicians, health professionals, bureaucrats or others choose which individual or unit should receive which intervention. Although the researcher usually has little or no control in the assignment of the intervention, he may still have considerable control over other aspects of the study such as assessment, such as the when and to whom of measurement.[17]

In palliative care research, quasi-experimental studies are often employed in the evaluation of educational programmes (i.e. the effectiveness of an education programme in cancer pain assessment and management) or in health services research, when randomization is not possible or practical, or is questionable for ethical reasons.[18]

A quasi-experimental study can be conducted in a variety of ways, using different study designs. Many of these designs (and their methodological problems) are very similar to those of observational studies except that the study factor is artificially manipulated, and so potentially the researcher has more information about, and potentially more control over, the intervention. These designs may involve one-group comparisons, multiple group comparisons or a combination of these.

### Designs without an external control group

#### One-group post-test only design

In the one-group post-test only design, each individual serves as its own control (Fig. 6.2). There are different variants of this simple design[17] that rarely

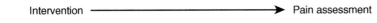

**Fig. 6.2** One-group post-test only design.

can reduce the plausibility of alternative explanations for the observed association. The simplest and weakest design (one group post-test only design) obtains a post-test assessment of an outcome of interest (e.g. pain) from an individual who experienced an intervention. This approach is commonly considered inadequate to evaluate the causal relationship between the intervention and the outcome. Even though it is regarded as very weak in research terms, it is important to mention, because most health professionals (and patients) during their daily work use this approach to decide on a causal relationship between an act (usually a therapy) and an outcome of interest. Perhaps it seems paradoxical that the situation which is regarded as the weakest in research terms is the one used to decide the effectiveness of many treatments for individual patients and families in day-to-day practice.

### One group pre-test/post-test design (before and after studies)

Adding a pre-test assessment before the intervention yields a one-group pre-test/post-test design (commonly called a before and after study) (Fig. 6.3). While this is stronger than a single assessment, this approach provides weak information on the nature of the association between intervention and outcome.

Although in clinical settings this approach is used to describe changes over time of an outcome of interest, these studies have important limitations. First, regression to the mean explains most of the variations observed in these studies,[19] and secular trends can affect the results, independently from the intervention under study. Thus, the lack of an external control does not allow the investigator to know if other events which happened at the same time might be contributing to the observed changes. For example, data on the consumption of opioids in Italy before and after the implementation of a new law aimed at facilitating opioid prescription for cancer pain have been used to state that: '… freedom of prescribing should not be seen as automatically leading to increases in opioid consumption'.[20]

This is probably truth, but the study design is too weak to allow these conclusions.

### Time series studies

There are many variants in the group of quasi-experimental studies with an internal control group, but the most interesting are the interrupted time series

Pain assessment ⟶ Intervention ⟶ Pain assessment

**Fig. 6.3** One-group pre-test/post-test design.

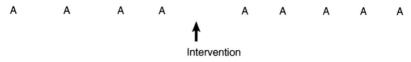

**Fig. 6.4** Time series.

studies (Fig. 6.4). In this design, multiple assessments (A in Fig. 6.4) are made within a single group before and after the intervention is implemented.

The advantage of this approach is that it is possible to take trends over time into account, and thus make a causal relationship more plausible between the intervention and a change in the outcome after it. This study design is often considered in health services research, because of problems identifying a control group. There are two main problems in this type of study. The first is that a bias can occur if other events able to affect the outcome occurred together with the intervention. The second is that it requires more complex statistical analyses.

## Designs with an external control group

With this study design, the groups (those who receive the intervention under study and the control group) are compared with each other, as in a simple observational study. The experimental group is usually formed from a convenience sample (different health districts) or from subjects who volunteer (not necessarily the patients). Usually the control group is selected to be as similar as possible to the intervention groups for all characteristics except the intervention. This study design, in all its variants, has the same characteristics of a randomized study except for the absence of a randomization procedure to allocate subjects to different interventions.

The investigator using this type of study should always consider how bias could have affected the results, as selection bias is built into all non-randomized studies. Selection bias refers to systematic differences in prognosis or responsiveness to the intervention between patients who receive the intervention under study (the experimental group) and those who do not (the control group). This limitation is the same as discussed earlier for cohort studies.

There are many variants in this group of study design, most of them rarely used in health research.[17] The most popular design uses a pre-test assessment in both the experimental group and the control group (Fig. 6.5). In this design, the association between the independent variables (the intervention) and the outcome (pain) is analysed by comparing the distribution of pain in the two groups (the experimental and the control group), taking into account baseline values.

The most important limitation of this study design is that, as discussed above, it is impossible to avoid selection bias. The question is how much the

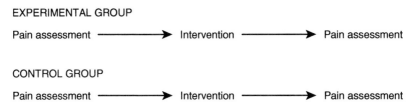

EXPERIMENTAL GROUP

Pain assessment ————————➤ Intervention ————————➤ Pain assessment

CONTROL GROUP

Pain assessment ————————➤ Intervention ————————➤ Pain assessment

**Fig. 6.5** Pre-test/post-test with external control group design.

selection bias, inherent in all non-randomized studies, can affect the results. The answer is based on the way participants are assigned to groups and on how much control the investigator has over the independent variable.[21] Designs in which participation of subjects is voluntary, especially when the intervention under study is a therapy, are very weak, as there is almost always a relationship between factors related to the preference for the intervention and the outcome under study. Other studies identify groups on the basis of factors not related to their preferences for the intervention, such as the geographical area of residence.

A number of designs that combine different design elements have been described.[17] For example, multiple assessments made before and after the intervention, within both the experimental group and the control group, can be viewed as a design that combines elements from a time series study (Fig. 6.4) and a design with an external control group (Fig. 6.5).

## Conclusions

It is commonly stated that RCTs represent the gold standard for the assessment of the effectiveness of health interventions. This statement, although generally true, is oversimplistic because it fails to take into account at least two issues.

◆ All clinical and epidemiological studies, including RCTs, are subject to bias. Randomized studies have the advantage potentially to protect the study from selection bias, because the units under study (usually patients) are allocated to the intervention by a random process. However, many other sources of bias can affect the results of a randomized study, including bias in the assessment of the outcome, contamination, drop-outs and those lost to follow-up. Furthermore, in many instances, substantial flaws have been observed in randomization procedures as well as in blinding. Few, if any, RCTs can be considered free of bias, and in many instances their internal validity is questionable, and possibly lower than that of a well designed and conducted non-randomized trial (Chapters 2 and 3).

◆ In the design of a study in order to answer a clinical question, three dimensions must be taken into account: feasibility; validity; and generalizability.

None of these can be ignored, and the choice of the study design will be the result of a compromise, where all the advantages and limitations of the various methodological options are thoroughly considered.

Clinical and health services research in palliative care is hampered by the objective difficulties encountered in the design of prospective studies, and, as a consequence, the amount and quality of the available evidence is far lower than in other areas. To fill this gap, RCTs will have only a marginal role, because of feasibility problems. What is needed is a new generation of high quality studies deploying all the available methodological tools, including randomization, when possible, in order to expand the pool of the available evidence on which clinical and health service decisions should be based.

# References

1. Sackett DL (1979) Bias in analytic research. *Journal of Chronic Diseases* **32**, 51–63.
2. Higginson IJ (1999) Evidence based palliative care. There is some evidence and there needs to be more. *British Medical Journal* **319**: 462–3.
3. Kleinbaum DG, Kupper LL, Morgenstern H, (ed.) (1982) *Epidemiologic Research*. New York: Van Nostrand Reinhold, pp. 40–50.
4. Costantini M, Viterbori P, Flego G (2002) Prevalence of pain in Italian hospitals: results of a regional cross-sectional survey. *Journal of Pain and Symptom Management* **23**: 221–230.
5. Higginson IJ, Costantini M (2002). Communication in end-of-life cancer care: a comparison of Team Assessment in three European countries. *Journal of Clinical Oncology* **20**: 3674–82.
6. Higginson IJ, Astin PA, Dolan S (1998) Where do cancer patient die? Ten-year trends in the place of death of cancer patients in England. *Palliative Medicine* **12**: 353–363.
7. Costantini M, Balzi D, Garrone E, Orlandini C, Parodi S, Vercelli M, Bruzzi P (2000) Geographical variations of place of death among Italian communities suggest an inappropriate hospital use in the terminal phase of disease. *Public Health* **114**: 15–20.
8. Zylicz Z, Smits C, Krajnik M (1998) Paroxetine for pruritus in advanced cancer. *Journal of Pain and Symptom Management* **16**: 121–4.
9. Zylicz Z, Malgorzata K, Alistar van Sorge A, Costantini M (2003) Paroxetine in the treatment of severe non-dermatological pruritus: a randomised controlled trial. *Journal of Pain and Symptom Management* **26**: 1105–12.
10. Higginson IJ, Webb D, Lessof L (1994) Reducing hospital beds for patients with advanced cancer. *Lancet* **344**: 47.
11. Costantini M, Fusco F, Bruzzi P (1996) Uno studio epidemiologico a Genova dal 1986 al 1990 sul luogo di decesso per neoplasia. *Informatore Medico Oncologico* **5**: 21–4.
12. Grimes DA, Schltz KF (2002) Cohort studies: marching towards outcomes. *Lancet* **359**: 341–5.
13. Albert SM, Murphy PL, Del Bene ML, Rowland LP (1999) Prospective study of palliative care in ALS: choice, timing, outcomes. *Journal of Neurological Sciences* **169**: 108–13.

14. Costantini M, Higginson IJ, Boni L, Orengo MA, Garrone E, Henriquet F, Bruzzi P (2003) Effect of a palliative home care team on hospital admissions among patients with advanced cancer. *Palliative Medicine* **17**: 315–21.

15. McCusker J, Stoddard AM (1987) Effect of an expanding home care program for the terminally ill. *Medical Care* **25**: 373–85.

16. Butters E, Higginson I, George R, Smits A, McCarthy MM (1992) Assessing the symptoms, anxiety and practical needs of HIV/AIDS patients receiving palliative care. *Quality of Life Research* **1**: 47–51.

17. Shadish WR, Cook TD, Campbell DT, (ed.) (2002) *Experimental and Quasi-experimental Designs*. Boston: Houghton Mifflin Company, pp. 103–206.

18. Black N (1996) Why we need observational studies to evaluate the effectiveness of health care. *British Medical Journal* **312**: 1215–8.

19. Bland JM, Altman DG (1994) Regression towards the mean. *British Medical Journal* **308**: 1499.

20. Mercadante S (2002) Opioid prescription in Italy: new law, no effect. *Lancet* **360**: 1254–5.

21. Morgan GA, Gliner JA, Harmon RJ (2000) Quasi-experimental designs. *Journal of the American Academy of Child and Adolescent Psychiatry* **39**: 794–6.

Chapter 7

# Outcome measurement

Irene J. Higginson and Richard Harding

## What do we mean by outcome measures?

Outcome measures are used to quantify a change in health status or quality of life (QoL), usually resulting from a treatment or service. The term is taken from a model developed by Donabedian[1] and others[2] who developed methods to assess the quality of health care, using ideas from manufacturing industry. This outlined that health care comprised the following:

◆ Structure/or inputs: resources in terms of manpower, equipment and money

◆ Process: how the resources are used (such as visits, beds, clinics, drugs or treatments given)

◆ Output: productivity or throughput (such as rates of clinic attendance or discharge, throughput—the rate that patients are seen)

◆ Outcome: change in health status or QoL that can be attributed to health care.

Usually, therefore, an outcome measure assesses a particular health status, QoL or need for care. Repeating measurements over a period of time describes the change in health status, QoL or need. Alternatively, some measures ask patients how much they have changed.

There are thousands of existing outcome measures, which cover different diseases, problems and aspects of treatment. Textbooks such as Bowling's *Measuring Disease,*[3] or those by McDowell and Newall[4] or Wilkin et al.[5] provide a critical assessment of measures, as well as good overviews of the topic. There are also web-based resources, such as the Quality Of Life Instruments Database which has information on >1000 patient outcome and QoL instruments, provides web links to authors' own pages describing these instruments and can be found at http://www.qolid.org. It has a structured presentation of frequently updated data on outcome measures, and aims to:

provide an overview of existing Patient Reported Outcomes (PRO) instruments, provide relevant and updated information on outcome instruments, facilitate access to the instruments and their developers, and facilitate the choice of an appropriate outcome measure.

## Why should outcomes be measured in research?

The success of any study of QoL, PRO or the effect of any intervention or treatment, or the assessment of need depends greatly on the choice of appropriate instruments. These must be selected according to the domains they measure and the populations and pathologies for which they were designed. Practical issues, such as the availability of different translations, copyrights and access to instruments, are also major criteria in the choice of instruments. Many studies have floundered because of their choice of inappropriate instruments; in some instances, data failed to be collected,[6] in others the measures failed to detect change.[7]

## Issues in choosing an outcome measure for a study

There are a number of key issues to consider when choosing a measure for a study. These include the psychometric properties of the measure—validity, reliability etc.—and the more practical aspects, such as whether there is a cost for using the measure and whether other studies report data from a similar measure, permitting future comparison.

### Validity

Validity assesses whether the instrument measures what you intend to measure, e.g. QoL. There are several questions to be considered when assessing the validity of measures:

- Does the measure appear to cover aspects that are relevant to the area of enquiry of the study, as perceived by patients, their families and relevant users (face validity)
- Are the domains covered appropriate, important and sufficient for the intervention and types of patients being studied? (content validity)
- Does the measure correlate with a 'gold standard' or superior measure? (criterion validity). If this is not known, because there is no 'gold standard', then an alternative question is whether the measure produces results that conform to a theory. For example, it might be hypothesized that a measure of weakness should correlate with a patient's stage of disease. This test, called construct validity, however, is only as accurate as the theory used.
- Validity is the single most important aspect of measurement, and without it there is no point proceeding.

### Reliability

Reliability assesses whether the measure produces the same results when repeated in an unchanged population. This includes inter-rater (or inter-observer) reliability, which tests for similar results with different observers, and test–re-test reliability, which tests for similar results when the measure is used at different points in time when the object of measurement remains unchanged. Statistical tests of this use Cohen's kappa, which measures the level of agreement controlled for chance agreement. Sometimes correlation or simple reporting of agreement is appropriate, but note that these do not control for chance agreement. In certain circumstances, kappa is not so helpful, particularly when there is a high level of chance agreement. Another test often used to assess reliability is whether individual items of the measure correlate with each other (called internal consistency). This can be assessed using a range of different statistics. Cronbach's alpha is probably the most common: this reports the average of correlations between all possible halves of the scale (e.g. even-numbered items versus odd-numbered items, first 10 items versus second 10 items). Split-half reliability and Guttman may also be reported. Note that if a measure has a very high internal consistency (e.g. a score of 0.9), although it is likely that the measure is reliable, it also suggests that many items in the measure are capturing similar aspects of care. Thus, some may be redundant, and the measure could be shortened, often making it more appropriate and practical. This is particularly important in palliative care.

Reliability is also tested when criterion and construct validity are tested. Measures shown to have some degree of criterion or construct validity must have some degree of reliability, otherwise they could not have provided sufficiently consistent results.

## Appropriateness and acceptability

Appropriateness and acceptability assess whether the measure is suitable for its intended use. This is crucial as inappropriate measures can lead to missing data. Large amounts of missing data will bias the results, and so measures must be able to be used by the majority of patients. There are several questions to be answered:

- ♦ Is the measure short/long enough for completion or administration in the intended setting and with the intended types of patients, families or informants?
- ♦ Is the format of the measure and questions acceptable and suitable for administration in the intended setting and with the intended informants?
- ♦ Has it been used in this or similar settings before, and was it successful?
- ♦ If the measure is a translation of an existing measure, will it work in this culture and language? Has it been translated into the language, and then back-translated into the original language? Has more than one translator been used? Has its conceptual as well as its semantic equivalence been assessed?

In studies, a researcher often uses a combination of measures. The appropriateness and applicability question should be applied to the whole battery of measures. Methods for testing questionnaires discussed in Chapter 5 will be useful in testing appropriateness and applicability. The appropriate order of measures should be considered at this stage. Given the frailty of many palliative care patients, it may be necessary to decide on the measures which are most essential to the study and order the questionnaires in such a way that these questions are asked of all patients, regardless of frailty.

## Responsiveness to change

Responsiveness to change is whether the measure can detect meaningful changes. This is sometimes called sensitivity to change. This is critical if the measure is to be of any use in detecting changes that occur as a result of a treatment or intervention. For example, will the measure discriminate between different degrees of severity, or detect the level of changes likely to result from treatment? Among patients who have a progressive or advanced illness, many QoL measures produce poor scores (so-called floor effects), because they rely heavily on function as part of the QoL assessment. Thus, changes in symptoms, family support or other important components of care are not detected. Responsiveness to change is difficult to test. This usually needs to be done by assessing patients over time, and seeing if the measure detects changes which either (1) the clinicians and/or patients and/or families feel are important; (2) are associated with events or treatment or service changes; (3) are observed by an independent observer; or (4) are observed on a 'gold standard' measure.

## Interpretability

Interpretability is whether the results from using the measure have clinical interpretation and relevance. When given a QoL score, or a series of QoL scores over time, the researcher needs to be able to consider what to do with this information, and what it will mean for those who actually experience the QoL and problems. For example, an overall QoL score of, say, 5 out of 10, means little to a patient or family. The patient and clinician need to understand what aspects are impeding QoL (e.g. symptoms, informational concerns, worries), so that they can see what difference the treatment is making. Outcome measures are often presented using mean scores. For example, the Factual Assessment of Cancer Therapy (FACT) fatigue subscale showed, among 1152 varied cancer patients in five randomized trials, a mean score of 28.2 [standard deviation (SD) 11.8]. However, the potential range of score is 0–52.[8] At what point is a problem considered as severe? What is a clinically important change? The study compared four groups, with differences in mean values of around 2 points, and the authors noted that a clinically meaningful improvement was ≥3 points.[8] Similarly, on the FACT-L, a change of 2–3 points was found to correlate with symptom changes.[9] Changes of one point on individual items of the Palliative Care Outcome Scale (POS) have been linked to clinical changes, and stability was found in patients deemed by staff as not changing.[10,11] Some screening scales have cut-off points to make a diagnosis or to determine 'a case' (e.g. depression scales), but for others whether the problem is rated as severe is more important. The researcher needs to consider how the data from the measure will be translated into something meaningful for patients, families, professionals and policy makers.

## Cost

Cost is unfortunately an issue which must be considered. Some measures do have a charge for use and, if this is the case, then a sufficient budget must be available. Most measures will have manuals and guides for which a charge will be required. The time taken to administer the measure will also have cost implications, as will the mode of administration, e.g. patient or researcher, computer based or pen and paper completion.

## Generalizability

This may be a factor if the researcher wishes to compare their data with those in other studies. For example, a number of studies have now recorded symptom profiles in different groups of patients with advanced disease including cancer, neurological conditions and HIV/AIDS. Where these have used the same scale, there is an opportunity to compare results with other populations. One problem with comparing prevalence data is the lack of standardized measures used.[12] Using measures similar to other studies makes systematic reviewing and meta-analysis much more straightforward and reduces heterogeneity (Chapter 8).

# Moving to a more person-centred and individualized approach in measuring outcomes

QoL measures are seen as ways of capturing patients' perspectives of their disease and treatment, their perceived need for health care and their preferences for treatment and disease outcomes. They are hailed as being 'patient-centred'. However, a main challenge in measuring outcomes, and particularly QoL, lies in their uniqueness to individuals. Many of the existing measures of QoL impose standardized models of QoL and pre-selected domains, which may make them measures of general health status rather than QoL. To what extent do they really represent the QoL of individual patients or groups of patients? Are they simply descriptions of patients' health status in relation to health professionals' or society's idea of what ought to constitute quality of life for people who are ill?

The failings of some QoL measures can be seen in some of the contradictory results obtained in research studies. Attempts to quantify and compare QoL across different populations of patients using standardized, generic measures have been confounded by the so-called 'disability paradox'. Patients who clearly have significant health and functional problems or intrusive symptoms do not necessarily produce QoL scores that researchers expect. For example, transplant patients, haemodialysis patients and peritoneal dialysis patients who report a wide variety of health problems are more likely to rate themselves as 'very happy' than the general population.[13] Patients with neoplasms rate their QoL in the top quartile of the World Health Organization (WHO) QOL questionnaire across all life domains, better than all other groups of patients including those attending a family planning clinic.[14] This paradox brings into question the value of using some of the very general QoL measures to assess outcomes in research.

## Choice of generic or specific outcome and quality of life measures

There are three main categories of outcome measure: generic measures, specific measures and patient-centred measures, which are considered below. Which measure, or group of measures, is chosen depends upon the aim of the study and the nature of the enquiry.

### Generic measures

These have been developed for application across broad populations and settings, both healthy and ill. These are very useful for comparing different diseases and health states because they assess a broad range of domains.[15] Thus they might be used to contrast outcomes from diabetes treatment, pinning a hip fracture, cancer treatment and coronary bypass surgery. Common examples of these measures include: the Short Form 36, or Short Form 12, developed in the USA as part of the Medical Outcomes Study, by Ware et al.,[16] the EuroQoL, which comprises six items,[17-19] the Nottingham Health Profile[20,21] and the Sickness Impact Profile.[22] Data from these measures, especially the EuroQoL, have been attached to data from the general population about preferences for different states of health to produce utility measures, such as quality-adjusted life years (QALY).[23-25] These provide a utility value of different health statuses enabling the number of QALY produced by different treatments to be compared.

Generic measures can have some value in palliative care research, particularly if the aim is to determine how palliative treatment compares with other treatments. They have the advantage of wide validation in general populations and different cultures, although they have not been validated specifically in palliative care settings. However, these measures are often strongly geared to measuring functional status and self-sufficiency, and so are not responsive to clinically important change amongst patients in both cancer and in palliative care, often producing floor effects. Most of these scales produce a single utility score, thereby not conveying information about specific problems.[15]

## Specific or targeted measures

These are measures which are specifically developed for a group of patients or a treatment. Most outcome and QoL measures are specific measures. They range from measures of QoL in cancer, such as the European Organization for Research into Treatment of Cancer 30-item Quality of Life Questionnaire (the EORTC QLQ-C30)[26] and the FACT,[8,9,15] to measures specifically addressing outcomes or QoL in palliative care—of which there are a growing number of measures. Three such measures are described in more detail below.

### The Palliative Outcome Scale (POS)

The POS was designed to cover systematically those domains considered important to palliative care.[10] It aims to address the resolution of emotional, social, psychological and spiritual problems; the provision of information; good communication; and support for the family. It was validated among 337 patients and 148 staff in eight palliative care services. It may be used prospectively as a core measure to assess palliative care, enabling consistent assessments of patients and their families. The scale consists of 12 items and builds from those included in a variety of measures including the STAS (below) and the McGill Quality of Life Questionnaire. The first 10 items address patient and family/caregiver psychosocial needs (including two items regarding patient pain and symptoms). All these items are scored using a Likert scale (0–4). The last two items address the patient's two main problems and, if completed by staff or families, the patient's performance status. All items refer to events of the previous 3 days. Specific modules of POS, for example addressing symptoms[27] or other non-cancer diseases, and variations to its items are being developed.

### The Support Team Assessment Schedule (STAS)[28,29]

This includes 17 items covering pain and symptoms: patient anxiety, insight and spiritual; family anxiety and insight: planning affairs; communication; home services; and support of other professionals. Development was by means of collaboration with five palliative care teams, and it was revised in light of presentations at professional meetings, observation of palliative care and interviews with patients and families. The STAS is reported to be being used by >100 registered users including home, hospital and hospice settings in at least nine countries. Time to complete ratings for one patient averages 2 min. Its reliance on professionals' assessments may be a weakness, but the STAS was validated to ensure that professional ratings reasonably reflected patient view.[30,31] Extra items, such as individual symptoms, can be added.[32–34]

### The Edmonton Symptom Assessment System[35]

This includes nine visual analogue scales: pain, activity, nausea, depression, anxiety, drowsiness, appetite, well-being and shortness of breath. Assessments are completed by the patient, and if this is not possible a family member or nursing staff completes the ratings.

There are also specific measures to assess carer needs. Palliative care aims to address the needs of both patients and their families and carers, and relevant measures are necessary to evaluate the effectiveness of services and interventions for this population, whose needs may exceed those of the patient.[36] Challenges to outcome measurement for carers and families are that existing measures generally appear to lack sensitivity to change, that carers with least need are most likely to access services thereby limiting potential for observable improvement,[37] and that very few outcome evaluations have been undertaken with this population and so the usefulness of existing measures is largely unknown.[38] Data from several measures for informal carers have been reported, which have been validated mainly in populations of carers of geriatric patients.

A further challenge in selecting appropriate outcome measures in evaluation studies is that carers' needs cross many domains including information, psychological support, fatigue, technical and nursing support and training, finance, occupational and physiotherapy, relationship and communication difficulties, and anticipatory grief. Therefore, measures that are global are unlikely to detect change in specific domains, while the number of measures comprising a battery of measures must be kept to a minimum. A further challenge in outcome measurement is that palliative care interventions for informal carers usually have a short period of time, in comparison with other groups such as mental health, gerontology and disability, in which to establish change in areas such as coping and psychological status. Therefore, the expectation of measurable improvement may be unrealistic. The measurement of aspects of coping (a key variable measured in caregiving evaluations) is also problematic. In a study of samples of patients with chronic diseases, a standardized coping measurement tool produced inconsistency in coping data, and this inconsistency was explained to be a result of the nature of coping.[39] The study concluded that the tool did not contribute to inconsistency but that low stability reflects a genuine behaviour pattern. Therefore, the use of measures of coping in outcome evaluations may be inappropriate if behavioural coping strategies are indeed changing over time.

Two examples of specific carer outcome measures are detailed below.

### Zarit Burden Inventory

The Burden Inventory was designed to assess the stress experienced by carers of older and disabled persons.[40] Caregivers respond to 22 questions about the impact of the patient's disabilities on their life. For each item, carers are asked to indicate how often they have felt that way: never, rarely, sometimes, quite frequently or nearly always. The burden interview is a composite measure, combining different aspects or dimensions of caregivers' reactions to their involvement. The burden interview is scored by summing the responses of the individual items. Higher scores indicate greater carer distress. The Burden Inventory should not be taken as the only indicator of emotional state, and other measures of depression should be used to supplement the measure.

### Coping Responses Inventory (CRI)

The CRI is a measure of eight different types of coping responses to stressful life circumstances,[41] measured by eight scales and 48 items. The first set of four scales measures approach coping; the second set of four scales measures avoidance coping. The first two scales in each set measure cognitive coping strategies; the third and fourth scales in each set measure behavioural coping strategies. Each of the eight dimensions or scales is composed of six items. Individuals select and describe a recent stress, and use a 4-point scale varying from 'not at all' to 'fairly often' to rate their reliance on each of the 48 coping items. Therefore, each of the eight scales can range in score from 0 to 18.

Other measures not specific to carers have been used such as the GHQ (General Health Questionnaire), a popular and well-validated measure of psychological morbidity),[42] and the SAI (State Anxiety Inventory), another often used measure of apprehension, tension, nervousness and worry.[43] However, the problems associated with the use of global measures in this population have been discussed above.

## Person-centred measures

It is possible to measure QoL using a patient-centred approach employing individualized measures. These address the concerns raised above that existing standardized measures may impose standardized modes of QoL on individuals.

Instead, they allow individuals to define what is important and their QoL themselves. Although less widely used than standardized measures, these are receiving increasing interest. Two common examples are given below.

**SEIQOL** (Schedule for the Evaluation of Individualised Quality of Life)[44] is an interviewer-administered questionnaire. Patients are asked to specify five areas of their life of most importance to them and then rate their current status in each of these areas on a 0–100 visual analogue scale. In the direct weighting version of the questionnaire, patients are then asked to rate the relative importance of each of the five areas using an aid called a sectogram. Results can be presented as a profile of the five areas (bar chart) or as a global QoL score. This measure has been used in palliative care.

**Patient Generated Index** (PGI)[45] is based on Calman's definition of QoL. It can be interviewer or self-administered (although some problems have been encountered with the postal, self-administered version). Patients are asked to specify the five areas of their lives that are most affected by their condition. They then rate how badly affected they are in these five areas on a 0–100 visual analogue scale. Patients are then asked to weight the relative importance of these areas by allocating a total of 60 'spending points' between the five areas, the most points being allocated to the area in which a health improvement would be of most importance. The severity ratings are multiplied by the proportion of points allocated to that area and combined to give a QoL index between 0 and 100.

However, these measures have their own problems. First, some patients have some difficulty understanding the system of direct weighting, which limits their use as postal questionnaires,[46] among patients who are very sick, which is very relevant in palliative care,[47] or among those who have compromised concentration spans for any reason. Secondly, patients may not readily volunteer some important aspects, particularly those related to mood,[48] and the information that an individual is willing to volunteer may change over time.[49] Finally, because of its individualized nature, interpretation and analysis of some of the data is complex. This can make comparison of groups of patients or change within individuals over time difficult.

## What about developing country contexts?

The need to select outcome measures according to context and the aim of research is universal. The example of sub-Saharan Africa demonstrates this clearly. UNAIDS estimates that in 2003 there were 26.6 million people in sub-Saharan Africa living with HIV, and that there were 3.2 million new infections and 2.3 million AIDS-related deaths.[50] Cancer rates in Africa are expected to grow by 400 per cent over the next 50 years.[51]

## Contextual dimensions to defining outcomes

The 'good death' varies both culturally and historically, and interplays with notions of religion, community and (pertinent to debates on the role of modern palliative care) the length of time from diagnosis to the end of life.[22] Therefore, outcome measures must take account of factors considered important by local populations, as well as considering the diversity of meanings attached to factors within diverse national populations. A further complexity is describing what constitutes palliative care need in resource-poor settings. Although the principles of palliative care are consistent around the world, the socio-economic environments, prevailing diseases, health care systems, technology and drug availability differ enormously, meaning that palliative care has different characteristics in different regions.[52] In considering the application of measures and processes to developing countries, the principles remain the same. It may be even more important to identify failure and identify success, as palliative care is in a rapid growth stage.

While the WHO definition of palliative care[53] is globally relevant, how it translates into specific needs and their relative importance varies greatly according to setting. A simple demonstration of this variation is offered by a qualitative study of palliative care needs between the UK and Kenya, which found Kenyans' primary concern was for pain control and that of UK patients was for emotional pain.[54] A survey of the needs for palliative care among terminally ill people in urban Uganda identified key needs as home care, pain and symptom control, counselling and financial assistance for basic needs such as food, shelter and school fees.[55] The WHO 5-country African palliative care project has assessed the needs of terminal patients as the first phase of its community, public health approach to palliative care.[56] These multicountry WHO data clearly show that beyond primary clinical need for pain and symptom control, patients' main self-reported needs are social support, financial difficulties, emotional concerns, spiritual need and food security.[57]

## The challenge of outcome measurement in sub-Saharan Africa

Research into palliative care in sub-Saharan Africa is embedded into a nexus of challenges: clinical, logistical, financial, social, political and research:

> Clinical and health service audit and research is desperately needed so that we can establish how best to deliver palliative care in the resource-poor setting, and to establish an information base relevant to the developing world.[58]

Research is a fundamental necessity in this resource-poor context, enabling the allocation of scarce resources to best effect.

Once the initial task of identifying appropriate goals and outcomes to be measured is achieved, the next stage of identifying feasible and acceptable data collection methods will need to be addressed. This task may be frustrated by both practical challenges and unfamiliarity with scoring.[52] A comparison of pain assessment methods by a hospice in Uganda found good completion rates for a verbal rating of specific individual pain (100 per cent completion for primary pain) but only 60 per cent completion of a hand-score for total pain experienced (P. Cartledge, R. Harding, L. Mpanga Sebuyira and I.J. Higginson, personal communication). A further multimethods evaluation of morphine procurement, prescribing and patient outcomes found incomplete use of pain measurement charts and pain scales, and weaknesses in assessment recording procedures (Logie and Harding, personal communication). Despite current weaknesses in the use of recording and data systems, there is a strong awareness of the need for the provision of technical skills and tools among African providers. Survey data from end-of-life HIV care providers in sub-Saharan Africa identified a need for technical assistance in quality assurance, monitoring and evaluation, and commonly requested relevant outcome measurement tools for use within their services.[57]

## Conclusion

Palliative care is at a rapid growth stage, and research is needed. Valid, reliable, responsive and appropriate measurement of outcomes is critical to any quantitative study, if meaningful results are to be obtained. Validated and appropriate measures can be found in palliative care for a range of contexts and should be reviewed and if possible used before new measures are considered.

## References

1. Donabedian A (1980) *The Definition of Quality and Approaches to its Assessment. Explorations in Quality Assessment and Monitoring.* Ann Arbor, MI: Health Administration Press.
2. Higginson I (1993) *Clinical Audit in Palliative Care.* Oxford: Radcliffe Medical Press.
3. Bowling A (1995) *Measuring Disease.* Milton Keynes, UK: Open University Press.
4. McDowell I, Newall C (1987) *Measuring Health: A Guide to Rating Scales and Questionnaires.* Oxford: Oxford University Press.
5. Wilkin D, Hallam L, Doggett M (1992) *Measures of Need and Outcome for Primary Health Care.* Oxford: Oxford University Press.
6. McWhinney IR, Bass MJ, Donner A (1994) Evaluation of a palliative care service: problems and pitfalls. *British Medical Journal* **309**: 1340–2.
7. Greer DS, Mor V, Morris JN, Sherwood S, Kidder D, Birnbaum H (1986) An alternative in terminal care: results of the National Hospice Study. *Journal of Chronic Diseases* **39**: 9–26.

8. Cella D, Kallich J, McDermott A, Xu X (2004) The longitudinal relationship of hemoglobin, fatigue and quality of life in anaemic cancer patients: results from five randomized clinical trials. *Annals of Oncology* **15**: 979–86.

9. Cella D (2004) The Functional Assessment of Cancer Therapy-Lung and lung cancer subscale assess quality of life and meaningful symptom improvement in lung cancer. *Seminars in Oncology* **31**: 11–5.

10. Hearn J, Higginson IJ (1999) Development and validation of a core outcome measure for palliative care: the palliative care outcome scale. *Quality in Health Care* **8**: 219–27.

11. Aspinal, F, Hughes R, Higginson I J, Chidgey J, Drescher U, Thompson M (2002) *A User's Guide to the Palliative Outcome Scale*. London: Palliative Care and Policy Publications.

12. Potter J, Higginson IJ (2002) Frequency and severity of gastrointestinal symptoms in advanced cancer. In: Ripamonti C, Bruera E, (ed.) *Gastrointestinal Symptoms in Advanced Cancer Patients*. London: Oxford University Press, pp. 1–15.

13. Evans RW (1991) Quality of life. *Lancet* **338**: 363.

14. Skevington S (1999) Measuring quality of life in Britain. Introducing the WHO QOL-100. *Journal of Psychosomatic Research* **47**: 449–59.

15. Cella D, Chang C-H, Lai J-S, Webster K (2002) Advances in quality of life measurements in oncology patients. *Seminars in Oncology* **29**: 60–8.

16. McHorney CA, Ware JE Jr, Raczek AE (1993) The MOS 36 item short-form health survey (SF-36): II. Psychometric and clinical tests of validity in measuring physical and mental health constructs. *Medical Care* **31**: 247–63.

17. Brazier J, Jones N, Kind P (1993) Testing the validity of the EuroQoL and comparing it with the SF-36 health survey questionnaire. *Quality of Life Research* **2**: 169–80.

18. Van Agt H, Essink-Bot M-L, Krabbe P, Bonsel G (1994) Test re-test reliability of health state valuations collected with the EuroQoL questionnaire. *Social Science and Medicine* **39**: 1537–44.

19. Hurst NP, Jobanputra P, Hunter M, Lambert M, Lochead A, Brown H (1994) Validity of EuroQoL—a generic health status instrument—in patients with rheumatoid arthritis. *British Journal of Rheumatology* **33**: 656–62.

20. Hunt SM, McEwen J, McKenna SP (1985) Measuring health status: a new tool for clinicians and epidemiologists. *Journal of the Royal College of General Practitioners* **35**: 185–8.

21. Hunt SM, McKenna SP, McEwen J, Williams J, Papp E (1981) The Nottingham Health Profile: subjective health status and medical consultations. *Social Science and Medicine* **15**: 221–9.

22. Walter T (2003) Historical and cultural variants on the good death. *British Medical Journal* **327**: 218–20.

23. Rosser R, Kind P (1978) A scale of valuations of states of illness: is there a social consensus? *International Journal of Epidemiology* **7**: 347–58.

24. Torrance GW (1987) Utility approach to measuring health-related quality of life. *Journal of Chronic Diseases* **6**: 593–600.

25. Kaplan RM (1993) Quality of life assessment for cost/utility studies in cancer. *Cancer Treatment Reviews* **19** Suppl A: 85–96.

26. Aaronson NK, Ahmedzai S, Bergman B, Bullinger M, Cull A, Duez NJ, Filiberti A, Flechtner H, Fleishman SB, de Haes JCJM, Kaasa S, Klee M, Osoba D, Razavi D, Rofe PB, Schraub S, Sneeuw K, Sullivan M, Takeda F (1993) The European Organization for Research and Treatment of Cancer QLQ-C30: a quality-of-life instrument for use in international clinical trials in oncology. *Journal of the National Cancer Institute* **85**: 365–76.

27. Sherry KL (2004) Symptom prevalence and the use of systematic symptom assessment. *Palliative Medicine* **18**: 75–6.

28. Higginson IJ, Wade AM, McCarthy M (1992) Effectiveness of two palliative support teams. *Journal of Public Health Medicine* **14**: 50–6.

29. Higginson IJ (1993) *Audit Methods: A Community Schedule*. Oxford: Radcliffe.

30. Higginson IJ, McCarthy M (1993) Validity of the support team assessment schedule: do staffs' ratings reflect those made by patients or their families? *Palliative Medicine* **7**: 219–28.

31. Higginson I (1993) Audit methods: validation and in-patient use. In: Higginson I, (ed.) *Clinical Audit in Palliative Care*. Oxford: Radcliffe Medical Press.

32. McKee E (1993) Audit experience: a nurse manager in home care. In: Higginson I, (ed.) *Clinical Audit in Palliative Care*. Oxford: Radcliffe Medical Press.

33. Edmonds PM, Stuttaford JM, Penny J, Lynch AM, Chamberlain J (1998) Do hospital palliative care teams improve symptom control? Use of modified STAS as an evaluative tool. *Palliative Medicine* **12**: 345–51.

34. Higginson I (1994) Clinical teams, general practice, audit and outcomes. In: Delamothe D, (ed.) *Outcomes into Clinical Practice*. London: BMJ Publishing.

35. Bruera E, Kuehn N, Miller MJ, Selmser P, Macmillan K (1991) The Edmonton Symptom Assessment System (ESAS): a simple method for the assessment of palliative care patients. *Journal of Palliative Care* **7**: 6–9.

36. Higginson IJ, Hodgson C, McDonnell M, Butters E (1997) Family anxiety in advanced cancer: a multicentre prospective study in Ireland. *British Journal of Cancer* **76**: 1211–4.

37. Harding R, Higginson IJ, Leam C, Donaldson N, Pearce A, George R, Robinson V, Taylor L (2004) Evaluation of a short-term group intervention for informal carers of patients attending a home palliative care service. *Journal of Pain and Symptom Management* **27**: 396–408.

38. Harding R, Easterbrook PE, Karus D, Raveis VH, Higginson IJ, Marconi K (2005) Does palliative care improve outcomes for patients with HIV/AIDS? A systematic review of the evidence. *Sexually Transmitted Infections* **81**, 5–14.

39. Schwartz CE, Daltroy LH (1999) Learning from unreliability: the importance of inconsistency in coping dynamics. *Social Science and Medicine* **48**: 619–31.

40. Zarit SH, Zarit JM (1990) *The Burden Interview*. #189, Part 3. Penn State, Gerentology Center, College of Health and Human Development.

41. Moos RH (1997) Coping Responses Inventory: a measure of approach and avoidance coping skills. In: Zalaquett CP, Wood RJ, (ed.) *Evaluating Stress: A Book of Resources*. Lanham, MD: Scarecrow, pp. 51–65.

42. Goldberg D, Williams P (1991) *A User's Guide to the General Health Questionnaire*. Windsor, UK: NFER-Nelson.

43. Spielbeger CD (1983) *State-Trait Anxiety Inventory (Form Y)*. Mountain View, CA: Consulting Psychologists Press, Inc.

44. McGee HM, O'Boyle CA, Hickey A, O'Malley K, Joyce CRB (1991) Assessing the quality of life of the individual: the SEIQoL with a healthy and a gastroenterology unit population. *Psychological Medicine* **21**: 749–59.

45. Ruta DA, Garratt AM, Leng M, Russell IT, MacDonald LM (1994) A new approach to the measurement of quality of life. The patient-generated index. *Medical Care* **32**: 109–26.

46. Macduff C, Russell E (1998) The problem of measuring change in individual health-related quality of life by postal questionnaire: use of the patient-generated index in a disabled population. *Quality of Life Research* **7**: 761–9.

47. Hearn J, Higginson IJ (1997) Outcome measures in palliative care for advanced cancer patients: a review. *Journal of Public Health Medicine* **19**: 193–9.

48. Vachon MLS, Kristjanson L, Higginson I (1995) Psychological issues in palliative care: the patient, the family, and the process and outcome of care. *Journal of Pain and Symptom Management* **10**: 142–50.

49. Higginson IJ, Priest P, McCarthy M (1994) Are bereaved family members a valid proxy for a patient's assessment of dying? *Social Science and Medicine* **38**: 553–7.

50. UNAIDS. AIDS Epidemic Update 2003, Sub-Saharan Africa 2004. wws.//unaids.org.wad/2003/Epiupdate2003_en/Epi03_04_en.htm#P64_1

51. Morris K (2003) Cancer? In Africa? *Lancet Oncology* **4**: 5–6.

52. Higginson IJ, Bruera E (2002) Do we need palliative care audit in developing countries? *Palliative Medicine* **16**: 546–7.

53. World Health Organization (2003) Palliative Care. www.who.int/hiv/topics/palliative/PalliativeCare

54. Murray SA, Grant E, Grant A, Kendall M (2003) Dying from cancer in developed and developing countries: lessons from two qualitative interview studies of patients and their carers. *British Medical Journal* **326**: 368–72.

55. Kikule E (2003) A good death in Uganda: survey of needs for palliative care for terminally ill people in urban areas. *British Medical Journal* **327**: 192–4.

56. Sepulveda C, Habiyambere V, Amandua J, Borok M, Kikule E, Mudanga B, Ngoma T, Solomon B (2003) Quality care at the end of life in Africa. *British Medical Journal* **327**: 209–13.

57. Harding R, Stewart K, Marconi K, O'Neill JF, Higginson IJ (2003) Current HIV/AIDS end-of-life care in sub-Saharan Africa: a survey of models, services, challenges and priorities. *BMC Public Health* **3**: 33.

58. Mpanga Sebuyira L, Moore J (2003) Palliative care: the 21st century challenge. *Health Exchange.*

Chapter 8

# Systematic reviews

Marjolein Gysels and Irene J. Higginson

## What is a systematic review?

Systematic reviews have developed in the context of the new norm of evidence-based medicine, which became established as a response to the growing awareness that decision making in clinical practice was not based on the findings of research.[1] Traditionally, clinical practitioners learned from textbooks and expert opinion rather than seeking information from an evidence base.[2] Even with an improved understanding of the reasons for the uptake of research findings, it is difficult to keep up with the evidence which is accumulating in a field. The volume of biomedical literature published annually is constantly expanding. Over 2 million articles in 20 000 journals are published annually.[2]

Expert opinion represented in the traditional discursive review has been shown to be subjective and therefore prone to bias and error.[3] Selective inclusion of studies that support the author's view is common. Observation showed that the number of times clinical trials are cited is related to their outcome. Trials that concur with the prevailing opinion were quoted more often than trials reporting unsupportive results. Reviews carried out according to the traditional methods also tend to reach opposite conclusions and miss small, but potentially important differences. In areas where opinions differ, conclusions reached from the evidence obtained may often be more influenced by the specialty of the author than by the actual data. 'Expert opinion' often lags behind the research evidence and is not infrequently inconsistent with it.[4]

There has therefore been an increasing focus on formal methods of systematically reviewing studies to produce explicit, replicable and up-to-date summaries of the effectiveness of health care interventions.[2] Systematic reviews apply pre-defined strategies to identify, appraise and synthesize research findings from primary studies to provide empirical answers to targeted clinical questions.[5] They are a fundamental scientific enterprise applying methods of systematic collation and analysis of research findings which reduce unmanageable amounts of information into meaningful, integrated packages of relevant evidence.[6,7] They are exhaustive compilations of studies on a particular subject with an evaluation of the validity of the studies included, following an open design to preclude bias.[5]

## Why do systematic reviews?

The findings from systematic reviews are needed in different institutions. In the medical profession, practitioners use systematic reviews to remain literate in broader aspects of medicine and to keep abreast of the primary research in a given field.[8] Doctors and nurses have to plan the use of available resources, or decide when to call upon knowledge generated by research, and how to apply the evidence to a specific case.[9] Reviews in an applied field of research such as the evaluation of health care can have serious consequences. In the past, the adoption of some life-saving therapies has been delayed due to the lack of scientific principles in reviews. The opposite has also happened, with some treatments continuing to be recommended long after controlled research has shown them to be harmful.[5,10]

Policy makers need systematic reviews to formulate guidelines and legislation regarding the use of drugs, treatments or the organization of care. Increasingly, decisions are attuned to patients' needs and wishes. Clinicians are required to involve patients in their care according to the doctrine of 'informed consent' so that these patients can make autonomous or at least shared decisions. Informed and critical use of health services is encouraged by initiatives to educate patients into more critical participants by providing them with evidence-based information which is both scientifically sound and understandable.[11]

In research, systematic reviews are considered worthwhile before starting new research. Through exploring what was done before, the new work can adjust its research questions to contribute more adequately to the existing body of evidence.[2] A systematic review can be thought of as a puzzle, and a single study as a piece of that puzzle.[12] The value of a new study is derived from how it fits with and expands previous work. Through systematically reviewing a field of interest, the puzzle's intricacies may be disentangled. The diversity of multiple reviewed studies provides an interpretative context not available in any one study. Systematic reviews may separate unsound or redundant work from innovative and carefully designed studies that deserve further consideration. Where gaps in evidence exist, they serve the function of alerting the research community to unexplored terrain.[2,6] They reveal the level of primary material to be developed and the urgency to combine findings, and consider them in their totality.

## Are systematic reviews relevant in palliative care?

Although still limited, the literature base in palliative care is growing. Just as in other areas of care, doctors, nurses and other clinicians, researchers, educators and policy makers are inundated with amounts of information which are difficult to manage. Systematic reviews are needed to integrate existing information efficiently and help provide data for rational decision making. Palliative care is a specialty that has been growing rapidly, and reviews are essential to bring together much of the literature, which may be scattered across health, social and other journals. The multiprofessional nature of palliative care, and therefore the wide range of different journals which might include relevant information, makes the need for systematic reviews even more urgent.

A further reason why systematic reviews are important in palliative care is because the systematic review represents an efficient scientific technique. Palliative care is beset with small studies, often with inadequate sample size. These are underpowered to detect differences which might really exist between intervention and control groups. This type II error would result in not rejecting a null hypothesis when it is in fact false (Chapter 2). According to Simon:

> An effective clinical trial must ask an important question and provide a reliable answer. A major determinant of the reliability of the answer is the sample size for trials. Trials of inadequate size may cause contradictory and erroneous results and thereby lead to an inappropriate treatment of patients. They also divert limited resources from useful applications and cheat the patients who participated in what they thought was important clinical research. Sample size planning is, therefore, a key component of trial methodology.[13]

Despite this aspiration, the truth is that palliative care studies often fail to recruit the intended sample size because of all of the well known difficulties of interviewing and recruiting people who are seriously ill.[14] A systematic review offers an efficient way of combining data from small studies so that the combined sample size may be sufficiently large to detect a difference. Thus, it could be argued that systematic reviews are more relevant in palliative care than many other areas of health care.

## When not to do a systematic review

In general, systematic reviews attempt to answer very specific questions. They are not good at answering very general questions of an exploratory nature. In these instances, a researcher might want to use some systematic elements in their literature searching and data extraction. This might include defining the databases, years searched, keywords and the types of information extracted from the studies. It might even involve preparing tables of the information.

However, a more exploratory enquiry where questions are not clear cannot be subject to the data extraction and methods of data synthesis or analysis in a systematic review. To use an analogy, it would be rather like collecting data randomly in a study without aims or objectives, and collecting different information from one patient to the next and expecting somehow to put these together in a systematic format. General explorations and more philosophical 'think' pieces are still highly suited to the traditional form of literature review.

Protocols for systematic reviews generally recommend that prior to developing the questions for the systematic review a brief general quick review is undertaken. The purpose of this initial review is to understand the scale and scope of the literature and the nature of potentially relevant studies so that the questions can be clearly formulated.

## When systematic reviews are useful

Systematic reviews are useful in answering a clearly defined question. The question may relate to effectiveness. For example, do tricyclic antidepressants reduce neuropathic pain, or are palliative care teams effective in improving pain, other symptoms and distress in families?[15,16]

Systematic reviews can also be used to answer questions not related to effectiveness but to understanding the nature of a problem. For example, what is the prevalence of pain, and in particular neuropathic pain, in patients with lung cancer?[17] Systematic reviews might also look at aspects such as what information is available about patients' preferences, for example preferences for place of care.[18] Systematic reviews are also useful when there is a sufficient body of literature to be brought together. This does not have to be extensive, but ideally there should be a number of studies which can be combined. It would be fairly futile, for example, to carry out a systematic review of only one, two or three studies. If the pilot reviewing suggested that there would be only one or two relevant studies, then the authors should reconsider their questions and whether a systematic review is the appropriate methodology.

## Defining the aims and questions

The focus of a review is born out of the need for information on the effectiveness of interventions in a certain area, especially when there is uncertainty regarding the potential benefits or harms of interventions, when there are variations in practice or when research is being planned. The guidance for supportive and palliative care for those affected by cancer, for example, produced by the National Institute for Clinical Excellence (NICE),[19] was a policy document to guide decisions about the commissioning and organization of services. The process of the development of the recommendations for action in the

Guidance Manual had to be supported by evidence about the effectiveness of different models of service delivery. The objective of a review in this area was to determine the current state of evidence on interventions, targeted at health care professionals or the structure in which health care professionals deliver their care, to improve the supportive and palliative care for those affected by cancer.

Each review question typically defines (1) the participants in the primary studies, in this case the population affected by cancer; (2) the interventions being considered: this was broadly stated as those which are meant to improve supportive and palliative care; and (3) the outcomes which evaluate the success of the intervention, i.e. those reported in the studies, including, for example, psychological morbidity, place of death, quality of life, etc. Once these three aspects of the review question have been defined, the inclusion criteria for eligible papers can be clarified, together with criteria for the research designs which will be considered eligible.

The area to be reviewed can be further separated into more specific research questions; this process is termed the 'operationalization of the review'. In the above example, the original scope question was operationalized into more refined questions, relating to: the effectiveness of communication training for health professionals caring for patients with cancer, and the best ways in delivering these; the role of interactive technology and videotape for patient education; the most appropriate instruments for the assessment of spiritual needs; and the patient group for which the patient-held record is the most suitable in cancer care.

## Systematic review methods

When planning any systematic review, a protocol, outlining the questions, the methods and planned analysis, must be prepared. It should include the features below.

### Searching the literature

The purpose of searching is to generate as comprehensive a list as possible of studies, both published and unpublished, to ensure that the process of identifying studies is not biased. The thoroughness of the literature search is one factor that distinguishes systematic reviews from traditional discursive reviews.

Search strategies are built up from a series of trial and pilot searches. These can also be refined by discussion and consultation with experts in the subject. For inspiration of adequate search terms, one can turn to articles in the same areas and see how they have been indexed. Constructing a combination of search terms should be done in a structured way; an effective strategy is breaking down the review question into facets (population, intervention, outcomes, designs).

For observational studies or qualitative research, many kinds of study designs exist, the names of which are not standardized. Imaginative searching with lots of synonyms is required.

The first source to consult is the electronic databases, such as the general health and medical databases (MEDLINE and EMBASE) or the databases which are available at the Cochrane Library (CDSR, DARE and CCTR). Also, databases with a more specific focus can be consulted (e.g. PSYCHINFO, CANCERLIT, CINAHL, etc.). However, one should bear in mind that no database is complete and they have their own geographical and language biases. The selection of keywords and the combinations of these is critical, and several pilots may be needed. It is therefore necessary to search several databases to maximize coverage. Electronic searches should find a balance between sensitivity or recall (ability to identify relevant articles), and specificity or precision (ability to exclude irrelevant articles). Searches with high recall tend to have low specificity (a large proportion are not relevant).

Searching in databases can be combined with hand searching which is an important way to identify very recent publications which have yet to be cited by other publications or included in electronic databases. Hand searching is also an important way of identifying references missed by electronic searches. Hand searching may then identify new keywords, which should be used in the search. Electronic database searches in MEDLINE have been shown to identify 17–82 per cent of known trials and 46–88 per cent of trials published in MEDLINE journals. Other sources are the 'grey literature' in which important findings can be reported but are in formats which have not been indexed in the main databases (e.g. discussion papers, dissertations, conference proceedings, etc.). Pharmaceutical companies have details of trials carried out with their support in a private database.

Contact with authors of publications is advisable in the case of missing or confusing data. Poor reporting also occurs in published articles.

## Selection of studies

Once the search is complete, a large number of potential articles will have been identified. The aim of study selection is to identify those articles that help to answer the questions being addressed by the review. The process of selection must be undertaken to minimize bias. Therefore, decisions about the inclusion and exclusion criteria for studies must be made before the review is commenced and be clearly documented in the protocol.

The inclusion and exclusion criteria should follow logically from the review question and be defined in terms of the population studied, if relevant, the interventions, the outcomes and the study design of interests. Only those studies which meet all of the inclusion criteria and none of the exclusion criteria should be included in the review. These criteria should be piloted to check that they are reliably interpreted and that they classify studies appropriately. The process of selecting the studies for inclusion in the review should be checked or independently carried out by a second reviewer. Decisions can sometimes be made on the titles, but more commonly the abstract and in some instances the full paper is needed to be able to make the appropriate decision.

The reviewers should clearly specify the process of including and excluding studies within the review, with all of the reasons for exclusion being clearly given. This can be presented in a flow chart or a simple summary table, or in the text.

## Hierarchy of evidence

Studies are usually assessed according to methodological quality, and this then allows the studies to be put into a broad hierarchy, depending upon the quality of the study.

For studies assessing whether treatments are effective the normal hierarchy is:

◆ Level 1—experimental studies [e.g. randomized controlled trials (RCTs) with concealed allocation into groups].

◆ Level 2—quasi-experimental studies (e.g. experimental studies without randomization).

◆ Level 3—controlled observational studies; this is often subgrouped into 3a cohort studies and 3b case-controlled studies.

◆ Level 4—observational studies without control groups.

◆ Level 5—expert opinion based on consensus, clinical observation, pathophysiology or bench research.

These designs are explained more in Chapter 6. However, different hierarchies may be applied for different types of questions. For example, if the systematic review question is to understand the prevalence of a particular problem, then whether studies are experimental or not is not relevant. An RCT is generally accepted as being the gold standard method of determining the effectiveness of a treatment or service, but not at determining the prevalence of a problem in a situation. In these instances, a different hierarchy is needed. For example, a hierarchy which we developed to assess prevalence studies[18] was:

◆ Level A—longitudinal study with standardized, systematic and pre-defined assessment of outcome of interest, >80 per cent response rate and multicentre.

◆ Level B—longitudinal study that falls short of criteria for Level A, cross-sectional, observational or retrospective study with >60 per cent response rate, standardized and systematic assessment of outcome of interest.

◆ Level C—response rate <60 per cent or no response rate given and/or inconsistent assessment of outcome of interest.

The hierarchy might be different depending upon the nature of the question asked, although for systematic reviews assessing interventions, common hierarchies are usually preferable.

In addition to grading the studies in a hierarchy, it is useful to assess the methodological quality of the studies. A variety of quality assessment instruments can be used. These might assess individual aspects of the study methodology, might include checklists based on a number of quality items, or might actually produce a score examining the quality of the study.

Table 8.1 shows an example of the quality criteria for assessment of experimental studies and Table 8.2 shows some of the quality criteria for the assessment of observational studies.

Although qualitative research methods do not fit into many of the standard hierarchies that are developed for the assessment of experimental treatments,

**Table 8.1** Quality criteria for assessment of experimental studies[20]

| |
|---|
| 1. Was the assignment to the treatment groups really random? |
|    Adequate approaches to sequence generation |
|       Computer-generated random numbers |
|       Random numbers tables |
|    Inadequate approaches to sequence generation |
|       Use of alternation, case record numbers, birth dates or weekdays |
| 2. Was the treatment allocation concealed? |
|    Adequate approaches to concealment of randomization |
|       Centralized or pharmacy-controlled randomization |
|       Serially numbered identical containers |
|       On-site computer-based system with a randomization sequence that is not readable until allocation |
|       Other approaches with robust methods to prevent foreknowledge of the allocation sequence to clinicians and patients |
|    Inadequate approaches to concealment of randomization |
|       Use of alternation, case record numbers, birth dates or weekdays |
|       Open random numbers lists |
|       Serially numbered envelopes (even sealed opaque envelopes can be subject to manipulation) |
| 3. Were the groups similar at baseline in terms of prognostic factors? |
| 4. Were the eligibility criteria specified? |
| 5. Were outcome assessors blinded to the treatment allocation? |
| 6. Was the care provider blinded? |
| 7. Was the patient blinded? |
| 8. Were the point estimates and measure of variability presented for the primary outcome measure? |
| 9. Did the analyses include an intention to treat analysis? |

**Table 8.2** Some quality criteria for assessment of observational studies

**Cohort studies**

- Is there sufficient description of the groups and the distribution of prognostic factors?
- Are the groups assembled at a similar point in their disease progression?
- Is the intervention/treatment reliably ascertained?
- Were the groups comparable on all important confounding factors?
- Was there adequate adjustment for the effects of these confounding variables?
- Was a dose–response relationship between intervention and outcome demonstrated?
- Was outcome assessment blind to exposure status?
- Was follow-up long enough for the outcomes to occur?
- What proportion of the cohort was followed-up?
- Were drop-out rates and reasons for drop-out similar across intervention and unexposed groups?

**Case–control studies**

- Is the case definition explicit?
- Has the disease state of the cases been reliably assessed and validated?
- Were the controls randomly selected from the source of population of the cases?
- How comparable are the cases and controls with respect to confounding factors?
- Were interventions and other exposures assessed in the same way for cases and controls?
- How was the response rate defined?
- Were the non-response rates and reasons for non-response the same in both groups?
- Is it possible that overmatching has occurred in that cases and controls were matched on factors related to exposure?
- Was an appropriate statistical analysis used (matched or unmatched)?

**Case series**

- Is the study based on a representative sample selected from a relevant population?
- Are the criteria for inclusion explicit?
- Did all individuals enter the survey at a similar point in their disease progression?
- Was follow-up long enough for important events to occur?
- Were outcomes assessed using objective criteria or was blinding used?
- If comparisons of subseries are being made, was there sufficient description of the series and the distribution of prognostic factors?

Source: York Centre for Reviews and Dissemination.

there is a growing body of work demonstrating how qualitative research can be included in systematic reviews (see below). There are also quality criteria for the assessment of qualitative studies, health economic studies, screening tools and measurement scales.[21] An example of a method score to assess both observational and experimental studies is shown in Table 8.3.

More recent developments in systematic reviewing have established methods to rate the importance of publications to the field of study. Making an assessment of the 'pertinence' of a study is essentially a subjective judgement and depends upon the aims and objectives of the systematic review. However, it can be done in a systematic way. Preparing such information helps the

**Table 8.3** Method score, to grade the quality of evidence

| | Score |
|---|---|
| **1. Aims/outcomes[1]** | |
| Defined at outset | 2 |
| Implied in paper | 1 |
| Unclear | 0 |
| **2. Sample formation[1]** | |
| Random | 2 |
| Quasi-random; sequential series in a given setting or total available | 1 |
| Selected, historical, other, insufficient information | 0 |
| **3. Inclusion/exclusion criteria[1]** | |
| Explicitly described in paper | 2 |
| Implied by patient characteristics, setting | 1 |
| Unclear | 0 |
| **4. Subjects described[1]** | |
| Full info | 2 |
| Partial info | 1 |
| No info | 0 |
| **5. Power of study calculated[1]** | |
| Yes | 2 |
| No | 0 |
| **6. Outcome measures[1]** | |
| Objective | 2 |
| Subjective/self-report | 1 |
| Not explicit | 0 |
| **7. 'Best' follow-up (up to 12 months)[1]** | |
| >90 per cent of subjects enrolled/approached available | 2 |
| 80–90 per cent of subjects | 1 |
| <80 per cent of subjects/no info | 0 |
| **8. Analysis[1]** | |
| Intention to treat/including all available data | 2 |
| Excluding drop-outs but evidence of bias adjusted or no bias evident | 1 |
| Excluding drop-outs and no attention to bias or imputing results | 0 |
| **9. Baseline differences between groups** | |
| None or adjusted | 2 |
| Differences unadjusted | 1 |
| No info | 0 |
| Cohort/descriptive study only/not applicable | 8 |
| **10. Unit of allocation to intervention** | |
| Appropriate | 2 |
| Nearly | 1 |
| Inappropriate or no control group | 0 |
| Cohort/descriptive study only/not applicable | 8 |
| **11. Randomization/method of allocation of subjects** | |
| Random | 2 |
| Method not explicit | 1 |
| Before exclusion of drop-outs or non-randomized | 0 |
| Cohort/descriptive study only/not applicable | 8 |

[1]Include only these items if the study is observational. The denominator for the method score so constructed is 22 for an experimental study and 16 for a non-experimental study (in which components 9–11 do not apply).

reviewers assess the weight of evidence in a paper and enables individuals to balance two separate (although not completely independent) sources of information—the paper's pertinence or 'signal' and its methodological weaknesses (or noise).[22,23]

Thus, in the analysis, it is possible to distinguish some papers where the design is of a poorer quality (a high 'noise' level), but the findings are important because they are very pertinent to the question under study (a strong 'signal'). Conversely, a paper may be of very high methodological quality but the signal is only of modest importance. Some individuals have conceptualized this by presenting the balance of signal to noise ratio.[24] In a field such as palliative care, this may be useful because it does not eliminate research simply because it is not at a certain level of evidence or because it has methodological weaknesses. It offers a complementary assessment to the usual statistical approaches incorporating the assessments of the reviewing team of the relevance of the studies.

When constructing a scale to assess a paper's signal, the reviewers will need to refer to their specific questions and the settings to which they wish the results of the systematic review to apply. An example of one such scale, which was constructed for the review of palliative care teams,[16] is shown in Table 8.4.

**Table 8.4** SIGNAL scores, grading the relevance of studies for UK palliative care services (PCS)

Study **relevance:**
5  Highly relevant to and based in UK PCS
4  Highly relevant to but not based in UK PCS
3  Some relevance to UK PCS
2  Limited relevance to UK PCS
1  Little relevance to UK PCS
0  No relevance to UK PCS

Study **implementation** to UK PCS:
5  Existing PCS staff can implement without further training or resources
4  Existing PCS staff can implement with limited further training or resources
3  Existing PCS staff can implement with substantial further training or resources
2  New staff required with limited or no training for further implementation
1  New staff required with substantial training for further implementation
0  Could not implement

Study **value** to UK PCS:
5  Extremely important finding for UK PCS—effect size immense
4  Highly important finding for UK PCS—effect size substantial
3  Fairly important finding for UK PCS—effect size moderate
2  Fairly unimportant finding for UK PCS—effect size limited
1  Of very limited importance for UK PCS—effect size minimal
0  Of no importance for UK PCS—no effect size

Relevance + implementation + value = SIGNAL out of 15.

This assesses three components: the relevance of the paper to the review question; the applicability of the research findings (e.g. could existing staff with or without further training implement them); and the overall value of the study, relating to the effect size of the findings in the paper, i.e. was a substantial difference or improvement shown? Because such signal scores are open to individual interpretation, care must be taken to ensure the reliability of the assessments.[25] It is important to remember that the ratings are, in effect, personal opinions and therefore not as objective as key data, outcomes or methodological adequacy.

## Data extraction

Data extraction is the process by which the reviewers obtain the information they need from the reported studies. Because this can be a subjective process and therefore prone to bias, the protocol should clearly define the data items to be extracted from each of the primary studies. It is best, if possible, to use a standardized data extraction form. There is no one correct way of doing this; the amount of information to be extracted should be directly related to the questions posed. Forms that are too detailed can be wasteful in reviewer time; forms which are too brief may omit important information and reviewers may have to reabstract the information from the studies when deficiencies are noted later. It is generally wise to pilot the forms on a sample of studies before the full extraction is under way.

If time is very short, then it may be that the data extraction form can be reduced to simple tables explaining the main features of the results. Note, however, that studies often contain different amounts of information, and sometimes none, about items which are of relevant interest. Caution is needed when using tables to ensure that the same types of information are extracted for each study.

Electronic forms are particularly useful in handling large amounts of data. Using database programs such as Access or FoxPro, electronic data collection forms can be designed without the need for expertise in computer programming. They have the advantage that information can easily be stored and retrieved. A further advantage is that these forms can be programmed to calculate conversions of data reported in various formats, e.g. calculating mean, standard deviation and standard errors.

The data extraction form should contain general information, the name and details of the paper, the country, the nature of the publication and the name of the reviewer who is extracting the data. Specific information will need to be extracted about the aims and objectives, the study population, the outcome measures and study design. If the study is an intervention one, then details of the form and delivery of the intervention and the control group are needed.

The forms should include information about the numbers of patients (in intervention and control groups if appropriate), study eligibility, methodology, drop-out rates and other factors affecting the validity that are relevant to the systematic review questions. The quality assessment checklist and any methodological scoring should also be added.

Because data extraction is prone to error and involves a degree of subjective judgement, instructions and decision rules about coding should be included in the data extraction form. This is particularly important when multiple reviewers are participating in a project. Ideally data extraction should be performed independently by at least two reviewers because this improves reliability. If this is not possible, then a random sample should be reviewed or separately extracted by another member of the project team. It is also wise to consult with other members of the team if the reviewer is uncertain about areas of data to be extracted, particularly the statistical analysis.

Very commonly, studies included in the review have been published in several different publications. It is important to identify serial publications where papers may report accumulating numbers of participants or increased length of follow-up. However, during data synthesis, it would obviously be misleading to include the results of several reports of the same study as if they were different. It is important in these instances to report studies which may include several papers, rather than individual papers. If there are preliminary and more definitive results, then the more definitive results should be included.

During the process of data extraction, it will become apparent that the papers do not provide all the information that needs to be extracted. This may be because such information was never collected, or because it has not been reported. Depending upon the nature of the missing information and the requirements of the analysis, in some instances the authors of the original papers can be contacted with a specific request for completion of the missing data. However, unfortunately, some studies may not be able to be included in all aspects of the review because of missing data. Where the primary studies do not display the exact data required for the meta-analysis, it may be possible to transform the data to a format that is suitable. To avoid mistakes in this process, data should be first collected in the form that they are reported and then transformed into the subsequent step with careful checking by individuals who are well versed in the statistical approaches that are being used.

## Data synthesis

The aim of the phase of analysis or synthesis of the data in a systematic review is the evaluation of the results of the included studies. It would be unusual if the question being asked and the factors affecting effectiveness are so simple that a quantitative (statistical) pooling of results would provide sufficient information, about whether the intervention does more good than harm, and if so how much and under what circumstances. A broader assessment is therefore necessary and a qualitative overview is required. This considers all the results, not only the methodological rigour, and therefore reliability of these studies, but it also helps to highlight and explore differences between studies.

A qualitative analysis of the evidence is therefore an essential step in the assessment of effectiveness of a health intervention. It is within this context that any quantitative synthesis should take place.

The effectiveness of a health care intervention is likely to depend on a large number of factors relating to who receives it, who delivers it and how, and in what context. One area reviewed as part of the NICE guidance for supportive and palliative care[19] was communication training for health professionals who care for patients with cancer. Given the wide variety of objectives, participants, designs, outcome measures and results used in the studies included in this review, a quantitative meta-analysis was impossible. Still, the synthesis of these studies raised interesting issues. Most importantly, the results confirmed that health professionals could be trained to communicate more effectively with patients who have cancer. There were four RCTs providing level Ia evidence that ensured the replicability of the interventions applied; the level IIIc studies with a less rigorous design offered a broader picture and allowed for comparison among training programmes. The synthesis of the findings from these evaluations showed that basic skills training is not enough and that positive attitudes and beliefs are needed to maintain skills over time in clinical practice and to handle emotional situations effectively.

## Quantitative analysis of data and meta-analysis

An assessment of the nature of the studies and the data collected in tabular format will help identify the comparisons that might be made and the outcomes which could be combined. Any quantitative synthesis should only take place in the framework of a general data synthesis.

Meta-analysis is not possible when the necessary data to perform this analysis cannot be obtained, when the data are extremely sparse or where the studies are extremely heterogeneous, in either the populations studied, the interventions considered, the quality of study or the different designs.

There are three important decisions in conducting any meta-analysis. First, which comparison should be made; secondly, which outcome measures should be included in the synthesis; and thirdly, which effect measure should be used to describe effectiveness.

The comparisons to be made may be between certain specific interventions and the controls, or specific populations. The outcome measures should be chosen depending upon their relevance to the question and also those for which there are suitable data to combine in the synthesis. Ideally, data will have been collected by the same or similar instruments, and the instruments will have similar underlying constructs.

There are a variety of different measures of effect which can be chosen. These are summarized in Table 8.5, and will depend upon the nature of data

**Table 8.5** Measures of effect for use in meta-analysis of intervention studies

**Effect measure (treatment effect, estimate of effect)**
The observed relationship between an intervention and an outcome—summarized as a $P$-value, odds ratio, relative risk, risk difference, number needed to treat, standardized mean difference or weighted mean difference.

**$P$-value (statistical significance)**
The probability that the observed results in a study could have occurred by chance. A $P$-value of <5 per cent (i.e. $P$ <0.5) is generally regarded as statistically significant.

**Effect measures for binary data**
- **Odds** The ratio of the number of people in a group who experience something (e.g. an event) to those who do not. Thus, if out of 120 people, 40 had the event (and 80 did not), the odds would be 40/80 or 0.5
- **Risk (proportion, probability or rate)** The proportion of people in a group who are observed to experience something. Thus, if out of 100 patients, 40 had the event, the risk (rate of event) would be 40/100 or 0.4.
- **Odds ratio (OR)** The ratio of the odds of an event in the experimental group to the odds of an event in the control group. An OR of 1 indicates no difference between comparison groups.
- **Relative risk (RR) (risk ratio, rate ratio)** The ratio of risk in the intervention group to the risk in the control group. An RR of 1 indicates no difference between groups.
- **Absolute risk reduction (ARR) (risk difference, rate difference)** The absolute difference in the event rate between two comparison groups. A risk difference of zero indicates no difference between comparison groups.
- **Number needed to treat (NNT)** The number of patients who need to be treated to prevent one undesirable outcome. It is the inverse of ARR.

**Effect measures for continuous data**
- **Mean difference** Difference between the means (i.e. the average values) of two groups.
- **Weighted mean difference (WMD)** Where studies have measured an outcome using different scales (pain may be measured in a variety of ways), the mean difference may be divided by an estimate of within-group standard deviation to produce a standardized value.

**Effect measure for survival data**
- **Hazard ratio** A summary of the difference between two survival curves. It represents the overall reduction in the risk of death on treatment compared with control over the period of follow-up.

Source: Definitions adapted from York Centre for Review and Dissemination

in the primary studies. Dichotomous or binary data are usually summarized using odds ratios, risk ratios, number needed to treat or risk differences. Continuous data are usually summarized as means, differences in means or standardized differences in means (effect sizes). Depending upon the nature of their distribution, data arising from ordinal scales may be dichotomized and treated as binary data, or if sufficiently normally distributed may be treated as continuous data.

A problem commonly encountered in systematic reviews considering palliative care is that a number of studies will have collected the outcomes using binary scales while others will have used continuous scales. There is then a problem in conducting a meta-analysis as there are different forms of effect reported. However, it is possible to calculate an effect size using the general formula for continuous data, that of mean difference divided by standard deviation, and to use a similar formula for binary data.

In this instance, for continuous data, effect size is defined as

$$\frac{\text{Mean difference}}{\text{Standard deviation}}$$

Mean difference is the change or difference in mean outcome value associated with the intervention. Standard deviation is the standard deviation of an individual outcome value in a group given similar treatment calculated as a weighted average in the intervention and control group. It thus represents the natural variability in the outcome measure in the population.

For binary outcomes (proportions), the definition is similar to that for continuous outcomes, although the 'standard deviation' is calculated in a different way. The natural measure of effect here is the change or difference in proportions. This change in proportions must be subject to the same scaling adjustment as for continuous outcomes, i.e. it must be divided by the standard deviation of an individual value for which the formula is $\sqrt{p} \times (1 - p)$. In this instance, therefore, effect size is defined as

$$\frac{\text{Difference in proportions}}{\sqrt{(\text{Proportion yes}) \times (\text{Proportion no})}}$$

Although the calculations for these two types of outcomes are different, in each case the effect size relates to the change in the summary measure caused by the intervention divided by the variability of measurements within that group. Providing that the distribution of results for continuous and binary outcomes is similar, these two types of outcomes can be combined so that all of the relevant variables can be included in the analysis.

Once the results of each study are summarized using the effect measures, an average value of the effect can be calculated across all studies. Typically, the pooled effect estimates a weighted average of the studies included in the meta-analysis. The weights assigned to individual studies are usually in inverse proportion to their variance. This approach gives more weight to the larger studies and less to the smaller studies. It is possible to weight studies in relation to other factors, for example quality. The pooling of results in this way can be carried out using either a 'fixed effect' or a 'random effect' statistical model. The random effects model is usually the more appropriate method to use when there is heterogeneity between the studies. This is because the random effects model produces wider confidence intervals of the combined estimate compared with the fixed effect so that the results are more conservative. The meta-analysis is often conducted using specialist software such as that provided free of charge by the Cochrane Collaboration which can be downloaded from their web site.

Following data synthesis, it is useful to express the results in a graphical format. The most commonly used method is that of the Forrest plot. This represents individual study effects with their confidence intervals as horizontal lines, the box in the middle of the horizontal line representing the mean effect. Other plots include the L'Abbé plot, which also compares the benefit in control and treatment groups, but in a scatter plot, rather than showing the mean effect.

## Exploring heterogeneity

Heterogeneity is the variation or differences between estimates of the effects in the component studies in a systematic review. It may also represent differences in the intervention outcomes measured, or other major components of the studies.

Heterogeneity should be explored in any study. A simple way to explore it is by reviewing the information presented in the Forrest plot. Heterogeneity here will show a very mixed pattern of results. It is also possible to explore heterogeneity by carrying out $\chi^2$ tests. The results of these are frequently presented at the bottom of the Forrest plot.

Other ways to explore heterogeneity is to stratify the analysis or to analyse subsets, e.g. analysing RCTs separately from other forms of study, or analysing certain interventions separately from others. Finally, heterogeneity can be explored using meta-regression. In this instance, statistical regression modelling attempts to determine, through regression analysis, the reasons for heterogeneity.[26] Such an approach is only possible when there are sufficient studies included in the review.

## Publication bias

The accessibility of research results depends on whether the study is published or not, when, where and in what format. This influences whether relevant studies can be identified and appropriate data extracted. It is commonly argued that it is more likely that studies with positive results will be published and those with negative results will not. The search strategy and approaches for searching the grey literature often aim to reduce publication bias. A variety of statistical and modelling methods are also available to deal with publication bias. Funnel plots are most commonly used to explore publication bias. These show the distribution of effect sizes, plotted against sample size. It is expected that the points show an inverted funnel shape, there being more variability in the reported effect size for smaller studies.

# Systematic review methods for qualitative studies

The rationale for systematic reviews to obtain evidence on the effectiveness of health care is derived from the move to evidence-based practice in the early 1990s.[27] Its orientation towards medical and quantitative studies is therefore not surprising. The framework with which to assess the quality of studies distinguishes between study designs according to their susceptibility to bias and it specifies the results from RCTs or the systematic review of several RCTs as the gold standard to judge the effectiveness of health care. However, a broader range of evidence from a variety of sources needs to be drawn on when other research areas, such as health services, are evaluated. The questions which are relevant in these applied fields need to be addressed by different types of research. Effectiveness, although an important part, is not sufficient for decision making in clinical practice and policy. Appropriateness of health care interventions or evidence of the factors that influence decision making among policy makers, health care professionals and consumers may be required to inform practice. In palliative care, for example, there is little robust evidence as the questions posed are too complex to be explained by the RCT. Issues such as the coordination of services for patients who have cancer, or the specific ways in which to deliver spiritual care to the terminally ill are more suitably studied by qualitative research. Its methodology uses context to develop an understanding of subjective meaning and lay knowledge.

The contribution of qualitative evidence to health care evaluation has recently been acknowledged by the NHS Centre for Reviews and Dissemination.[28] However, questions remain as to how to integrate this type of evidence more systematically in reviews.

The established framework of the method of systematic review should be modified to accommodate research from a different paradigm, while remaining rigorous and explicit regarding its focus, selection, criteria for assessment and the ways of combining the empirical data.[29] The aim of searching the literature is to achieve as comprehensible a list as possible of relevant studies on a topic. This is particularly difficult as there is no equivalent of the Cochrane controlled trials register or other registers of clinical trials for qualitative research. Relevant literature is spread over a variety of databases or published in journals covering diverse topics. Poor reporting occurs more often in qualitative research, and study designs and terminology are frequently less standardized and discipline specific. Imaginative searching is required, with several trial searches yielding low precision. Filtering out irrelevant articles happens in stages, on the basis of the full texts, appraisal for relevance or assessment for methodological value.

A major concern in making the role of qualitative research in systematic reviews more systematic is the development of criteria to assess the validity of qualitative studies. Models developed for quantitative evidence using standards of validity, reliability and objectivity are unsuitable for qualitative approaches, and the categorization of qualitative research into hierarchies is not relevant. In this way, qualitative research will continue to be seen as inferior to quantitative research. As many researchers, practitioners and policy makers working in health care are not familiar with the assumptions and epistemologies on which qualitative research methods are based, the need has often been expressed for guidance to discriminate between strong and weak evidence. Due to the nature of the qualitative approach, 'there is no absolute list of criteria as to what constitutes good qualitative research'.[30] Rather, what is judged good or bad requires the invocation of criteria that are more tailored to the particular features of the work in question[30] (Chapter 11).

More work is needed on how to synthesize and present the findings from secondary investigation of empirical studies undertaken from a variety of theoretical approaches and research methods. The data to be synthesized could be the themes which emerged from content analysis for example, or quotations lifted from transcriptions of interviews. These products of interpretation are impossible to reconcile with the aim of generalizability which systematic reviews pursue. Tables summarizing the main findings, organized according to types of studies, are helpful in highlighting similar or contradictory findings. However, new ways should be developed to synthesize qualitative data. One such possibility is the role for theory-led synthesis of findings across studies, seeing the crucial role theory plays in informing the interpretation of data.[31] Triangulation may provide another approach for the systematic comparison of data obtained from different perspectives coming from different studies. Meta-ethnography is an attempt to deal with the complexities from ethnographic studies, similar to a meta-analysis of interpretative studies. Its aim is the translation of multiple qualitative studies into one another's terms.

## Conclusion

In this chapter, we have discussed the role of the systematic review method in palliative care research and described its essential steps. Given its holistic approach, it is important to collate and synthesize insights and experimental results from a variety of different disciplines. The systematic review method can address the question of effectiveness more accurately than single studies. In some areas in palliative care, systematic reviews have been effective in drawing together findings from separate studies and in showing the benefits for particular interventions, such as in specialist palliative care, psychological support and methods of information provision for patients.

However, palliative care poses its own specific challenges to secondary research. Due to the relatively recent interest in palliative care as a discipline, its research base is still limited and gaps in the evidence need to be addressed urgently. The complexity of the issues presented in palliative care and the methodological problems resulting from this in carrying out high quality trials is another barrier in reaching definite conclusions. Systematic review methodology is still being developed and adapted to the needs of new groups of people making use of them, to multiprofessional areas of research and to different types of research designs. The need to include qualitative study findings or integrate ideas from different research paradigms is also leading to the rethinking of the technique.

However, even in the face of a limited research base including many inconclusive findings, the systematic review is a valuable research tool, which can be employed to propose future research agendas, or highlight the methodological or ethical obstacles to carrying out research with seriously ill patients. The greatest merit of the systematic review lies in its explicitness. Judgements and assumptions are open to scrutiny and comment. Different parties, be they researchers, practitioners or policy makers, consulting the evidence assembled by a systematic review can therefore critically consider the value of the conclusions reached in the light of what they intend to use them for. Systematic reviews can be a pivotal tool in developing a productive relationship between research, policy and practice.

## References

1. Donald A (2001) Research must be taken seriously. *British Medical Journal* **323**: 278.
2. Chalmers I, Altman D (1995) *Systematic Reviews*. London: BMJ Publishing.

3. Mulrow CD, Linn WD, Gaul MK (1989) Assessing the quality of a diagnostic test evaluation. *Journal of General Internal Medicine* **4**: 288–95.

4. Hearn J, Feuer D, Higginson I, Sheldon T (1999) Systematic reviews. *Palliative Medicine* **13**: 75–80.

5. Chalmers I, Hedges LV, Cooper H (2002) A brief history of research synthesis. *Evaluation and the Health Professions* **25**: 12–37.

6. Mulrow CD (1994) Rationale for systematic reviews. *British Medical Journal* **309**: 597–9.

7. Petticrew M (2001) Systematic reviews from astronomy to zoology: myths and misconceptions. *British Medical Journal* **322**: 98–101.

8. Haynes B, Haines A (1998) Barriers and bridges to evidence based clinical practice. *British Medical Journal* **317**: 273–6.

9. Mulhall A (2001) Bridging the research–practice gap: breaking new ground in health care. *International Journal of Palliative Nursing* **7**: 389–94.

10. Haines A, Donald A (1998) Making better use of research findings. *British Medical Journal* **317**: 72–5.

11. Stocking B (1993) Implementing the findings of effective care in pregnancy and childbirth. *Milbank Quarterly* **71**: 497–522.

12. Cooper HM (1984) *The Integrative Research Review: A Systematic Approach.* Beverley Hills, CA: Sage Publications.

13. Simon R (1991) A decade of progress in statistical methodology for clinical trials. *Statistical Medicine* **10**: 1789–817.

14. Higginson IJ (1999) Evidence based palliative care—there is some evidence and there needs to be more. *British Medical Journal* **319**: 462–3.

15. Hanks GW, De Conno F, Cherny N, Hanna M, Kalso E, McQuay HJ, Mercadante S, Meynadier J, Poulain P, Ripamonti C, Radbruch L, Roca i Casas J, Sawe J, Twycross RG, Ventafridda V (2001) Morphine and alternative opioids in cancer pain: the EAPC recommendations. *British Journal of Cancer* **84**: 587–93.

16. Higginson IJ, Finlay IG, Goodwin DM, Hood K, Edwards AGK, Cook A, Douglas HR, Normand CE (2003) Is there evidence that palliative care teams alter end-of-life experiences of patients and their caregivers? *Journal of Pain and Symptom Management* **25**: 150–68.

17. Potter J, Higginson IJ (2004) Pain experienced by lung cancer patients: a review of prevalence, causes and pathophysiology. *Lung Cancer* **43**: 247–57.

18. Higginson IJ, Sen-Gupta GJA (2000) Place of care in advanced cancer: a qualitative systematic literature review of patient preferences. *Journal of Palliative Medicine* **3**: 287–300.

19. Gysels M, Higginson IJ (2000) *Improving Supportive and Palliative Care for Adults with Cancer: Research Evidence.* London: National Institute of Clinical Excellence. www.nice.org.uk/pdf/csgsresearchevidence.pdf. Accessed 20 June 2004.

20. Verhagen AP, De Vet HCW, de Bie RA, Kessels AGH, Boers M, Bouter LM, Knipschild PG (1998) The Delphi List: a criteria list for quality assessment of randomised clinical trials for conducting systematic reviews developed by Delphi Consensus. *Journal of Clinical Epidemiology* **51**: 1235–41.

21. Hearn J, Higginson IJ (1997) Outcome measures in palliative care for advanced cancer patients: a review. *Journal of Public Health Medicine* **19**: 193–9.

22. Edwards A, Russell I, Stott N (1998) Signal and noise in the evidence base for medicine—going beyond hierarchies of evidence? *Family Practice* **15**: 319–22.

23. Edwards A, Hood K, Matthews E, Russell D, Russell I, Barker J, Bloor M, Burnard P, Covey J, Pill R, Wilkinson C, Stott N (2000) The effectiveness of one-to-one risk communication interventions in health care: a systematic review. *Medical Decision Making* **20**: 290–7.

24. Edwards A, Elwyn GJ, Hood K, Rollnick S (2000) Judging the 'weight of evidence' in systematic reviews: introducing rigour into the qualitative overview stage by assessing signal and noise. *Journal of Evaluation in Clinical Practice* **6**: 177–84.

25. Higginson IJ, Finlay I, Goodwin DM, Cook AM, Hood K, Edwards AGK, Douglas HR, Norman CE (2002) Do hospital-based palliative teams improve care for patients or families at the end of life? *Journal of Pain and Symptom Management* **23**: 96–106.

26. Goodwin DM, Higginson IJ, Myers K, Douglas H-R, Normand C (2003) Effectiveness of palliative day care in improving pain, symptom control and quality of life. *Journal of Pain and Symptom Management* **25**: 202–12.

27. Rosenberg W, Donald A (1995) Evidence based medicine: an approach to clinical problem-solving. *British Medical Journal* **310**: 1122–6.

28. NHS Centre for Reviews and Dissemination (2001) *Undertaking Reviews of Research on Effectiveness: CRD's Guidance for those Carrying Out or Commissioning Reviews*, Vol. 4. York: Centre for Reviews and Dissemination, University of York.

29. Hawker S, Payne S, Kerr C, Hardey M, Powell J (2002) Appraising the evidence: reviewing disparate data systematically. *Qualitative Health Research* **12**: 1284–99.

30. Popay J, Rogers A, Williams G (1998) Rationale and standards for systematic review of qualitative literature in health services research. *Qualitative Health Research* **8**: 341–51.

31. Williams F, Popay J, Oakley A (1999) *Welfare Research: A Critical Review*. London: UCL Press.

# Section 4

## Qualitative research methods

Chapter 9

# Qualitative methods of data collection and analysis

Sheila Payne

## Introduction

This chapter provides an introduction to qualitative methods of data collection and analysis. These are among the most useful and frequently used methods in palliative care research. Their popularity might suggest that they are simple to use and unproblematic, but it is important to understand the science and assumptions that underpin each approach to data collection and analysis. The purpose of this chapter is to offer palliative care practitioners and researchers guidance on how to design and conduct qualitative research studies. However, it is not intended to be a detailed 'how to do' text. Readers are recommended to seek specialist texts in relation to specific methodological procedures, and advice from experienced researchers.

The chapter starts by offering a definition of qualitative methods. It then goes on to discuss how to make decisions about the design of qualitative studies. In my view, it is essential to have a focused research question(s) or hypothesis to guide the design of all research, be it qualitative or quantitative in approach. A major part of the chapter is devoted to considering data collection methods, both those that involve elicited data from interviews and focus groups, and those that focus on collecting spontaneously occurring data such as from normal conversations and written texts. The final part of the chapter focuses on a number of different qualitative methods of analysing data, without transforming them into numbers.

## What are qualitative methods?

Qualitative research methods draw on a range of epistemologies (theories of knowledge) which has implications for how data are collected and from whom, and how data are regarded during analysis, and what claims are made for the findings and even how the different methods should be evaluated. Qualitative research has been defined by Denzin and Lincoln[1] as:

> a situated activity that locates the observer in the world. It consists of a set of interpretive, material practices that make the world visible. These practices transform the world. They turn the world into a series of representations, including field notes, interviews, conversations, photographs, and recordings, and memos to the self (p. 3).

This definition of qualitative research implies that researchers are active participants in the creation of data and in its analysis. Qualitative research methods are a very broad category of approaches to data collection and analysis. It has been suggested that there are two major types of qualitative research: experiential (which focuses on how people understand their world) and discursive (which focuses on how language is used to construct the world).[2] The former type is best known in palliative care from analytical methods such as grounded theory, phenomenology and thematic analysis. They are based on the assumption that it is possible to make inferences about experience from verbal accounts. The discursive approaches are less well known in palliative care and they are concerned with the analysis of language and talk. They are based on the assumption that language serves to shape the world in which people live and is not merely reflective of it. Discursive approaches do not assume that it is possible to draw direct inferences about how people feel or think from their verbal accounts. The important point is that language is not regarded as a transparent medium for the relay of information. How language is *used* is regarded as social behaviour, for example people may use language to threaten, cajole, persuade or appeal.

Whatever methods of research that are used, it is important that they are rigorous and credible, and allow access to the processes and understandings that they seek to explore. Qualitative methods can be regarded as a toolkit of methods[3] or more fundamentally as a range of approaches which are based on different philosophical positions (epistemologies). What they are *not* is a single method which is set in opposition to a quantitative research method.

## When should qualitative methods be used?

All research should seek to address one or more specific research questions or hypotheses. For pragmatic reasons, by focusing on specific objectives, the research is more likely to be achievable in the constraints of finite resources such as time, money and energy, from the perspective of researchers but also from the perspective of palliative care patients who may have limited tolerance of research procedures which are time consuming or very taxing. Focusing on a specific research question is scientifically and ethically important because the more focused the question, the more likely the answer is to be valid, trustworthy and useful. Novice researchers may find this one of the most demanding aspects of designing their research, but it is essential that the research questions are clearly spelt out before embarking upon data collection. The wording of the research question should make it clear 'what, who, when and how' will be researched (Table 9.1). In Table 9.1, a number of possible research questions and methods of answering them are offered. Typically, research questions that seek to explore processes and/or meanings lend themselves to qualitative research methods. If the project is predominantly concerned with 'what, how many or how often' questions, these may lead to the adoption of quantitative methods of inquiry. If instead you want to ask 'why' questions, then qualitative designs may be the methods of choice.

**Table 9.1** Examples of research questions and possible methods of data collection

1. What evidence is there that involving palliative care patients in planning palliative care services improves quality of life and satisfaction for contributing patients, and quality of services for others?
   *This question could be answered by doing a systematic review of the literature*

2. How many people from different ethnic minority groups are invited to contribute to planning palliative care services?
   *This question could be answered by conducting a questionnaire or structured interview survey*

3. What do palliative care patients think about 'user involvement' initiatives?
   *This question could be answered by conducting semi-structured interviews or focus group discussions*

4. Is written or electronic information best for helping palliative care patients express choices and contribute to service planning?
   *This question could be answered by conducting an experimental study such as a randomized control trial*

5. What are family carers' experiences of 'user involvement' groups in palliative care services?
   *This question could be answered by conducting qualitative interviews to elicit carers' understanding and experience using a grounded theory analysis*

6. How do health and social care professional's conceptualize 'service users'?
   *This question could be answered by interpretative phenomenological analysis of interview data*

7. How do policy documents invoke 'user involvement'?
   *This question could use policy documents to explore terms in a discourse analytical study*

8. Why do some people more than others wish to express their views and participate in user involvement groups?
   *This question could be answered by asking participants for biographical accounts and using narrative analysis to explore relationships between illness, self concept, assertiveness and perceptions of choice*

In some qualitative methods, the research question may become more defined and specific during the course of data collection and analysis, such as grounded theory analysis. In action research, which may be based on positivist or constructionist epistemologies, it is common for a series of research questions to be asked, as this method uses sequential stages involving cycles of 'change' followed by data collection and data analysis from which subsequent questions arise and further 'change' is planned and implemented. Typically, qualitative methods of inquiry research are not aimed at testing hypotheses, although Silverman[4] has argued that they are appropriate in areas where there is a well established knowledge base.

There are four ways in which research projects can incorporate qualitative methods.

## As a prelude to using quantitative methods

Prior to developing a questionnaire or structured measure of nausea in palliative care patients, it might be helpful to interview a number of patients and professionals to ensure that a full range of issues associated with nausea are included. The use of qualitative methods in this case is designed to benefit the quantitative research which tends to be regarded as the 'real' research.

## Concurrently with quantitative methods

These are described as mixed methods designs and are increasingly advocated in health services research (Chapter 12). For example, in a study of the impact of death on fellow patients in a hospice, a structured checklist was used to elicit 'positive' and 'negative' experiences, and in addition patients were invited to talk freely about their experiences in a short interview.[5] The advantage of combining approaches is that they may help to explain counterintuitive results or offer different perspectives. However, the disadvantage is that in using both qualitative (interviews) and structured (standardized measures) approaches, you increase the burden of data collection on patients. Moreover, patients may interpret what they think you want to know from the nature and order in which you collect data. For example, if you ask questions first about their pain rather than their financial status, this may indicate that you are privileging physical symptoms rather than their social situation. It may also be difficult to know how to interpret responses which appear to be contradictory such as a low score on a standardized anxiety measure from a person who appears behaviourally anxious. There may also be incompatibility in the epistemological positions which gives rise to tensions in sampling methods. For example, random sampling of a defined population may result in fewer very old people, because there are less of them alive, but they might be the ones who are most helpful in providing data about health care services, because they are most likely to have used them.

## After using quantitative methods

In this variant of mixed method design, qualitative methods may be used following a quantitative study such as a survey. For example, following a survey of community nurses in the south of England to determine the extent of their involvement in delivering bereavement support, semi-structured interviews were used to explore the reasons for the diversity of practice and what factors influenced this.[6] Qualitative research has the advantage of capturing diversity and inconsistency which is difficult to achieve when categories (in content analysis) have to be mutually exclusive and are pre-determined.

## Alone

Qualitative methods may be used as a stand-alone design. These can be employed in major ethnographic studies such as those described in Chapter 13 by Seymour or in smaller research projects. The advantage is that the methods of sampling, data collection and analysis are congruent with the selected epistemological position.

This chapter is predominantly concerned with the latter type of stand-alone qualitative research designs. These have been described as 'big Q' compared with 'small q' use of qualitative methods, where open-ended, inductive approaches are defined as 'big Q', and the use of qualitative techniques such as asking open questions within the framework of a predominantly structured quantitatively designed study, as 'small q'. In this chapter, the main focus is on 'big Q' qualitative research.[7] This means that it will be about the collection of non-numerical data and those analytical procedures that do not start by transforming phenomena into numbers. These methods are based on a variety of epistemologies. The differences between qualitative and qualitative paradigms are often presented simplistically as a dichotomy between positivism and social constructionism. However, in some of the social science literature, the term positivism tends to be regarded as a form of abuse.[8] Instead, it is perhaps more helpful to think of realist researchers espousing a continuum of epistemological positions from those who seek an ultimate 'truth' out there in the world to those who reject notions of 'truth' and 'knowledge' altogether. The point I am arguing in this chapter is that there is not a single epistemological position taken by qualitative researchers but that the research question should be compatible with the epistemological assumptions of the selected method of analysis. For example, some types of discourse analysis make the assumption that it is possible to identify ways of talking about phenomena and concepts which are available to a number of people within a social group or culture, and those discourses may be potentially available to be drawn upon by some groups but not others. In a study exploring the views of patients nearing the end of life and their health professionals about how a 'good death' was construed, patients and professionals drew on similar (being pain free) and different notions of a 'good' death, for example suddenly (patients), in one's sleep (patients) and surrounded by family members (professionals).[9]

## Collecting data for qualitative analysis

Most methods of data collection are not inherently quantitative or qualitative.[10] What is crucial is how phenomena are collected and how they are transformed. For example, an interview may be used to collect verbal information which will be transformed through analytical procedures, such as content analysis, into numerical codes, or alternatively through a process of inductive categorization such as in grounded theory analysis, into textual conceptual categories. The origins of these data elicited in an interview context, in this case talk, will be the same, although the approaches of the researcher will be rather different as they will design either structured (for content analysis), or semi-structured and unstructured interviews (for grounded theory analysis). Depending upon the epistemological stance of the researcher, some but not all qualitative researchers regard themselves as part of the process of data collection and analysis. There is no assumption made that data are neutral 'objects' waiting to be 'discovered' and collected out there in the world. The separation between 'researcher' and 'researched' may be minimized or rejected altogether.

## Types of qualitative data

In the following section, methods of collecting data that are suitable for qualitative analysis in palliative care are discussed, and the processes of transforming the data for analysis are examined. There are three common types of qualitative data:

◆ Language in the form of written text or spoken words

◆ Observations of behaviours (this includes communication which is made up of both talk and non-verbal interactions)

◆ Images which may be dynamic events (captured digitally, on videos or films), photographs, drawings, paintings or sculptures.

It is important to recognize the difference between *elicited* data, that which is specifically requested and collected by researchers for the purpose of answering the research question, and *spontaneously* (or naturally) occurring data. Most data used by qualitative researchers is elicited for the purpose of the project by talking to patients or professionals during interviews or focus groups, for example. However, in certain approaches to qualitative analysis, for example in discourse analysis, it might be possible, and indeed preferable, to use existing sources such as policy documents or case notes. The reasons for this will be explained in the section on data analysis.

## Ways of gathering qualitative data

### Interviews

In the context of palliative care, interviews are a suitable method of collecting elicited data for a number of reasons. First, they build upon the experience of both patients and professionals in terms of previous clinical interviews, and patients are generally pleased to have the opportunity to talk with an attentive person in a face-to-face situation. Participating in interviews requires the ability to talk and understand the questions, and may be less demanding for patients than completing questionnaires or trying to write. However, for certain patients such as those who are very breathless or have difficulty in speaking (such as those with head and neck cancers), interviews may be very tiring. Language and comprehension difficulties may exclude patients who have intellectual disabilities, low educational attainment or simply because they do not understand the language or accent of the interviewer. Typically, face-to-face interviews are popular with researchers because they tend to generate a higher response rate than other methods and there is likely to be less missing data than in questionnaires (Chapter 5). However, they are expensive and time consuming, especially when interviews are conducted in patients' homes.

Interviews vary in the extent to which they are controlled by the researcher's agenda. In *structured interviews*, the researcher asks closed questions requiring yes/no answers, or provides pre-determined answers which respondents are invited to endorse or reject. The interview schedule is prepared much like a questionnaire and interviewers are often carefully trained to ensure consistency in their style of asking and responding to questions. An example of this is the 'Voices' questionnaire[11] used to elicit data from family members or others who have known a deceased person over their last year of life. This approach to interviewing is unsuitable for in-depth qualitative analysis using grounded theory analysis, although the addition of open-ended questions might produce data amenable to content or thematic analysis. *Semi-structured interview* formats pre-define to some extent the research agenda, but enable respondents some freedom to present a range of views and offer new insights. Interview schedules may be loosely specified, for example as a list of topics to be covered, and these are often described as aide memoirs. In a study examining health professionals' and health managers' understanding of palliative care in South London, an agenda of topics was used to guide the interviews.[12] *Unstructured interviews* are open-ended and typically invite participants to talk about a topic or tell their story with minimal prompts. Copp undertook a series of open interviews with patients about their experience of dying in a hospice in England.[13] This method of interviewing is most appropriate if a phenomenological analysis is to be used.

Research interviews are different from clinical interviews because they are not intended to lead to clinical interventions or diagnosis. In common with clinical interviews, researchers will need skills which encourage respondents to feel comfortable, relaxed and able to talk freely. Researchers need to learn how to explore topics using probes to elicit full accounts (specific advice on interview techniques for qualitative research is obtainable elsewhere[14-16]). Research interviews may be conducted face-to-face or via the telephone, and are usually dyadic interactions. While telephone interviews may be more cost effective and time efficient, they are likely to be most suitable for short structured interviews, which are likely to yield less extensive or 'rich' data (Chapter 5). Because it is more difficult to establish a rapport with the respondent, they may not be suitable for some sensitive topics, such as interviews with bereaved people. They are probably most appropriate for eliciting data from health and social care professionals, especially if a specific time is arranged beforehand. Telephone interviews may exclude certain people such as those with hearing problems or those without access to private telephones.

## Focus groups

The use of focus groups has become increasingly popular to elicit data from a group of people. In focus groups, the purpose is to encourage interaction between the participants so that a range of views may be elicited and discussion is generated. Decisions must be made at the outset whether focus group participants should be similar or not, and strangers or already known to each other. These are likely to relate to the research question and topic area, and the sampling strategy. For example, in some cultures, women may feel uncomfortable discussing sexual health problems in mixed gender groups. Asking palliative care nurses to discuss working practices in the presence of their managers may result in few data because of pre-existing power relationships. Focus groups are generally run by a facilitator, whose role is to introduce topics, encourage participation and address respondent comfort and safety issues, while an observer has the role of recording the nature and type of participation by group members. The number of participants may vary from six to 12 depending upon the topic and group. There needs to be a balance between the desire to have a range of views represented and the difficulties of managing a large group, and making sense of the resultant audio-recording. It may be preferable to have smaller groups if topics are likely to be very personal or elicit strong emotions, such as with bereaved people. However, participants should be reminded that the purpose of the focus group is to discuss a research issue rather than being a therapeutic intervention. More detailed information about conducting focus groups is available from Hennink and Diamond.[17]

## Group discussions

Group interviews are rather like other types of interviews in that the researcher directs the questioning and responses are made to the interviewer. They are not the same as focus groups because participants are not encouraged to engage with each other, by challenging, debating and arguing about issues. They are commonly used in group settings such as palliative care day centres, and are a cost-effective way to collect data.

## Obtaining spontaneously occurring data

Sometimes the focus of the research may be on talk that is not elicited specifically for the purpose of the project. For example, in studies of doctor–patient or nurse–patient communication, both spontaneous (in clinics) and elicited (using actors) interactions have been recorded to understand how professionals and patients convey information to each other or make clinical decisions.[18,19] Discourse analysts may use public speeches or broadcast media (radio or television) to investigate how health messages are delivered or how politicians present palliative care policies to the public[20,21] (Chapter 14).

## Documentary data

Written texts including public documents (e.g. government policy documents, hospice procedure manuals, minutes of management meetings, patient medical or nursing records, newspaper or magazine articles, and websites) and private accounts (diaries, stories, biographies and letters) may all provide valuable data (Chapter 14). These documents may be elicited specifically for the research, such as diaries or stories of patients' experience, or they may be 'naturally' occurring data such as ward diaries or patient case records. Of course, obtaining access to some of these types of data may raise ethical issues about confidentiality. It is also important to regard these sources of data as potentially problematic because they may have been produced to serve different purposes other than the research. For example, Quested and Rudge[22] conducted a discursive analysis of the 'Last Offices' section of a procedure manual of a hospital in Australia to examine how nursing practices served to transform the living patient into the dead body. Their analysis indicated how the language used in the procedure manual reflected wider cultural views on the transition between life and death, and the embodied individual and the dead corpse. Their study helped to reveal how the institutional language and culture of the hospital shaped the way nurses acted towards their dead patients. Documentary analysis may be used to supplement other types of data collection (such as interviews) or as a primary source of data.

## Observations

One of the challenges of research within palliative care contexts is that patients may become too unwell to participate in any type of data collection procedures. Observations may therefore be one of the few methods that can yield direct data in such situations. Researchers may observe social interaction, and their written records are described as field notes. Ethnography is an approach to data collection and analysis which relies heavily on observations made by researchers within social situations. There is a long tradition of ethnographic studies about people nearing the end of life in hospitals,[23–25] in clinics[26] and in hospices.[27] See Chapter 13 for more details and a fuller discussion of the types of participant and non-participant observations, how data are recorded in field notes and ethical issues in the use of this method.

## Images

Researchers may also collect elicited or spontaneous images such as drawings, photographs and paintings (e.g. patient's art work or family photographs). For some people such as children, who find it difficult to express themselves verbally, images such as paintings may provide an insight into how they feel or are dealing with their experiences. Technological developments mean it is also possible to record behaviour using video and digital cameras much more unobtrusively than in the past. These images represent useful ways to gather examples of elicited and spontaneous behaviour.[28,29]

## Recording data

Talk and behaviour are ephemeral and need to be 'captured' to permit researchers to work on them. Elicited and spontaneous talk is generally audio-recorded, while behaviours may be digitally/video recorded or written down by the researchers as field notes. Whatever method of recording is selected, it is helpful to use the best quality equipment that can be purchased to ensure a high standard of recording and to aid the transcription process.

# Transforming and processing data for analysis

Qualitative research designs typically generate large amounts of data from relatively few sources. Qualitative researchers may quickly become overwhelmed by the large volume of data collected. It is therefore essential to establish consistent and reliable systems to manage data, whether data are to be stored electronically or in paper form. This ensures that during analysis, data can be retrieved when required, and also provides an audit trail (part of the process of establishing quality). To this end, researchers should consider the use of qualitative data analysis software if they have a reasonably large data set and/or if more than one person is going to be involved in the process of analysis. There are many different software packages, and each has characteristic advantages and disadvantages. In my view, they are potentially useful in facilitating the manipulation, indexing and retrieval of data, but do not alter the need for a deep, intensive engagement with the data during the intellectual process of coding and interpretation. The disadvantage of some packages is that they are labour intensive in terms of their input and coding requirements, and may inadvertently serve to structure data analysis in prescribed ways (e.g. as hierarchical or linear structures).

In my view, all data (even those described by researchers as 'raw' unanalysed data) have been transformed in some way. Written text needs to be selected, edited and usually scanned electronically prior to analysis. Verbal accounts are generally transformed into written text by the process of transcription. Many textbooks on research methods devote little space to considerations about transcription, but this is the first stage of the analysis and critical decisions need to be made at this point about the style of transcription to be used. It is not merely something that is delegated to a secretary! O'Connell and Kowal highlight the decisions to be made about the extent of transcription to be undertaken.[30] They define four elements:

- The verbal—the words (are local dialects, slang or jargon to be transformed into conventional written English?)
- The prosodic—the volume, pitch and intonation used in speech
- The paralinguistic—for example, the coughs, laughter or crying which may accompany speech
- The extra-linguistic—for example, hand, eye or body movements which accompany speech.

Decisions about how speech will be transcribed are dependent upon the nature of the analysis to be conducted (for a discussion of these decisions in the context of palliative care, see Ingleton and Seymour[31]). For example, if a grounded theory analysis is planned, it is important to transcribe the speech of both the interviewer and interviewee but not usually necessary to transcribe prosodic, paralinguistic or extra-linguistic elements. Discourse analysis, however, requires more complete and detailed transcriptions because the researcher is often concerned with not only what is said but how it is said. It may be important to know things such as when speech is overlapping or how long the pauses are between speakers. Perhaps the most detailed, and therefore time-consuming, transcription procedures are necessary for conversation analysis where specific and precise notation systems are available.[32–34] In designing a qualitative study, an estimation of the cost and time needed to complete transcription procedures should be included.

I often suggest that novice researchers undertake at least a few transcriptions themselves because this allows them to become aware of the level of analysis required and gives an insight into the hard work involved. Even if the majority of transcriptions are done by others, it is necessary to listen to all the audio-tapes and carefully check through the transcriptions for errors and omissions. It has been argued that researchers should conduct analysis directly from the spoken word rather than from transcriptions, because it allows access to the prosodic and paralinguistic features. For example, irony is difficult to 'capture' in written transcriptions, but the tone of voice or an accompanying giggle may indicate the intention of the speaker which is not directly evident from the words alone. There are also arguments about the use of punctuation and how the text is presented on paper. For example, Coffey and Atkinson suggested that parsing text into clauses retains more of the emotional resonance of the spoken words.[35] This type of transcription gives the written text a poetic appearance. In conclusion, transformation of spoken language to written text should be regarded as the first stage in the interpretative process.

## Analysing data qualitatively

It is tempting for novice researchers to seek 'cookbook' recipes or procedures to guide them in the process of data analysis. However, as Clark argues, qualitative analysis is more than a slavish adherence to prescribed procedures, it is an intellectual exercise, done rigorously but with imagination, of engaging comprehensively and deeply with original data sources.[3] Analytical methods should be regarded as dynamic and flexible. Research methods, just as in palliative care services, evolve over time and can be adapted to particular contexts, but all changes and modifications made by researchers should be made explicit and justified in presenting the research. Before going on to introduce various methods of qualitative data analysis, I start this section with a consideration of the status afforded to the responses of participants and the implications which are drawn from talk, and the purposes of the analysis of talk from differing perspectives. I will start by differentiating between two major conceptual approaches in qualitative methods of analysis:

- Those approaches which are concerned with inferring *meaning* from data and draw inferences about what people think, feel and do. These have been labelled as 'experiential' approaches. They include methods of analysis such as thematic analysis, framework analysis, grounded theory analysis, narrative analysis and phenomenology.

- Those approaches which are concerned with how talk is *used* in social situations and that do not make inferences about how people feel or think. These are labelled as 'discursive' approaches. They include methods such as conversation analysis, analysis of institutional interaction and discourse analysis.

The conventional status afforded to interview data, for example when using grounded theory analysis or thematic analysis, is that responses are construed as evidence of what people think and feel and how they *understand* their world.[36,37] These insights are assumed to have stability over time and are inferred as being characteristic of that individual. Qualitative researchers working with these methods feel able to draw conclusions about the state of mind of individuals on the basis of their talk. They are interested in exploring the influence of previous experiences and personal understanding on the emotional and cognitive reactions displayed in talk. Thus, from this perspective, talk is seen as representing the contents of people's minds and providing direct access to thoughts and emotions. The social situation of the interview is regarded as largely unproblematic.

In comparison, discursive approaches regard interview responses as evidence about how people *use* language to construct that particular situation at that particular time. Discursive approaches makes no assumptions about consistency of responses in other situations, no inferences about intra-psychic processes (how people think or feel), and explain talk as representing a repertoire of ways that people have of dealing with questions in social situations, such as that of an interview. In discursive approaches, analysis of talk is concerned with individuals' attempts to deal with their current situation (e.g. in an interview maintaining their credibility as a 'good' patient, trying to 'help' the interviewer or complaining). To illustrate these differences, I will use an example taken from an interview with a woman with advanced ovarian cancer[16] (Table 9.2).

An experiential approach to this interview using a method such as thematic analysis or grounded theory analysis might start by identifying segments of text which are then given descriptive labels (called categories in grounded theory).

**Table 9.2** Interview transcript

| |
|---|
| *Interviewer*: Can we start at the beginning of your treatment for cancer. How did you know that there was something wrong with you? |
| *Interviewee*: Well, last August, I went up North, went on holiday up to Yorkshire and that was the first time. I had a job to sit down with it. I was constipated and I thought it was that. And of course, naturally, I didn't go to the doctor because I thought it was because I was constipated that it was pressing on it. Anyway, this went on. And I haven't been able to sit down for quite a while, you know. If I have been sitting down in the evening, I have sat on the floor with my hands resting on the chair. Well, sitting on the side, you know, and if I have sat anywhere I have sat on my side and then, oh, when would it be about, well it was before Easter because I went to the doctor before Easter, didn't I? |
| *Interviewer*: um |
| *Interviewee*: And I told him, you know, about this that I was constipated and that. He gave me some Isogel and he said try it for a month. |

For example, it can be observed that the interviewee refers to a number of dates/times which locate her story in a temporal sequence, and this could generate a category called 'Significance of timing' and further instances of this category could be searched for in subsequent parts of the same interview and in further interviews with other patients. Her description of the symptoms of constipation is taken to represent a 'real' account of her experiences and as indicative of her feelings *at the time* before diagnosis of cancer, although it is clear that the interview presents a retrospective account of her experiences.

An alternative discursive approach to this interview might focus on the interactional aspects of the situation. (A caveat is that interviews are not often used in discourse analysis, and that the transcription style in this example is inappropriate, because a much more detailed transcription indicating overlapping speech and other performance details would be required.) However, returning to this example, the researcher sets the context with the key words '*beginning*' '*cancer*' and '*know*'. This interview draws on a shared taken-for-granted understanding about 'medical' discourses used in clinical interviews, such as the need to provide a history which is located in time and place, a description of (physical) symptoms and a justification of the actions and non-actions she undertook. The analysis might identify how this is achieved in the interaction. For example, the woman justifies her actions by saying:

> naturally, I didn't go to the doctor because I thought it was because I was constipated.

This is offered as a moral justification of 'not wasting a doctor's time on trivial complaints'. Thus the purpose of the analysis is to identify the way talk (*what* and *how*) is *used in the interview* situation to create an account; no inferences are made about underlying motives or feelings experienced at the time these symptoms occurred.

# Examples of types of qualitative data analysis

It is not possible in a chapter to do justice to the diversity of methods of qualitative analysis. I therefore intend to just provide brief introductions to some common methods and to encourage readers to seek detailed specialist texts for fuller accounts. Each of the methods described is itself a subclass in which there are a number of different specific analytical approaches and many lively debates. The first examples can be largely regarded as experiential approaches based on a continuum from realist to social constructionist epistemologies. The features of these methods are summarized in Table 9.3.

## Content analysis

This method of analysis may be used to generate either quantitative or qualitative data. It involves establishing mutually exclusive and pre-determined categories (usually single words such as pain or depression) which are then identified, and counts of the frequencies of them in an interview transcript or other text are made.[38] This yields categorical data which may be incorporated into other statistical data analyses. Alternatively, the frequencies may be reported qualitatively with examples taken from the text. The advantage of this method is that there are clear analytical procedures and it is possible to achieve good inter-rater reliability between different coders. However, it tends to decontextualize the text, and evidence of greater frequency alone cannot be taken to infer importance. There may be many reasons why particular words occur more or less frequently, for example due to individual differences or sensitivity of topics. Content analysis should be considered if you wish to convert open textual responses to numbers, perhaps to combine with other numerical data, or if you wish to count discrete entities.

## Thematic analysis

This method of analysis tends to be used as a 'catch-all' term to include procedures similar to content analysis but without necessarily the intention of converting the data into frequencies. It involves the identification of patterns of similarity in the text which are relevant to the research question.[39] In thematic analysis, themes are generally searched for following data collection rather than being established *a priori*. Coding of themes may focus merely on manifest content such as specific phrases like 'family caregivers' or may include identification of

**Table 9.3** Summary of the features of common qualitative research methods

| | Types of data | Sample size | Features of coding | Results of analysis |
|---|---|---|---|---|
| Content analysis | Open-ended questions in questionnaires, structured interviews | Larger data sets | Pre-determined categories, mutually exclusive | Frequency counts |
| Thematic analysis | Semi-structured interviews, focus groups, written texts, images | Medium to smaller data sets | Inductive categories including manifest and latent themes | Descriptive accounts summarizing common phenomena across individuals |
| Grounded theory analysis | Semi-structured or unstructured interviews, focus groups | Smaller data sets, theoretical sampling | Inductive coding, constant comparative analysis, theoretical saturation | Generation of new theory, analytical and complex accounts of the data |
| Narrative analysis | Stories from verbal accounts (e.g. oral histories) written accounts (e.g. diaries, autobiographies biographies) | Smaller data sets | Experiential—focus on life changes, events and meaning Discursive—focus on employment of linguistic features | Experiential—descriptive and analytical account of stories and experience Discursive—account of the way language is used to create a story, moral accounts convey messages |
| Discourse analysis | Naturally occurring or 'spontaneous' text (e.g. medical records) or talk (e.g. public speeches) | Medium to smaller data sets | No specific procedures but include: reading; coding; interpenetration; and writing | Discursive approaches—detailed accounts of how language is used in shaping social interaction Foucauldian discourse analysis—detailed analytical accounts of role of language in the social construction of reality |

latent content such as coding segments of text making references to the role of family caregivers even when this actual phrase is not included. There are a number of specific methods such as framework analysis and template analysis which use similar methodological principles, although the actual procedures vary. These methods are popular because they appear to 'capture' the subtlety and complexity of qualitative data and present it in intuitively coherently accounts. They enable researchers to group apparently similar responses across individuals and represent meanings in the data. They have the advantage of requiring less intensive and time-consuming processing of data than methods such as grounded theory analysis. Thematic analysis should be considered when the aims of analysis are descriptive accounts which summarize phenomena across individuals.

## Grounded theory analysis

This method was first described by Glaser and Strauss,[40] but has subsequently evolved in rather different ways following the writings of Glaser[37] or Strauss and his colleagues.[36] There are lively debates about the justifications and 'correctness' of modifications to grounded theory analysis and what should be regarded as the 'essential' principles and procedures, and whether simpler or merely descriptive analysis should be labelled as a 'grounded theory approach'. The aims of grounded theory analysis are to develop inductive theory which is closely derived from the data, rather than deductive theory which is supported by hypothesis testing. It is a popular method of qualitative analysis because the procedures appear to be coherent and logical (Table 9.4). It is based on the assumption that it is possible to allocate labels (categories) to segments of text (meaningful units) during the process of coding. Subsequent coding is based on a process of constant comparative analysis where the coding of each transcript is compared with previous codes and these are modified by new insights as they are 'discovered'. Analysis, coding and sampling are concurrent, rather than sequential activities. In some versions of grounded theory analysis, it is considered appropriate to delay a formal literature review until data collection and preliminary analyses are undertaken. However, researchers should be sufficiently aware of the literature as to be sure that their research will contribute new knowledge. Awareness of the empirical and theoretical literature is essential during the latter stages of the analysis to ensure that new theoretical constructs are linked to existing work. Some of the major analytical constructs of grounded theory analysis include theoretical sampling and theoretical coding, as the aim of this type of analysis is to develop explanatory theory not merely describe data. The disadvantages of this method is that it is likely to be very time consuming, and palliative care patients may not live long enough to contribute

**Table 9.4** Suggested procedures in conducting a grounded theory analysis

| Process | Activity | Comments |
|---|---|---|
| 1 | Collect data | Any source of textual data may be used but semi-structured interviews or observations are the most common. |
| 2 | Transcribe data | Full transcriptions of interviewer and interviewee talk. |
| 3 | Develop initial categories—open coding | Categories are developed from the data by open coding of the transcripts. Open coding means identifying and labelling meaningful units of text which might be a word, phrase, sentence or larger section of text. |
| 4 | Saturate categories | 'Saturation' means gathering further examples of meaningful units as one proceeds through the transcripts until no new examples of a particular category emerge. |
| 5 | Defining categories | Once the categories have been saturated, formal definitions in terms of the properties and dimensions of each category may be generated. |
| 6 | Theoretical sampling | From the categories which have emerged from the first sample of data, choose theoretically relevant samples to help test and develop categories further. |
| 7 | Axial coding—the development and testing of relationships between categories | During axial coding, possible relationships between categories are noted, hypothesized and actually tested against data which are being obtained in ongoing theoretical sampling. |
| 8 | Theoretical integration | A core category (or in some cases more than one main category) is identified and related to all the other subsidiary categories to determine its explanatory power, and finally links with existing theory are established and developed. |
| 9 | Grounding the theory | The emergent theory is grounded by returning to the data and validating them against actual segments of text. A search for deviant cases may be used to test the emergent theory. |
| 10 | Filling in gaps | Finally, any missing detail is filled in by the further collection of relevant data and a hypothesis derived for further testing of the new theory. |

Adapted from Bartlett and Payne.[41]

to further episodes of data collection (called respondent validation). More seriously, it has been criticized because it segments the text and potentially decontextualizes data. Grounded theory analysis should be considered if you wish to build new theories to explain phenomena, not just describe them.

## Narrative analysis

Narrative analysis represents a group of methodological approaches which focus on the tendency of people to tell stories about their condition or lives (autobiography). Reminiscence and recounting biographies are commonly used within palliative care to help people gain a sense of meaning, and may contribute to feelings of life closure. Telling stories either verbally (e.g. oral histories) or in writing (e.g. diaries) is suitable for use in palliative care. People tend to report these activities as pleasurable and helpful. Narratives characteristically have a plot, actors and are sequenced over time. In narrative interviewing, researchers seek to elicit stories told in participants' own words and at their own pace. Therefore, there are likely to be few questions asked except an invitation to 'tell your story' and prompts to encourage people to continue or clarify issues. A narrative is a re-creation and interpretation of events which the teller shapes to their audience. Narrative analysis may focus on the linguistic factors of the story, the emplotment, the structure and function of the story telling.[42-44] Analysis generally aims to maintain the integrity of the account by focusing on features of the story as told by each participant, rather than making comparisons across a number of individuals. For example, Ellis-Hill[45] explores how the experience of being a carer at various points throughout a person's life cycle was used (or not) in their suddenly acquired role of being a carer of a person following a stroke. She argued that for some people, previous experiences of caring for children or older family members contributed to their self-concept as a carer, while others resisted this identity and role. Narrative analysis should be considered if you wish to explore how people talk about their lives or if you are interested in the linguistic features of emplotment.

## Discourse analysis

The term discourse analysis tends to mean rather different things depending upon the disciplinary background of the writer. In this section, I am going to be describing discursive approaches from the perspective of psychology. According to Willig,[8] there are two major positions: what she describes as 'discursive psychology' which is derived from ethnomethodology and conversation analysis and is concerned with how everyday social interactions are negotiated and managed; and 'Foucauldian discourse analysis' which draws upon post-structuralist writers including Foucault to examine how language constitutes social and psychological experience. For a more detailed account of the differences in these approaches, see Parker[46] or Willig.[8] Palliative care researchers have tended not to use discursive analysis, but a good example is provided by Quested and Rudge whose analysis of 'Last Offices' in the procedure manual of a hospital in Australia reveals how nurses enact the transition between life and death in their behaviours and language towards the live patient and dead body.[22] For example, references to live people are always gendered. To refer to a person as 'it' is regarded as dehumanizing, but corpses are rarely described in gendered terms. Discourse analysis is ideally based on naturally occurring text (e.g. medical records, minutes of meetings, policy documents) and talk (e.g. public speeches). Many discourse analysts have resisted formalized coding procedures,[22] and there is less guidance on 'how to do' this method, but it requires researchers to take a different approach to interpreting or 'reading' text. This focuses on how language is used rather than what people are saying. Language is regarded as social action. Analytic procedures include careful reading, coding, interpretation and writing, while continually questioning the text.[8] Foucauldian discourse analysis tends to examine power relationships within society. The disadvantage of discursive approaches is that because they focus predominantly upon language, they may have little interest in changing behaviours or psychological states, which is often the concern of palliative care practitioners. Discursive analysis should be considered if you are interested in exploring how different versions of reality are produced, negotiated and evoked in normal conversation and in texts. These are powerful techniques to challenge taken for granted ways of knowing, and can ultimately reveal competing power positions in society.

## Assessing the quality of qualitative methods

There are a number of criteria for assessing the quality of qualitative research (Chapter 11). Researchers need to demonstrate the methodological rigour of their work and be clear and explicit in the claims made when research is written up or presented. A number of devices have been proposed to enable researchers to do this, such as maintaining an audit trail of key analytical decision making, often in the form of a research diary or in memo writing (in grounded theory analysis), and using reflexivity to allow the researcher to acknowledge their role in the creation of the analytical account.[47] Triangulation has also been proposed to support the claims made.[31,48] This may take a number of forms such as methodological triangulation, theoretical triangulation or respondent validation, but it should not be regarded as a panacea. Finally, researchers using qualitative methods need to address issues of transferability. What claims can be made for the research findings and who can they be applied to?

## Conclusions

Undertaking qualitative research can be regarded as an adventure.[8] It can be at times challenging, exciting, frustrating and enjoyable. To make the most of an adventure, it is important to be well prepared, well equipped and adequately funded, to design your route, set goals and targets in a realistic time structure, be flexible in accommodating the unexpected, be open to new experiences, discoveries and ways of seeing the world, and finally to be rigorous and accurately record your experiences to benefit others. Clark has argued that qualitative methods are more than a toolkit;[3] they require intellectual engagement, innovation, ethical sensitivity, reflexivity and the ability to write. It is hoped that this chapter will inspire and guide your journey.

## Suggested further reading

Denzin NK, Lincoln YS (2000) *Handbook of Qualitative Research*, 2nd edn. Thousand Oaks, CA: Sage.

Marks D, Yardley L, (ed.) (2004) *Research Methods for Clinical and Health Psychology*. London: Sage.

Mason J (1996) *Qualitative Researching*. London: Sage.

Seale C (1999) *The Quality of Qualitative Research*. London: Sage.

Silverman D (2000) *Doing Qualitative Research*. London: Sage.

Smith JA, (ed.) (2003) *Qualitative Psychology: A Practical Guide to Research Methods*. London: Sage.

Smith JA, Harre R, Van Langenhove L, (ed.) (1995) *Rethinking Methods in Psychology*. London: Sage.

Willig C (2001) *Introducing Qualitative Research in Psychology*. Buckingham: Open University Press.

## References

1. Denzin NK, Lincoln YS (2000) *Handbook of Qualitative Research*, 2nd edn. Sage: Thousand Oaks, CA.
2. Reicher S (2000) Against methodolatry: some comments on Elliott, Fischer and Rennie. *British Journal of Clinical Psychology* 39: 1–6.
3. Clark D (1997) What is qualitative research and what can it contribute to palliative care? *Palliative Medicine* 11: 159–66.
4. Silverman D (1993) *Interpreting Qualitative Data*. Sage: London.
5. Payne SA, Langley-Evans A, Hillier R (1996) Perceptions of a 'good' death: a comparative study of the views of hospice staff and patients. *Palliative Medicine* 10: 307–12.
6. Birtwistle J, Payne S, Smith P, Kendrick T (2002) The role of the district nurse in bereavement care. *Journal of Advanced Nursing* 38: 467–78.
7. Kidder LH, Fine M (1987) Qualitative and quantitative methods: when stories converge. In: Mark MM, Shotland L, (ed.) *New Directions in Program Evaluation*. San Francisco, CA: Jossey-Bass.

8. Willig C (2001) *Introducing Qualitative Research in Psychology*. Buckingham: Open University Press.

9. Low JTS, Payne S (1996) The good and bad death perceptions of health professionals working in palliative care. *European Journal of Cancer Care* 5: 237–41.

10. Payne S (1997) Selecting an approach and design in qualitative research. *Palliative Medicine* 11: 249–52.

11. Addington-Hall J, Walker L, Jones C., Karlsen S, McCarthy M (1998) A randomised controlled trial of postal versus interviewer administration of a questionnaire measuring satisfaction with, and use of, services received in the year before death. *Journal of Epidemiology and Community Health* 52: 802–7.

12. Payne S, Sheldon F, Jarrett N, Large S, Smith P, Davis C, Turner P, George S (2002) Differences in understandings of Specialist Palliative Care amongst service providers and commissioners in South London. *Palliative Medicine* 16: 395–402.

13. Copp G (1997) Patients' and nurses' constructions of death and dying in a hospice setting. *Journal of Cancer Nursing* 1: 2–13.

14. Rubin HJ, Rubin IS (1995) *Qualitative Interviewing: The Art of Hearing Data*. Thousand Oaks, CA: Sage.

15. Kvale S (1996) *InterViews: An Introduction to Qualitative Research Interviewing*. Sage: London.

16. Payne S (1999) Interview in qualitative research. In: Memon A, Bull R, (ed.) *Handbook of the Psychology of Interviewing*. Chichester: John Wiley, pp. 89–102.

17. Hennick M, Diamond I (1999) Using focus groups in social research. In: Memon A, Bull R, (ed.) *Handbook of the Psychology of Interviewing*, Chichester: John Wiley, pp. 113–44.

18. Perakyla A (1989) Appealing to the experience of the patient in the care of the dying. *Sociology of Health and Illness* 11: 117–34.

19. Perakyla A, Silverman D (1991) Reinterpreting speech-exchange systems: communication formats in AIDS counselling. *Sociology* 25: 627–51.

20. Potter J, Wetherell M (1987) *Discourse and Social Psychology: Beyond Attitudes and Behaviour*. Sage: London.

21. Potter J (1997) Discourse analysis as a way of analysing naturally occurring talk. In: Silverman D, (ed.) *Qualitative Research: Theory, Method and Practice*. Sage: London, pp. 144–60.

22. Quested B, Rudge T (2003) Nursing care of dead bodies: a discursive analysis of last offices. *Journal of Advanced Nursing* 41: 553–60.

23. Glaser BG, Strauss AL (1965) *Awareness of Dying*. New York: Aldine Publishing Company.

24. Field D (1989) *Nursing the Dying*. London: Tavistock/Routledge.

25. Seymour JE (2000) *Critical Moments: Death and Dying in Intensive Care*. Buckingham: Open University Press.

26. The A-M (2002) *Palliative Care and Communication: Experiences in the Clinic*. Buckingham: Open University Press.

27. Lawton J (2000) *The Dying Process. Patients' Experiences of Palliative Care*. London: Routledge.

28. Heath C (1997) The analysis of activities in face to face interaction using video. In: Silverman, D, (ed.) *Qualitative Research: Theory, Method and Practice*. London: Sage, pp. 183–200.

29. May J, Ellis-Hill C, Payne S. The use of video research techniques on a hospital ward for older people: ethical, practical and methodological issues. *Qualitative Health Research* (in press).

30. O'Connell DC, Kowal S (1995) Basic principles of transcription. In: Smith JA, Harre R, van Langenhove L, (ed.) *Rethinking Methods in Psychology.* London: Sage, pp. 93–105.

31. Ingleton C, Seymour J (2001) Analysing qualitative data: examples from two studies of end-of-life care. *International Journal of Palliative Nursing* 7: 227–34.

32. Atkinson JM, Heritage J (1984) *Structures of Social Action, Studies in Conversation Analysis.* Cambridge: Cambridge University Press.

33. Psarthas G, Anderson T (1990) The 'practices' of transcription in conversation analysis. *Semiotica* **78**: 75–99.

34. Psarthas G (1995) *Conversation Analysis. The Study of Talk-in-Interaction.* Thousand Oaks, CA: Sage.

35. Coffey A, Atkinson P (1996) *Making Sense of Qualitative Data.* Thousand Oaks, CA: Sage.

36. Strauss A, Corbin J (1990) *Basics of Qualitative Research: Grounded Theory Procedures and Techniques* Newbury Park, CA: Sage.

37. Glaser BG (1992) *Emergence vs Forcing: Basics of Grounded Theory Analysis.* Mill Valley, CA: Sociology Press.

38. Joffe H, Yardley Y (2004) Content and thematic analysis. In: Marks D, Yardley L, (ed.) *Research Methods for Clinical and Health Psychology.* London: Sage, pp. 56–68.

39. Boyatzis RE (1998) *Transforming Qualitative Information.* London: Sage.

40. Glaser B, Strauss A (1967) *The Discovery of Grounded Theory: Strategies for Qualitative Research.* New York: Aldine.

41. Bartlett D, Payne S (1997) Grounded theory—its basis, rationale and procedures. In: McKenzie G, Powell J, Usher R, (ed.) *Understanding Social Research: Perspectives on Methodology and Practice.* London: Falmer Press, pp. 173–95.

42. Labov W (1972) The transformation of experience in narrative syntax. In: Labov W, (ed.) *Language in the Inner City: Studies in the Black English Vernacular.* Philadelphia: University of Philadelphia Press.

43. Ricoeur P (1984) *Time and Narrative 1.* Chicago: University of Chicago Press.

44. Reissman C (1993) *Narrative Analysis—Qualitative Research Methods Series No. 30.* London: Sage.

45. Ellis-Hill C (1998) New world, new rules: life narratives and changes in self-concept in the first year after stroke. Unpublished PhD thesis, University of Southampton.

46. Parker I (1992) *Discourse Dynamics: Critical Analysis for Social and Individual Psychology.* London: Routledge.

47. Appleton J (1995) Analysing qualitative data: addressing issues of validity and reliability. *Journal of Advanced Nursing* 22: 993–9.

48. Floss C, Ellefsen B (2002) The value of combining qualitative and quantitative approaches in nursing research by means of method triangulation. *Journal of Advanced Nursing* **40**: 242–8.

Chapter 10

# Ethical and practice issues in qualitative research

Frances Sheldon and Anita Sargeant

## Introduction

Researchers embarking on a qualitative research project in palliative care face a series of interesting ethical and practice challenges, which are reiterated throughout the process of research, from devising the proposal to dissemination. This chapter aims to help researchers think through some of those challenges, so that they are not defeated by them and work from a clear ethical base.

Qualitative research in palliative care raises a number of questions. The first is concerned with a key debate about the researcher as a participant and their influence in the process of the research and, in particular, the extent to which this is accepted and how this is dealt with. The second is concerned with the interpersonal relationships with participants, gatekeepers and colleagues which are crucial in qualitative research, both theoretically and practically, because most qualitative research requires social interaction. This raises questions about how these relationships are built and maintained, and whether there are necessary compromises in that continuing process. The third is particularly relevant in palliative care, and is concerned with the impact of data collection and analysis on the researcher, if they are part of this process and of whether ways can be identified to safeguard and sustain the researcher. Palliative care research often tackles what are commonly regarded as particularly sensitive issues, and the next question is concerned with how we decide what is a 'sensitive issue' and for whom it is sensitive (Chapter 3). The final question considered here arises when professionals want to research their own professional practice and looks at what needs to be to be taken into account. How do we deal with issues of consent with people with deteriorating conditions? How do we ensure anonymity with the small samples so common in qualitative research?

The use of the interview and observational methods pose some particular challenges, and the continuing process of negotiation, which is inherent in qualitative research, is a minefield. Debating these issues is vital if we want to conduct research which is ethical, viable and contributes to the well-being of patients and those who care for them, whether these are family and friends or staff.

One early issue that many researchers employing qualitative approaches for the first time have to tackle is the privileged position of quantitative 'objective' approaches. The common description of the randomized controlled trial as the 'gold standard' for research reflects the way such approaches have dominated clinical research, and are embedded in the way that the general public think about research (Chapter 2). However, as Pope and Mays[1] point out, the most appropriate research method is the one that best explores the research question (Chapter 9). So new qualitative researchers have to stop apologizing and place themselves firmly in the mindset of qualitative research.

Entwhistle et al.[2] suggest that qualitative researchers need to be very aware of how different settings affect data collection; the acceptability of different ways of collecting data to different social groups; how research participants experience different forms of data collection; and whether some data collection methods particularly influence how, for example, older people or women respond: and they make a plea for further research on these issues.

## 'Sensitive' research

Given that palliative care is an acceptable research area and that it is also in general perceived as a sensitive research area, it is legitimate to ask how these general sensitivities may be approached, whether there are particular aspects of the general field needing special consideration and whether qualitative research methods are more inappropriately invasive or intrusive than other methods. The nature of the taboo around discussion of death, dying and bereavement in Western society has been much debated. Contrasts have been drawn between the withdrawal from most of the dying and bereaved and their consequent isolation, and the intense media interest in the stories of prominent people who die or of traumatic deaths.[3,4] Bereavement researchers[5] have alerted us to the cultural taboos on male expressions of emotion in Western Europe which meant that the most distressed bereaved men were under-represented in bereavement studies there. In turn, this led at one time to the widespread acceptance of a model of grief for both genders based to a large extent on female experience. So culture and gender must be considered in relation to any research project, even if they are not the specific focus. In a multicultural society such as the UK, it is inappropriate to exclude some research participants from general studies of service provision in palliative care or attitudes to death and dying because they are from a particular ethnic minority or do not speak English.

In his classic text, Lee[6] identifies three broad areas in which research may be perceived as threatening—the threat of intrusion, the threat of sanction and political threat. Under the category of intrusive threat, he draws on survey research to suggest that research into personal finances and sexual behaviour produces most unease, and it is interesting that financial pain is often found to accompany the end of life, yet is one of the most under-researched areas in palliative care.[7,8] Lee[6] comments:

> In part disclosing private information in interviews is likely to be problematic because privacy produces pluralistic ignorance. That is, because individuals only know about their own behaviour, it is difficult for them to judge how 'normal' that behaviour is compared to other people (p. 5).

He characterizes bereavement research as not so much private as emotionally charged, and recognizes too the potential pain or discomfort for the researcher involved in such an area, here reflecting his own cultural bias. An example of unexpected sensitivity emerged in a study by Young of the role of friendship for women who were dying.[9] She asked her participants to nominate one friend whom she might also interview. This for many was an impossible task. It was disloyal to other friends to single out one particularly. For some it was disparaging of their relationship with their husband. So in any private or emotionally charged area, and these are likely to be culturally determined, the premise must be for the researcher to understand that every question, even relating to seemingly innocuous demographic information such as number of children, can be potentially threatening. It is this perception of the intrusiveness of research with people who are dying that is behind so much of the gatekeeping by professionals in relation to patients.

The threat of sanction is most likely to arise in palliative care research in relation to legal and ethical issues such as surveying doctors' participation in euthanasia. Here careful attention to ensuring anonymization may produce a more accurate picture. Clear agreements about the terms and conditions of a research contract, especially around intellectual property and dissemination issues, will reduce the perception of political threat, which may arise with funding by government or major charities.

Common qualitative methods themselves have the potential to be intrusive. A respondent to a postal survey can toss it into the wastepaper bin, but it is harder to avoid a question which suddenly touches on a sensitive subject from a pleasant interviewer who is sitting on your sofa. Brannen[10] points out some problematic areas. First, in qualitative research which is so often exploratory, it is not always possible to be sure at the start of the research process what aspects of the topic will prove to be most significant, nor will the respondent always be clear before an interview which will feel the most sensitive question.

Consent has to be developmental and based on trust. It is clear, however, that an interview can be helpfully cathartic as well as distressing.[11] Secondly, qualitative interviews are often investigating meaning or phenomena which are fluid and context driven. Brannen[10] observes:

> Respondents' accounts of sensitive topics are frequently full of ambiguities and contradictions and are shrouded in emotionality. These form an integral part of the data set and therefore need to be confronted and taken account of in their interpretations.

Reflexivity, defined by Steier[12] as a 'turning back onto a self', is an important safeguard in tackling these dangers, which will be discussed in the next section. Whether the respondent is providing one interview or is engaged in a series over time, proper attention to closure is essential. This should include making available a source of support, for example a counselling service or palliative care professional other than the researcher, that the respondent can contact if the interview has raised distressing issues which continue to be troubling. Here the division between the research role and the practitioner role for a practitioner–researcher needs to be particularly clear. The nominated source of support also needs to be prepared for any potential contact.

## Who am I? The role of reflexivity

Negotiating and managing the potential ethical quicksand and research relationships requires an active engagement with reflexivity and consideration of the self in the process. Reflexivity is more than a reflection on the research process, it is an active critical engagement in a cyclical ongoing process which requires an exploration of yourself, your values and biases as they inform the data collection and social processes used, but equally of the environment and processes within which the research is taking place. Indeed this material is in itself data. Young provides an interesting example of this in her reflexive account of the complexity of her feelings and responses while researching the role of friendship for women who were dying.[13]

Using yourself as the tool of the research raises issues about how to engage in the reflexive cycle and how to negotiate between the different aspects of the self that become engaged in the data collection and subsequent analysis. Peshkin[14] suggests we engage with our subjectivity and the different 'I's within us, i.e. those different aspects of ourselves which inform our knowledge and research practice. The social worker 'I' or the nurse 'I' are likely to operate concurrently with the researcher 'I' and the educator 'I'. If you are a practitioner undertaking research in your own work environment or a related area, the different subjectivities of your own life history with which you interpret the world around you will be drawing your focus to different aspects of the context and informing the questions you ask and pursue. It is important that these are recognized and their influence addressed and recorded. By making our biases, values and prior knowledge explicit, there is a greater transparency to the process of data collection and interpretation.

There will be times when one or other aspect of yourself will be in conflict with another. It is at this point that reflexivity is crucial in finding a way through. There will also be times when observing closely people's distress and dying as a researcher can have a much more profound effect than it does as a practitioner. This is in part because there is a different aspect of your subjectivity actively engaged during the research observations, or when listening to the personal stories of participants.

## Supervision, safety and support

Supervision provides one arena where these biases, values, prior knowledge and emotional pain can be examined and understood. Throughout the research process from proposal to dissemination, the supervisor has to keep before the researcher–practitioner the questions 'Who are you—researcher or practitioner?' 'How are you thinking as a researcher?' 'How is this different from the way you approach problems/issues as a practitioner?' This iterative process within supervision is designed to help practitioner–researchers incorporate this mindset for themselves so that it can act as an automatic check on conceptualization and action. Similarly, supervision should enable academic researchers to understand the particular values and biases that they bring. However, supervision is of course much more than this. Good supervision will provide the structure which enables the research to be completed rigorously and on time. Jones[15] suggests that effective structure is an ethical requirement which should have wider benefits for organizations and research participants beyond the two main players. In qualitative as in quantitative research, supervisor and student or principal investigator and academic researcher need to agree jointly on a structure which is not so tight as to stifle the essential creativity that each can bring.

If, in qualitative research, researchers themselves are part of the process, then some understanding of the impact of the research on them, and of their emotional and practical support and safety needs, is vital to enabling researchers to develop both themselves and the project. Practical aspects of personal safety have been surprisingly neglected until comparatively recently. As soon as research moves out of the laboratory or in-patient area and into the community, this must be considered. Kenyon and Hawker[16] sought responses from researchers in the social and human sciences, about undertaking lone social research. Of their 46 respondents, both male and female, 13 had had no negative experiences, though they were still interested to comment. Four had experienced serious assaults and 19 had felt isolated, vulnerable or frightened in the field. Many had changed their behaviour as a result—avoiding one-to-one interviews, interviewing only in public spaces or refusing to 'cold call'. Cartwright and Seale[17] note how a substantial minority of their interviewers expressed their dislike of 'cold calling' and one withdrew from the survey because of a distressing experience directly related to it. An interesting aspect of Kenyon and Hawker's study was that their respondents often used relatives or friends as the contact point for information about their whereabouts and any safety concerns, feeling that they would have a more personal interest in their welfare than work colleagues.

Now most universities and large research organizations do pay attention to safety issues for their researchers in the field. For example, Simons and Kendrick[18] have produced a video for health and social researchers outlining good practice, with sections on assessment, prevention, identifying and responding to threat, and follow-up. The importance of knowing the geographical area and any potential risks from the research participants are emphasized, as is the agreement of an action plan with colleagues for moments of danger, of the researcher's expected location being known to others at all points, the importance of safety over completion of the task and the use of the mobile phone as an essential piece of equipment. All qualitative researchers undertaking fieldwork should take their own responsibility for assessing and preventing risk, but they should also challenge their research supervisors or employers to support them in this. For example, a woman may interview a bereaved man at home in the evening. He may in his distress find it very difficult to perceive where the boundaries are between a research interview and an empathetic personal concern for his most intimate feelings. Such issues also apply to male researchers.

However, practical concerns are not the only factor to take into account in maintaining a safe researcher and safe research in palliative care. We have already noted that this field embraces many topics that are perceived as particularly sensitive. Researchers are members of a particular society and may well share common understandings and perceptions of that society. So their feelings and perceptions about death, dying and bereavement are important, and have to be specifically considered in the course of the research. There may be different emphases depending on whether the researcher has been a professional practitioner in the field, or comes to it as an academic researcher with no previous experience of these issues. Practitioners working in the palliative care setting that an academic researcher is investigating will have developed their own defences to cope with their daily encounters with distressed people and may not understand the challenges for a researcher new to the field.

For example, an academic researcher and an administrative assistant were making an introductory visit to a new palliative care research site, an inpatient unit where they were investigating how palliative care was delivered. As part of the tour of the unit, the accompanying nurse took them into the mortuary where there was the body of a patient who had recently died. The nurse saw this as just a normal part of a familiarization visit. The researchers were faced with an aspect of the reality of what they were researching in a way that felt very challenging. Also they were very aware of their ethical framework and the importance of patient consent, and here they were in contact with someone who could no longer give consent. For them, this raised issues of ethics and of the dignity of the dead person.

As a practitioner–researcher you can become more sensitive to the 'everydayness' of the world you have taken for granted for so long and become part of. You are also less able to step in and make a difference clinically. In addition to examining these issues in supervision, keeping a research journal can be of help in following thoughts and feelings, and engaging these with observations in the field and interpretations. Support which needs to be considered in a sensitive research area such as palliative care may be securing confidential consultancy which is specifically available to the researcher to explore the aspects of the research which may have affected them emotionally. Not every supervisor has the skills to undertake psychological support, and even if they have it may be wise to separate out to some degree the management of the research from these human personal responses. Researchers may fear that job references may be affected if they show too openly the impact of the distress that they have witnessed. These issues need consideration by all parties at the start of the process and checking as it proceeds.

## Negotiating roles and relationships

Undertaking observations and interviews within any field of practice raises a variety of ethical and practice-related issues. These must be considered when planning the research and be negotiated during its process through to the ending, within the site of study and in the writing and publication of reports or journal articles.[19–22] How you build and maintain research relationships is crucial, from getting approval to undertake the research to then gaining continuing access to participants through the potential gatekeepers. Gender, race, age, sexuality, personality, professional background and general presentation will affect perceptions and relationships. In many respects, this is similar to the everyday practice of establishing working relationships. Interviews with nurse specialists revealed how they adapted their approaches and language using different aspects of themselves and their personalities in building and maintaining relationships with their patients and their carers, whilst remaining authentic and honest.[23] This is no different from how most qualitative researchers enter into and maintain their relationships in the field. A degree of flexibility is usually required to build and maintain trusting relationships whilst at the same time managing how you present yourself in order to 'fit in' and to reduce the amount of disruption caused by being present in the site.[24]

It is not possible to perform two roles, practitioner and researcher, without it potentially causing some confusion or changed awareness for both the participants and the researcher. Where good relationships exist and there is trust, participants that know the researcher's practice background often expect the researcher to behave in a manner representative of their practice discipline, for example nurses often expect researchers with a previous nursing background to behave in a particular way, often asking for assistance and sometimes advice. As for the researcher, it is often a surprise to find that you can slip easily into seeing the world through the lens of a practitioner once more rather than through the lens of a researcher.

For example, a nurse researcher found herself unexpectedly being positioned as 'an expert knower' during a period of field work with community palliative care nurses. The researcher was asked about her knowledge and experience of managing nerve pain by a community nurse in the car journey in between observed visits. For the researcher, this required a conscious balancing of needs including: social friendliness and engagement in the conversation about that particular situation, building and maintaining a trusting relationship with the nurse, being seen as credible but not wanting to influence the decision making of the nurse and the process of care.

There is a risk that the longer you spend in the 'known' field, the more comfortable you become. For the nurse researcher in the example, thinking as a researcher occasionally became briefly blurred by the emergent thoughts associated with being a practitioner and entering back into a problem-solving mode and out of the questioning observational mode. It can be difficult to remain immersed yet retain the ability to stand back and question the 'taken for granted' in an environment in which the language and behaviours appear familiar. However, it is also recognized that to build and maintain the trust of participants or colleagues in your role as a researcher, you must also help out with some of the requests for assistance, and engage in the everyday social conversations, since a degree of reciprocity often develops and exists over time which can facilitate the research process.[25,26]

Researchers should negotiate their role before entering the site of study, and not undertake tasks associated with their professional practice. Often researchers undertaking observational studies in palliative care or other health care settings have chosen to become general helpers or volunteers, enabling them to participate and blend in whilst observing the often taken for granted and unseen aspects of care, decision making and the experiences of patients without the responsibility of professional practice.[21,25,27] The potential for role confusion from the participants' perspective also raises important concerns over how 'informed' informed consent is. The potential for exploitation of participants' interactions is found in the relaxed 'everydayness' of having developed good and trusting relationships with colleagues and participants, to the point that they forget about the ongoing research process. It is therefore vital that the researcher consider how to ensure they are identified as different so that participants remain aware of their role.[28,29]

Finch[30] raised these ethical concerns when she noticed that other women were more ready to share their experiences with her because she shared not only the same gender but similar social circumstances. As a researcher, this offered her greater access to privileged information, yet made her ethically uncomfortable. Therefore, as a practitioner undertaking research in your own field, even if it is not your own work place, there is an increased potential to acquire more privileged and intimate information because some participants may identify with you in terms of either your professional position or other personal characteristics.

Existing relationships will also raise these same ethical dilemmas. How do you know when to listen and record and when just to listen and let go of what you have heard? As a researcher you can come to be seen as a safe person to talk to, a friend. You may hear conversations and information that few would be privy to and which may also include hearing about unlawful events or observing unprofessional practice. There may indeed be a fine line between overt and covert research depending on how open you are as a researcher and the tactical decisions that are made. How you respond to these issues and judge whether to use the information gained needs to have been given consideration prior to commencing the study, and incorporated, where necessary, in the information provided to potential participants, although not everything can ever be predicted or prepared for.

## Engaging in ethical research practice

The introduction of research governance in the UK and the need to gain ethical approval from Research Ethical Review Committees will require the researcher to be able to address these issues at the time of submission of their research protocol and during the undertaking of the process itself, since there is now a requirement for all research in the UK to be appropriately supervised.[31,32] Using an ethical framework to guide research has been recommended as a way to manage the difficult ethical situations that may arise when carrying out research with vulnerable people and where observing or hearing about potential unprofessional or substandard practice may occur.

The choice of ethical framework may be dependent upon a particular professional code of ethics. However, the adoption of a universal principle-based ethical framework such as that of Beauchamp and Childress[33] can provide a sound basis for ethical decision making as issues arise. The principles of beneficence, non-maleficence, respect and justice underpin the everyday work of palliative care, and can be seen to underpin most ethical social interactions that a researcher is engaged with. Having an ethical framework can improve the openness and integrity of the research process. As informed consent is sought, it is carried out in a manner that makes explicit the researcher's ethical responsibilities to the participants and the research process.[34]

Unless participants are offered complete confidentiality and anonymity, you must decide whether to make explicit in the information sheet that you give to them what you will do if you see or hear things that concern you about practice. The challenge lies in balancing the competing ethical demands of any professional codes of conduct with the ethical requirements of confidentiality and anonymity, in relation to informed consent. An ethical framework can assist in finding a way through the difficult to decide situations. Could anyone be harmed by what you have heard or seen? What good will be achieved by acting upon what has been seen or heard? Can the situation be managed by the researcher in a respectful and just way? Some ethics committees require that the researcher choose their allegiance to professional ethical guidance or more general research ethics where you have had a professional background and are carrying out research in a related area. This can lead to a sense of compromise. However, where you are both practitioner and researcher in your own work setting, the role of professional ethical guidance must be made explicit in the process.

## Opting in—ensuring consent is informed

The practicalities of obtaining informed consent remain a struggle in the real world of palliative care where the complexities of rapidly changing situations occur. In the UK, the Data Protection Act 1998 requires that all potential participants must be informed of the ongoing research although they cannot be approached by the researcher. Potential participants have to agree to their names and contact details being given to the researcher before they can be approached to discuss the research and choose whether to become involved. This can add a significant time delay before someone becomes a participant, and in palliative care time is often important. As a researcher, you cannot assume to access the names and details of unknown potential participants unless they are already within the public domain. It is very possible that, from a research perspective, you are having to gatekeep your own access to the personal information presented to you as 'helpful' colleagues try to offer you notes or talk to you about a particularly interesting person.

The degree of trust charged to you as a researcher, or by your association with certain health care professionals, can find you trying to pursue the ethical route to informed consent by presenting the appropriate information when the person you are talking with does not want to engage with it. The person perceives you as trustworthy and would rather get on and tell you their story or have you 'watch and learn'. Sometimes people spill out their stories in a manner which would be rude to disrupt until an appropriate moment to explain about the research.[22,25] For others, the presentation of a consent form can cause concern because of its formalized nature, or association with unpleasant procedures. This may leave people unwilling to sign it, and less willing to participate. Being ethical requires diplomatic negotiation with those who do not wish to engage in the required rigorous process of consent yet wish to participate in the study.

Engaging with the concept of consent as an ongoing process, rather than as a one-off event, is recommended to ensure consent remains informed and understood throughout the course of the research. This can be practised by periodically checking participants' understanding of the research as well as their awareness of their right to withdraw their involvement at any time. This approach incorporates a clearer ethical balance in the research process over time.[29,35]

A balance, however, must also be struck between constantly reminding and drawing attention to the research with the need for the researcher to 'fit in' and blend into the back ground to enable 'everyday' activities to continue relatively unchanged. This is central to managing the ethical and practical concerns within the context of the study. Decisions sometimes have to be made in the moment or on the run, which is one of the reasons why researchers need to maintain a reflexive engagement with the process.

Achieving informed consent can be problematic with observational research undertaken in an open environment. However, this can be counterbalanced by observing agreed 'episodes' of practice or care, for which specific consent has been obtained. Increasing regulation and formalization of the process of gaining and recording informed consent, and the need for overt research practice will affect the use of naturalistic observational and interview techniques. The art of managing these ethical decisions, whilst maintaining as much of the naturalism as possible, is to be found in the sensitivity of balancing social norms and interactions with the need for openness and ethical transparency.[36]

## From the outside looking in, from the inside looking out

The benefits and disadvantages of researching the 'known' world of your own area of practice have to be weighed up. Undertaking research with fellow colleagues in an environment that the researcher is known in can offer a range of possibilities. The researcher does not have to negotiate entry to the group or gain the trust of gatekeepers because they are already an insider with inside knowledge, and are known to the participant group. This can cause difficulties in that the researcher is not free of group ties, the expectations of colleagues and team commitments, so may not be seen as a researcher.

Prior knowledge from the inside world of palliative care allows for the incorporation and development of practice perspectives into theory. Insights can be gained with a fresh view without having to ask potentially distracting questions of the participants. However, asking the 'naïve' questions is less possible, and seeing the often taken for granted aspects of palliative care, such as its routines, can be more difficult to achieve. The existing relationships with colleagues can enable interviewees to feel more trusting and talk more openly than perhaps they would to an unknown interviewer, therefore acting as a very rich source of information and data. This may have the opposite effect where there is an imbalance in the relationship with the researcher in terms of their prior position, where participants may not feel comfortable to relay negative concerns. Colleagues or patients and their carers may feel obliged to participate, for fear of letting the group down or because of perceived peer pressure. Ethics committees rightly raise concerns over the freedom to choose to participate without coercion of any kind.

Understanding the language, the jargon used on a daily basis and the culture of the palliative care setting is extremely helpful and prevents increased distractions of everyday practices by the continual asking of questions by the outside researcher. It enables exploration and explanations for meanings and processes that have developed over time within the context. Where the outsider has the advantage is in questioning the linguistic assumptions of taken for granted meanings, and exploring the culture from a less subjective perspective. The outsider is less likely to experience role conflicts and is often more able to ask the difficult questions. However, learning to understand a new culture and language takes time, and the subtleties of the language used may be lost on the outsider.[37]

Similar issues can be encountered when a researcher with a background in palliative care undertakes research in an unknown palliative care environment. The researcher balances between being both an insider and an outsider. As an outsider to the participants, the researcher must build trust and develop relationships, especially with gatekeepers, yet at the same time they understand the language and practices although some of the jargon may be different as will some of the practices and routines in a setting with its own institutional culture. This offers a potentially insightful and creative balance between the known and the unknown. The researcher can ask some of the naïve questions from an outsider's perspective, and yet assume a greater degree of understanding of the everyday as an insider.

The issue of power is never far away from the dynamic of the research relationship, and recommendations have been made for some research within palliative care to be multiprofessional so that the power dynamics between different professional groups which may affect the interviewing process can be minimized.[38] Although many feminist researchers[30,39,40] suggest ways to reduce the influence of power within the research process, power continues to exist at different points within the process and within the different relationships, and it would be naïve to suggest otherwise. Hierarchical perceptions held by participants about the position and power of the researcher and their professional background will influence access to the research site and to future participants and interview interactions. The power of the organization can encourage or limit research participation.

Lack of understanding about the complex issues involved in qualitative research methodologies or a lack of appreciation of qualitative research as a valuable approach to gathering rich data by the members of Research Ethics Review Committees can detrimentally affect and delay the acceptance of qualitative research proposals.[19] Although protection and maintaining ethical standards is a vital aspect of the role of the Research Ethics Review Committees, a lack of awareness and an understanding of palliative care issues can deny individuals their right to choose to participate and the opportunity of having their voices and experiences heard and valued. Lee and Kristjanson[41] recommend that ethics committees engage in facilitative approval processes, where advice is sought from methodological experts in the field and there is dialogue with all parties. Researchers should ensure an openness, honesty and balance of the potential harm with the potential benefit of participation of those involved, and clarity in the dynamic of consenting procedures and ability to withdraw in their proposals.

Where you undertake research in your own setting, power dynamics and expectations are already established, which may influence colleagues' or patients' decisions to participate or not. Where you undertake research at a different palliative care setting, your presentation and background may influence the perception of potential participants and gatekeepers. Power is not simply organizational or hierarchical; the personal power of the researcher and participants also influences how the research relationship unfolds and the interactions during participant observations and interviews. Power is dynamic, and may need to be negotiated, and its balance may change over the duration of the research process. How organization, hierarchical and personal power is managed and negotiated will have a bearing on the outcomes of the research data.

## Issues in recording data

Transcription and anonymization are two issues meriting some attention in palliative care research. Most qualitative interviews are audio-recorded or occasionally video-recorded and then transcribed, though Mason[42] cautions against thinking that the recording constitutes an 'objective' record. Field notes can assist with recording some of the non-verbal aspects, and judgements still come into play about writing down some verbalizations which are not words. For most Masters and doctoral students, transcribing personally is the only practical possibility for reasons of cost. Through listening to the transcripts, they may re-contextualize, get in touch with their feelings again and hear more than when in the middle of the interview. It is more likely in a larger study that transcribing will be performed by a secretary, who may for the first time hear a dying person express panic and fear about the moment of death. Here again the issue of the personal impact of distressing material and the importance of support systems needs to be considered.

Anonymization can present greater problems for qualitative researchers, often working with small samples and rich individualized data, than for quantitative researchers.[10] Kite[43] raises the implications of anonymization for all participants in the research process. She highlights the potential for confusion unless there is very careful tracking of the allocation of false names. More importantly, she questions whether researchers may be doing violence to participants by changing names and details as they try to represent participants' worlds. In the world of qualitative research where people are characterized as active 'participants' rather than passive 'subjects', it is becoming more common to ask participants to choose a false name for themselves, and some may wish to retain their real name. Personal details of individuals in a sample may be changed, but with caution.

In a survey in a defined geographical area of the attitudes to a particular issue of Macmillan nurses employed there, only one was male. The researcher scrutinized the data for evidence of gender-based responses. Having found no examples, she made it clear that all participants would be described as female. Had there been examples, it might have been much more difficult to protect his identity, since the stratagem of describing him as female would have prevented a true account of the findings. In another study, the researcher had taken pains to anonymize the three organizations she had studied in the text, but in an introduction recorded her thanks to particular key people in each organization who had helped her to gain access. It was not difficult to link them with material in the text.

## Conclusion

The importance of social relationships founded on trust within an ethical framework cannot be overemphasized in qualitative research. Lee suggests that such trust may develop if mechanisms are in place to block possible negative repercussions from the research, and that it is emergent:

> building over the course of the research relationship of increasing levels of fellowship, mutual self-disclosure and reciprocity.[6]

He identifies too the value of an imaginative cast of mind when researching sensitive topics, which may result in innovative methodological solutions. Provided this is underpinned by rigorous reflexivity, the outcome should be more ethically focused research practice in palliative care.

## References

1. Pope C, Mays N (1995) Researching the parts other methods cannot reach: an introduction to qualitative methods in health and health services research. *British Medical Journal* **31:** 42–5.
2. Entwhistle V, Tritter JQ, Calnan M (2002) Research experiences of cancer: the importance of methodology. *European Journal of Cancer Care* **11:** 232–7.
3. Armstrong D (1987) Silence and truth in death and dying. *Social Science and Medicine* **24:** 651–7.
4. Pickering M, Littlewood J, Walter T (1997) Beauty and the beast: sex and death in the tabloid press. In: Field D, Hockey J, Small N, (ed.) *Death, Gender and Ethnicity*. London: Routledge.
5. Stroebe M (1998) New directions in bereavement research: exploration of gender differences. *Palliative Medicine* **12:** 5–12.
6. Lee RM (1993) *Doing Research on Sensitive Topics*. London: Sage.
7. Sykes NP, Pearson S, Chell S (1992) Quality care for the terminally ill: the carer's perspective. *Palliative Medicine* **6:** 227–36.
8. Soothill K, Morris S, Harman J, Francis B, Thomas C, McIllmurray MB (2001) The significant unmet needs of cancer patients: probing psychosocial concerns. *Health and Social Care in the Community* **9:** 597–605.

9. Young E (1999) Collaborating with 'the media' to recruit for palliative care research. Paper given at the Joint Meeting of the Forum on Palliative Care of the Royal Society of Medicine and the Palliative Care Research Forum on Ethnography and Palliative Care Research. 12th January 1999. Royal Society of Medicine.

10. Brannen J (1988) The study of sensitive subjects. *Sociological Review* **36:** 552–63.

11. Hutchinson S, Wilson M, Wilson H (1994) Benefits of participating in research interviews. *Image* **26:** 161–4.

12. Steier F, (ed.) (1991) *Research and Reflexivity.* London: Sage.

13. Young E, Lee R (1996) Fieldworker feelings as data: 'emotion work' and 'feeling rules' in first person accounts of sociological fieldwork. In: James V, Gabe J, eds. *Health and the Sociology of Emotions.* Oxford: Blackwell Publishers Ltd.

14. Peshkin A (1988) In search of subjectivity—ones own. *Educational Research* **7:** 17–22.

15. Jones A (1999) Significant relationships: planning for effective research supervision. *Nurse Researcher* **6:** 5–17.

16. Kenyon E, Hawker S (1999) Once would be enough: some reflections on the issues of safety for lone researchers. *International Journal of Research Methodology* **2:** 313–327.

17. Cartwright A, Seale C (1990) *The Natural History of a Survey: An Account of the Methodological Issues Encountered in a Study of Life Before Death.* London: King Edward's Hospital Fund for London.

18. Simons L, Kendrick T (2002) *Safety Issues for Research in the Community.* Southampton: University of Southampton School of Medicine.

19. Ramcharan P, Cutcliff J (2001) Judging the ethics of qualitative research: considering the 'ethics as process' model. *Health and Social Care in the Community* **9:** 358–66.

20. McEvoy P (2001) Interviewing colleagues: addressing issues of perspective, inquiry and representation. *Nurse Researcher* **9:** 49–59.

21. Lawton J (2001) Gaining and maintaining consent: ethical concerns raised in study of dying patients. *Qualitative Health Research* **11:** 693–705.

22. Lawton J (2000) *The Dying Process: Patients Experiences of Palliative Care.* London: Routledge.

23. Aranda S (1999) Being authentic and being a chameleon: nurse–patient interaction revisited. *Nursing Inquiry* **6:** 75–82.

24. Punch M (1998) Politics and ethics in qualitative research. In: Denzin N, Lincoln Y, (ed.) *The Landscape of Qualitative Research: Theories and Issues.* London: Sage.

25. Seymour J (2001) *Critical Moments—Death and Dying in Intensive Care.* London: Sage.

26. Kite K (1999) Participant observation, peripheral observation or apart-icipant observation? *Nurse Researcher* **7:** 44–55.

27. Hockey J (1990) *Experiences of Death: An Anthropological Account.* Edinburgh: Edinburgh University Press.

28. Seymour J, Ingleton C (1999) Ethical issues in qualitative research at the end of life. *International Journal of Palliative Nursing* **5:** 65–73.

29. Merrel J, Wiliams A (1994) participant observation and informed consent: relationships and tactical decision-making. *Nursing Research Nursing Ethics* **1:** 163–72.

30. Finch J (1993) 'It's great to have someone to talk to': ethics and politics of interviewing women. In: Hammersley M, (ed.) *Social Research: Philosophy, Politics and Practice.* London: Sage.

31. Central Office for Research Ethics (COREC) (2002) Changes Affecting Procedures for Applications to NHS Research Ethics Committees. http:www.corec.org.uk/

32. Department of Health (2001) *Research Governance Framework for Health and Social Care*. London: Department of Health.

33. Beauchamp TL, Childress JF (1994) *Principles of Biomedical Ethics*. New York: Oxford University Press.

34. Cerinus M (2001) The ethics of research. *Nurse Researcher* **8**: 72–89.

35. Beaver K, Luker K, Woods S (1999) Conducting research with the terminally ill: challenges and considerations. *International Journal of Palliative Nursing* **5**: 13–7.

36. Sargeant A (2001) The Complexities and Uncertainties of Getting Started: Negotiating The New Dilemmas Facing Researchers In Palliative Care. Paper Presented at The Social Aspects Of Death, Dying And Bereavement Conference University Of Leicester November 8th 2001.

37. Bonner A, Tolhurst G (2002) Insider–outsider perspectives of participant observations. *Nurse Researcher* **9**: 7–19.

38. Ingleton C, Field D, Clark D (1997) Multidisciplinary case study as an approach to the evaluation of palliative care services: two examples. *International Journal of Palliative Nursing* **3**: 335–9.

39. Fine M, Weis L, Weseen S, Wong L (2000) For whom? Qualitative research, representation and social responsibility. In: Denzin N, Lincoln Y, (ed.) *Handbook of Qualitative Research*, 2nd edn. London, Sage.

40. Reinhartz S (1992) *Feminist Methods in Social Research*. New York: Oxford University Press.

41. Lee S, Kristjanson L (2003) Human research ethics committees: issues in palliative care. *International Journal of Palliative Nursing* **9**: 13–8.

42. Mason J (1996) *Qualitative Researching*. London: Sage.

43. Kite K (1999) Anonymising the subject: what are the implications? *Nurse Researcher* **6**: 77–84.

Chapter 11

# Evaluating qualitative research

Michele Crossley

## Introduction

In recent years in Britain, qualitative methods have become increasingly important in health service research, largely in terms of the pursuit of 'evidence-based' health care. This has led to recognition of the importance of understanding the views of 'users' or 'consumers' of health care and, relatedly, of health care professionals involved in the 'delivery' of such care. Increasingly, there is widespread recognition amongst purchasers and providers of health services that many health problems and processes of care cannot necessarily be evaluated through use of traditional quantitative research-based studies because these are unable to provide adequate insight into the meanings and perceptions of those centrally involved in health care.[1,2]

This issue is obviously of central importance to any evaluation of palliative care services. Probably more so than in any other area of health care, in evaluating the services offered to dying people, it is necessary to find out how 'users' themselves feel about and perceive their care, and, relatedly, the perceptions of health professionals responsible for providing such care. The intrinsic nature of palliative care is such that people encountering such services (patients, relatives and health professionals) are forcibly faced with existential issues of profound significance—often unanswerable questions related to life, death, meaning and spirituality—what, when I was once in a conversation with a HIV/AIDS patient, he referred to as 'all the big ones'. Any adequate evaluation of palliative care services is forced to take these considerations into account—they are, in a sense, the 'bread and butter' of such care. In order to do this, it is difficult to see how such concerns could be researched effectively in anything other than a qualitative framework.[3]

Despite the growth in qualitative research, however, and the obvious importance attributed to its utility in health service research, it is only recently that attention has been paid to the development of standards for assessing the quality of qualitative research.[2] This is important because the pursuit of 'evidence-based' health care has led to growing enthusiasm for the use of systematic reviews and the development of a framework for establishing a 'hierarchy of evidence' with regard to ways of establishing the 'effectiveness' of health care (Chapter 8). As most of these reviews have focused almost exclusively on quantitative research, they reinforce the view that evidence from quantitative research, in particular, randomized controlled trials, represents the highest level of research evidence[2] (p. 342). In order to appreciate the important role played by qualitative methods and theories in evaluating the 'evidence' base of health care, it is therefore necessary to highlight the aims and objectives of such perspectives, which differ from quantitative approaches, and to articulate the criteria relevant to an assessment of their quality.

It is important to appreciate the fundamental philosophical differences between quantitative and qualitative approaches (Chapter 9). These have previously been outlined by Popay *et al.*[2] and consist of epistemological (the type of knowledge that different methods generate) and ontological (the type of reality or object to which different methods are relevant) differences. In the context of research questions related to health service research, these differences are of fundamental importance and must be articulated in any evaluation of qualitatively based research studies. One of the main aims of this chapter is to make clear the different criteria relevant to the evaluation of qualitative research approaches. The importance of these differences for palliative care research cannot be overemphasized. If these differences are not upheld, the true potential of qualitative research in the field of palliative care runs the risk of being subsumed by a hegemonic quantitative paradigm. For palliative care, this would be disastrous because this is not just a question of methods, but of preserving a philosophical challenge which has massively humanitarian implications in terms of how we look after dying people. It may seem somewhat 'old hat' to refer to Kubler Ross's and Dame Cicely Saunders' classic work on death and dying and their insistence that we 'simply listen to the dying patient'. However, maybe it is necessary to return right back to those early and simple messages. These palliative pioneers were fighting against a predominantly biomedical system which produced 'passive patients' who were denied individual autonomy and decision making during the final stages of their life.[4] In today's climate, it is necessary to reiterate the original aims and objectives of palliative care services.

## What are the different criteria relevant for assessing qualitative research?

This question has been addressed in recent years by a number of researchers with specific regard to health care research.[2,5] This chapter attempts to provide a distillation of these findings, summarizing four essential criteria appropriate to the evaluation of qualitative research. These include: the 'primacy of subjective meaning' and associated implications regarding issues of 'generalizability' and 'representativeness'; the importance of sustained integration between theoretical and empirical material; the importance of reflexivity; and impact. The ways in which these criteria differ from those sought in quantitative research are highlighted. In addition, the criteria are discussed specifically in terms of their relevance to palliative care research.

## The 'primacy of subjective meaning': implications for issues of 'generalizability' and 'representativeness'

The actual methods associated with qualitative research in health services include individual interviewing of various kinds (structured, semi-structured or in-depth), focus group interviewing, participant observation, ethnography and the analysis (discursive or narrative) of diaries or published/unpublished autobiographical accounts (Chapter 9). In palliative care, these methods are most likely to be used in order to gain insight into patient and health professional experiences with regard to the experience of dying, and the care received and provided during this process. Such research is likely to cover sensitive areas such as people's hopes, expectations, fears, worries and beliefs.

It is with regard to such issues that one criterion of qualitative research can be said to underpin all others—this is what Popay *et al.*[2] characterize as the 'primacy of subjective meaning'. This constitutes the 'primary marker' of standards in qualitative research related to the appropriateness and quality of health care. If such research is to inform policy and practice, it is absolutely necessary that it elucidates the 'subjective meanings' experienced by the various parties involved in the research [2] (p. 344). Hence, one of the key questions to ask in evaluating a piece of qualitative health service research is: 'Does it illuminate the subjective meaning, actions and context of those being researched?'[2] (p. 345).

This prioritization of 'subjective meaning' from a qualitative point of view relates to important differences between quantitative and qualitative approaches with regard to their deliberations regarding sample size and, relatedly, the representativeness and generalizability of findings. For instance, in quantitative research, sample size is often used to guarantee the strength of the claims made. This is because one of the main aims of quantitative research methods is to determine factors or relationships which exist between certain phenomena within a specific sample, and then to ascertain probabilistic generalizations that such relationships also exist within a larger population (Chapter 4). Hence, the greater the number of subjects within a survey or experimental sample, the better able the researcher is to generalize to the rest of the population. This, however, is not the aim of qualitative research which is, instead, the elucidation of 'subjective meanings'—the experiences and situations faced by those comprising the focus of investigation. In fact, from a qualitative point of view, the greater the sample size, the less the researcher is able to 'respect the specificities of each subject's response and the meanings of the response to the subject'[6] (p. 12). In a sense, the bigger the sample size, the more the aims of qualitative research are compromised, because the possibility of providing in-depth description and exploration is diminished.

The different aims of qualitative research also have important implications not just for sample size, but in terms of the actual selection of a sample in the first place. Again, unlike in quantitative research, this is not a matter of 'randomness' and, thus ultimately, of 'representativeness', but more an issue of 'relevance'[2] (p. 346). In qualitative research, it is often preferable to employ 'theoretical' sampling in which small numbers of people are chosen for their special attributes, or people who are extreme or typical exemplars of the phenomena of interest[5] (p. 218). Of course, if this is the case, the process by which individuals or cases were theoretically or purposefully sampled needs to be carefully described. The key question in assessing standards for qualitative sampling is: 'Does the sample produce the type of knowledge necessary to understand the structures and processes within which the individuals or situations are located?'[2] (p. 346). Once more, the questions relating to sample selection highlight that qualitative research has 'a different relationship' from the context of research than is the case with most quantitative research[2] (p. 346). Whereas the latter seeks to develop methods and produce findings that are independent of context, qualitative research 'seeks to maximise the use of context as a means of locating lay knowledge and understanding subjective meaning'[2] (p. 346).

In relation to these objectives, it is therefore important to emphasize that one overarching hallmark of good quality qualitative research is its ability to provide an in-depth description of the phenomena being investigated. Popay et al.[2] (p. 347) characterize this as the 'richness' of the picture the research produces. Using Geertz's[7] distinction between 'thin' and 'thick' description, Popay et al. point out that the former merely states a set of facts that are independent of intentions or circumstances. In contrast, 'thick' description provides the context of an experience, states the intentions and meanings that feed into the experience and exposes the experience as a process. It is basically a matter of whether or not the research account provides an in-depth, as opposed to a superficial, description of the phenomena under investigation. Such description is also important for further analytical inquiry. As Denzin and Lincoln[8] highlight, 'thick description' potentiates 'thick analysis and interpretation'. This is what good quality qualitative research should seek to achieve.

There is no doubt that a qualitative approach with in-depth focus on the particular serves as a continuous stumbling block for critics of such approaches, mainly because it continues to be perceived as a 'lack' of generalizability. However, this 'lack' is such only because the philosophical aims and objectives of quantitative research are implicitly being used as a benchmark. The kind of claims made by qualitative researchers are simply of a different order from those used in quantitative research. If any claims to generalization are made within qualitative research, they refer to 'logical generalisations based upon a theoretical understanding of a similar class of phenomena rather than probabilistic generalisations to a population'[2] (p. 348). This brings us to the next essential criterion for assessing the quality of qualitative research: theoretical sophistication and evidence of sustained integration between theoretical and empirical material.

## Evidence of sustained integration between theoretical and empirical material

Theoretical sophistication is of particular importance in assessing the quality of a piece of qualitative research. As Yardley points out, awareness of the relevant literature and previous related empirical work is essential for all research, whether quantitative or qualitative, but in much qualitative research the 'sophistication of the interpretation of the data is particularly crucial'[5] (p. 219). Whereas quantitative researchers rely on procedures such as random sampling and standardized measurement to ensure the 'horizontal generalization' of their findings, qualitative researchers, 'aspire instead to the theory building work of "vertical generalisation" i.e. an endeavour to link the particular to the abstract and to the work of others'[5] (p. 219). Accordingly, in qualitative research it is necessary to show a 'fairly extensive grounding' in the philosophy of the approach adopted because such understanding then becomes evident in the profundity and depth of analysis achieved.

Yardley provides an example from some of my own research[9] in which I conducted an empirical analysis of the emotional problems faced by people living with a long-term HIV diagnosis. In that research, my main concern was to show how the shattering of 'routine temporal assumptions' underpinned the trauma experienced by many of my research participants. In order to do that, I drew upon previous phenomenological work such as Sartre's and, in doing so, presented in Geertz's terms, an in-depth 'thick' description of the data combined with theoretical analysis. Both data and theoretical ideas were reciprocally used to illuminate each other. At the same time, however, it is important that the analysis remains sensitive to the data and does not simply 'impose' theoretical ideas. This relates to the next issue: reflexivity.

## Reflexivity

The search for reliability in quantitative research rests on the assumption that it is possible to produce 'objective' knowledge that is independent of the researcher (hence the concern with the 'inter-rater reliability' of research tools) and independent of the particular time and location in which the research was conducted (hence the concern with test–re-test reliability). This all feeds into the aim of 'replicating' and thus generalizing research results. However, from a qualitative standpoint, data are never pure and research knowledge cannot be objective because it is always shaped by the purposes, perspectives and activities of those who create it[2] (p. 347). For instance, from a qualitative point of view, the use of 'inter-rater reliability' measures as a check on 'objectivity' is totally meaningless. Yes it is possible to train two people to code something in the same way, but this does not exclude the element of subjectivity in data interpretation—it is just that a certain form of interpretation has been agreed by two (or more) people[5] (p. 219).

As Parker[6] (p. 11) argues, good qualitative research will never make the claim that it is perfectly replicable. It may be possible to repeat the work that has been described, but that repetition will necessarily be a different piece of work: 'different at the very least by virtue of the change in the researcher, informants and meanings of the research tool over time'[6] (p. 11). Qualitative research treats all data as the product of interaction. This means that the onus is on the researcher to render transparent the processes by which the data have been collected, analysed and presented. For instance, it may be important to discuss the experiences or motivations which led the researcher to undertake a particular investigation in the first place, or consider the way in which the research (and therefore the final results) was influenced by external funding pressures[5] (p. 223). These are all issues that are systematically excluded from quantitatively based research investigations in pursuit of 'objectivity'. However, from a qualitative point of view, refusal to address such questions constitutes a refusal to deal with the way in which so-called 'objective' data have been influenced by the research process. Once more, the aim in qualitative research is 'not so much replicability as *specificity*'[6] (p.11).

Hence, an essential criterion for assessing the quality of qualitative research is its 'variability rather than standardisation'[2] (p. 346). Has the researcher considered the ways in which the data have been shaped by the research questions they have asked? To what extent does the researcher show evidence of having responded to 'circumstances as they exist' rather than having 'attempted to create a situation in which the variables of interest can be controlled'? In accordance with such objectives, there should be 'some evidence of adaption and redesign in the writing up of research'[2] (p. 346). Yardley[5] (p. 222) likewise refers to the 'transparency and coherence' of the research description and argument. The researcher should pay adequate attention to the 'fit' between the research question, the philosophical perspective, the methods and analysis used in the study. All of this should be bound together in a well written narrative, the quality of the narrative constituting an integral part of the research itself.

As Yardley argues, paying attention to the way in which the researcher influences the research process and people studied during the course of investigation bears some resemblance to traditional clinical practice, insofar as clinicians are encouraged to take account of the personal and ethical issues arising from the potential for mutual influence. It is with regard to such ethical problems that Owens and Payne[3] (p. 160) suggest that qualitative methods have a particular appeal for conducting research with dying people. Qualitative methods have often been especially conscientious in addressing the ethics of research studies with particular regard to matters such as ownership of the research and potential power imbalances. Such issues are likely to have an 'especial imperative' in terms of research in palliative care. As Owens and Payne[3] (p. 158) make clear:

> To the person who is dying, every minute may be precious, too precious to spend participating in research of indifferent value to themselves or others. Moreover, the person who is dying is typically already in a relatively powerless position; actions and procedures which are central to their survival may be in the hands of relatively powerful others—physicians, nurses, family members and so on.

## Impact

The final, and arguably the decisive, criterion by which any piece of research must be judged is in relation to its impact and utility[5] (p. 223). However, as Yardley argues, there are many varieties of usefulness, and the ultimate value of a piece of research can only be assessed 'in relation to the objectives of the analysis, the applications it was intended for, and the community for whom the findings were deemed relevant'[5] (p. 223).

In the context of health service research, and with specific application to palliative care research, it may be argued that the aim of qualitative research is to facilitate further understanding of the beliefs, thoughts and activities of the patient, relatives and health professionals, as a way of addressing the appropriateness of care within specific settings. From this perspective, one would expect qualitative research to have some clear implications for policy and practice, indicating the relevance of the research to a variety of stakeholders[2] (p. 349).

Having said that, however, it is important not to fall into the trap of assuming that the impact of a study rests solely with its ability to present direct implications for policy and practice. Theoretical sophistication and the theory-building work of 'vertical generalization' has already been discussed as an important characteristic of good quality qualitative research. Theoretical worth is therefore often of primary importance in qualitative research. As Yardley[5] argues, some analyses are important because they draw on empirical or theoretical ideas to open up new ways of understanding and thinking about a topic. Some pieces of theoretical academic work may be extremely esoteric and appear to have very little practical import. However, such ideas may eventually have a wider impact in terms of their application in other areas by different researchers.

In addition to practical and theoretical considerations, it is also important to consider the 'political' and critical potential of qualitative research. Some qualitative researchers would argue that one of the main aims of such research is to be inherently political insofar as there is an attempt to challenge traditional and established modes of thinking and researching a particular phenomenon. For instance, in the context of health service and palliative care research, this may involve challenging the way in which health professionals and researchers orient towards and routinely manage issues of health, illness and death[1] (Chapter 7) (which has specific relevance to palliative care).

## Conclusion

A number of important criteria are relevant for appraising the quality of qualitative research. These involve asking the following questions of a piece of research:

- Is 'subjective meaning' and the action and context of those being researched articulately conveyed?
- Is there sustained integration between empirical and theoretical material?
- Does the researcher engage with issues of reflexivity?
- Does the researcher adequately assess the critical impact of the research?

These criteria are important in evaluating the quality of qualitative work, both generally within health service research, but also with more specific application to palliative care.

## References

1. Crossley M (2000) *Rethinking Health Psychology*. Buckinghamshire: Open University Press.
2. Popay J, Rogers A, Williams G (1998) Rationale and standards for the systematic review of qualitative literature in health services research. *Qualitative Health Research* **8**: 341–51.

3. **Owens G, Payne S** (1999) Qualitative research in the field of death and dying. In: Murray M, Chamberlain K, (ed.) *Qualitative Health Psychology: Theories and Methods*. London: Sage.

4. **Saunders C, Baines M** (1983) *Living with Dying: The Management of Terminal Disease*. Oxford: Oxford University Press.

5. **Yardley L** (2000) Dilemmas in qualitative health research. *Psychology and Health* **15**: 215–28.

6. **Parker I** (1994) Qualitative research. In: Banister P, Burman E, Parker I, Taylor M, Tindall C, (ed.) *Qualitative Methods in Psychology: A Research Guide*. Buckinghamshire: Open University Press.

7. **Geertz C** (1973) *The Interpretation of Cultures: Selected Essays*. New York: Basic Books.

8. **Denzin N, Lincoln Y** (1994) *Handbook of Qualitative Research*. London: Sage.

9. **Davies ML** (1997) Shattered assumptions: time and the experience of long-term HIV positivity. *Social Science and Medicine* **44**: 561–71.

Chapter 12

# Mixed methods for evaluation research

## Christine Ingleton and Sue Davies

Evaluation is central to research on health services, and the importance of systematic evaluation is now widely recognized. Yet, in spite of this attention, there is still little unanimity on the precise meaning of the term, and a universally appropriate and comprehensive methodological approach has proved elusive. Whilst the precise meaning of evaluation is difficult to articulate, it is possible to identify some themes within the literature. A wide variety of models and methods exist in the evaluation field and, within this chapter, we intend to provide a brief overview of the most commonly used approaches. Given the complex nature of palliative care, we will argue that a systematic evaluation of either the effectiveness of palliative care interventions or the quality of care delivery often requires the use of both quantitative and qualitative methods of data collection and analysis. We shall provide examples of how applying mixed methods in evaluation and case study research can 'open up' a new field of study and help us to understand issues relevant to palliative care in an ever-changing context.

## What is evaluation research and how does it differ from 'traditional' research?

In spite of the ambiguity around the term, evaluation generally involves some kind of judgement about the worth or value of something, usually against a set of specified criteria. Within the context of health care, it involves:

> The critical assessment, on as objective a basis as possible, of the degree to which entire services or their component fulfil stated goals.[1]

Evaluation research is a form of applied research that embraces a wide range of methodologies. It includes:

> ... defining the objectives of health care initiatives and procedures, monitoring inputs, ascertaining the extent to which the anticipated outcomes are achieved and identifying the existence of any unintended consequences of the planned intervention.[2]

Evaluation research therefore moves beyond the presentation of findings to a series of judgements and recommendations in relation to the intervention, service or policy under consideration. The specific techniques of an evaluative study will be determined by a range of factors, including the purpose of the evaluation, the methodological persuasions of the investigators and the resources available. However, mixed methods are increasingly used to gather information for evaluative inquiry in order to provide as complete a picture as possible. As Clarke points out, evaluation research is not just about measuring the effectiveness of health care, it is also about illuminating the processes of care.[2]

One of the most widely used distinctions in evaluative research is between formative and summative approaches. Formative evaluation is concerned with describing the nature of an intervention and how it works, with the intention of improving the development of a service or programme. For example, in the following quote, Clark et al.[3] explain why a combination of research methods and data sources was used in a formative evaluation of Macmillan Carer schemes:

> This paper reports on a descriptive study of seven pilot Macmillan Carers Schemes in England. The schemes sought to provide practical and emotional help to cancer patients and families living in their own homes. The study was conceived as participatory and formative in character. Its overall design and conduct were carried out in close liaison with both the sponsoring charity (Macmillan Cancer Relief) and with local managers and staff. Since it focused on, at that time, a recently initiated and still experimental service that could vary in the particular manner of its organisation at local level, the primary aim was descriptive. Such an approach called for a variety of quantitative and qualitative methods, drawing on a range of sources. Techniques of randomisation or comparison were not feasible given the circumstances described above. Instead the researchers present aggregate data generated by the evaluation and in particular fields of enquiry relating to service activities and user satisfaction[3].

Summative evaluation is concerned with the effectiveness and value of an intervention or programme. Addington-Hall's study of the effects of palliative care coordinators on patient quality of life is an example of a summative evaluation as the focus was on measuring the effect of the service in relation to the stated objectives.[4] Evaluation research helps managers to make choices and supports decision making.[5] Consequently, it becomes an explicitly political activity through its potential to influence policy making.[6] In this way, evaluation research differs from more traditional research approaches that attempt to maintain an apolitical stance. Perhaps the most widely used framework for evaluation in health care settings is that described by Donabedian, who suggests that evaluation may focus on three different attributes of an intervention or programme, namely structure, process and outcome.[7]

**Structure** refers to what may be termed the 'environment of care' and here the emphasis is on factors such as the nature and type of facilities available and the number of staff members and their qualifications and backgrounds. The under-lying assumption is that if organizational factors and resources meet specified standards, then the care provided will be good and patients/clients will bene-fit. In a case study analysis of a single hospice unit, Ingleton *et al.*[8] examined the 'environment' of care using a survey of key stakeholders and document analysis of policies and procedures, and strategic service frameworks.

**Process** evaluation is concerned with how services are actually organized and delivered. Quantitative data such as the number of patients referred to a specialist palliative care unit and the average length of stay within a hospice may provide an *indication* of the effects of process. However, evaluation of a process usually involves more than the routine monitoring of referral patterns and throughput. An examination of process may consist of looking at the activities of both the providers and recipients of care. Process evaluation is best served by qualitative methods, and case study designs that include obser-vation, interviews and documentary analysis. For example, Small and Rhodes[9] conducted interviews with people with motor neuron disease (MND), their carers and a range of professional services and supporting organizations in order to look at the concerns of people with MND about how services were delivered.

**Outcome** evaluation is concerned with measuring the impact of an inter-vention or programme. In this context, the evaluative criterion is effectiveness. For example, Bredin *et al.*[10] conducted a multicentre randomized controlled trial of a nursing intervention for breathlessness in patients with lung cancer. Six hospital centres from around the UK volunteered to join the study and several outcome measures were used to assess the effects of the intervention. The intervention aimed to increase fitness and tolerance of restricted lung function and reduce functional disability while acknowledging the meaning of breathlessness in the context of a life-threatening illness.[11] The results con-firmed findings from an earlier study and showed that interventions based on psychological support, breathing control and coping strategies can help patients deal with their breathlessness. Considering the difficulties of random-izing very ill patients to an 8-week intervention study, the completion and results of the study should be considered an accomplishment in the context of palliative care evaluation research.

The influence of Donabedians's framework is evident in much of the litera-ture on standard setting and quality assurance in health care. However, the limitations of focusing upon either structure, process or outcome variables as a means of evaluating an intervention have been highlighted: in particular, the importance of being able to attribute patient outcomes to an antecedent process has been recognized.[12,13] There are a number of challenges in attempting to make links between the 'process of care' and patient outcomes, not least the multidisciplinary nature of care and the intervening effects which other influences may have on a patient's health status.

## Approaches to evaluation research

As with all research, discussion about the most appropriate way to evaluate health care has tended to centre on the qualitative/quantitative debate (Chapter 9), and this rigid distinction has not always been helpful. Competing priorities and calls for greater accountability in the use of resources have led to demands for 'hard', structured evidence of effectiveness in order to justify expenditure on particular interventions and technologies. Indeed, many researchers would subscribe to the view that a key prerequisite for conducting rigorous evaluation of effectiveness is to make a comparison between two or more alternatives using techniques of randomization to avoid bias. However, as Bond[14] points out, experiments are only feasible where: the programme/service under trial is a simple one with clearly defined aims; there is a need to establish its effectiveness; inputs are specific and measurable; people can agree on how outputs should be measured; randomization is both practically and politically feasible and administratively possible; clinical objectives do not intrude; non-cooperation can be kept within acceptable bounds; and results are likely to be useful and timely.

In addition, the value of experiments has been subjected to criticism not only in evaluation research but also in social science as a whole. Serious questions have been raised about the ethics of denying a purportedly advantageous service to some people in order to fulfil the randomization requirement demanded by an experimental design. Likewise, quasi-experimental methods (Chapter 6) have also been criticized in recent years because of difficulties evident in interpreting treatment-related selection. Thus the failures of the experimental model in the context of service evaluation are well recognized. These failures include acknowledgement of the lack of harmony between the requirements of the experimental model, the demands of conducting 'real world' evaluation and problems associated with asking the 'wrong' sorts of question. In an editorial, Corner et al.[15] make the important observation that pursuit of the 'gold standard' of controlled clinical trials can sometimes lead to us asking rather meaningless questions. They draw on an evaluation of the work of clinical nurse specialists in palliative care to illustrate this point:

> In palliative care in general and in nursing in particular, there has been a preoccupation with questions regarding the benefits that may arise from referral to a specialist palliative care service, or to a nurse specialist …. In any case, the pursuit of the perfect clinical trial in this context may risk falling into a trap already described of answering

rather meaningless questions since it is unlikely that specialist nursing is of no value. More relevant, is to design studies that can help answer questions such as 'How does specialist nursing benefit patients? Or 'In what ways are specialist nurses effective or ineffective?[15]

The authors call for imaginative solutions that combine disciplinary perspectives and traditions to form a 'new language of thinking' about, and resolving the question of, health care evaluation. The following quote illustrates how they adopted a flexible, responsive and ethically sensitive approach to their evaluation study:

> The changeable nature of the research environment when working with health professionals and people who have advanced cancer and may be dying requires a responsive approach whereby the study design can be adapted and refined as problems arise. In our research we had to tackle issues such as health professionals so concerned by the potential burden for patients and families that they unwittingly prevented participation in the study. Our experience suggested widespread willingness (and indeed enthusiasm) from patients and families to participate in this kind of research, but extraordinary care is needed to not put further stress into these contexts. There was also significant attrition from the study as people became too ill to continue to work with the research team. These special problems made the research team develop new strategies for maximising insights. Multiple methods, conventional and less conventional were employed. Methods of collecting prospective information were devised wherever possible so that these did not require close and time-consuming involvement of patients who were very ill or in crisis. Yet the viewpoint of service users was recognised as the most important gauge of outcome or benefit. Specialist nurses, the focus of the evaluation, were thought of as collaborators in this research, since these were the individuals who were under close scrutiny[15] (p. 275).

Despite the well-rehearsed limitations of the randomized controlled trial, much of palliative care evaluation has been based upon the biomedical, 'positivist' and 'post-positivist' models of scientific research, arguably because they are the most familiar to medical researchers. Critics of quantitative research methods argue, however, that they provide only superficial information and may fail to take account of the variability in response to a programme or intervention. Such critics argue that qualitative methods, which incorporate the views of different 'stakeholders', give a more comprehensive picture. A middle view, and one adopted by an increasing number of researchers in palliative care,[13,15–17] suggests that all approaches to evaluation research have strengths and limitations and that the most appropriate methods will be determined by the particular focus of the evaluation, the source of funding, the resources available and the main interests of those involved.

A number of writers differentiate between traditional approaches to evaluation, which attempt to measure effectiveness against pre-determined objectives or goals, and 'goal-free' evaluation which attempts to describe the consequences of an intervention or programme for various stakeholders without pre-specifying goals. These have been variously described as 'stakeholder' evaluation,[18] 'pluralistic evaluation'[19] and 'illuminative evaluation'.[20] Hence pluralistic evaluation offers an 'ethnography' (see Chapter 13) of the way a service or a programme has developed and an explanation of this development in terms of the pluralistic interests of the participating groups. It also attempts to draw conclusions about the 'successes' (or failures) of the service on a range of criteria interpreted in various ways. Importantly, 'success' (or failure) is viewed as a pluralistic notion, and not a unitary measure.[19] As a consequence, pluralistic evaluation embodies the principles of triangulation (see below) and draws on case study approaches (see below) with an accompanying reliance on eclectic methods such as in-depth interviews, observation and documentary analysis.

Working within an interpretivist tradition, Guba and Lincoln[21] develop this distinction further in suggesting a four-generation evaluation framework. According to this, first-generation evaluation is treated as a scientific process characterized by a concern with measurement; second-generation evaluation is an approach characterized by description of patterns of strengths and weaknesses with respect to certain stated objectives; third-generation criteria are decided by experts and performance is measured against pre-set standards; and fourth-generation criteria are based upon a constructivist paradigm which aims to develop judgemental consensus among stakeholders. Guba and Lincoln[21] suggest that each succeeding generation represents a step forward in our knowledge about the most appropriate way to evaluate services and procedure.

This approach to evaluation typically draws upon naturalistic methods of enquiry such as in-depth interviews and participant and non-participant observation. The 'openness' of naturalistic inquiry enables the evaluator to be responsive to the differing and sometimes disparate views of the various stakeholders. This model embraces the following fundamental emphases:

- ♦ Identification of issues and concerns based on direct, face-to-face contact with key stakeholders
- ♦ Direct, personal contact and observation of service activities before formally designing the evaluation protocol to increase the evaluator's understanding of what is important and what can/should be evaluated
- ♦ An iterative approach which entails designing the evaluation based on issues that emerged in the preceding three steps
- ♦ Reporting information in direct, personal contact through themes and portrayals that are easily understood and rich with description
- ♦ Matching information reports and reporting formats to specific audiences with different reports and different formats for different audiences.

Guba and Lincoln[21] present this framework in a rather unproblematic way and as an approach that could be seen as a panacea for the ills of the 'measurement era'. However, the likelihood that all stakeholders involved in a project will reach consensus through lengthy dialogue has been questioned.[13] In addition, the approach fails to take account of the real competing concerns, politics and asymmetries of power that exist in any organization or service.

By way of summary, Table 12.1 offers a descriptive categorization of the main types of evaluation discussed above.

The basis of much mixed-method evaluation is the use of case studies to 'frame' the research and the application of the technique known as triangulation. We will turn to these next.

## Case studies

Case studies are valuable where broad, complex questions have to be addressed in complex circumstances.[22] In essence, the choice of case study design would be guided by a desire to uncover contextual issues, believing them to be pertinent to the area of study. This is in stark contrast to an experiment which deliberately divorces a phenomenon from context and thus the context is expressly 'controlled'. Case studies frequently employ multiple methods of data collection which can include observation, surveys, interviewing and also the analysis of documentary sources. While surveys tend to collect a small amount of information from a large sample of respondents, the case study is concerned with collecting a large amount of information about a small number of 'cases'. The case study approach has been used widely in palliative care research, and much of the formative evaluation work that has been carried out has tended to focus on particular cases. For example, an organizational case study of a single hospice might include the following elements: interviews with patients, informal carers, staff and local purchasers; observations of episodes of care in the home, day unit or in-patient area; observation of staff and management meetings; focus groups with volunteers and fundraisers; and documentary analysis of policy and strategic documents, correspondence and minutes of meetings. The aim of such a case study[23] is to understand the day-to-day work of the hospice and quality of its services through an analysis of how it relates to other services in the locality, matters of strategic planning and the views of those who support its work in the wider community. This kind of organizational case study offers the opportunity to gain a more 'holistic' view of the hospice in its wider context.

A perceived strength of the case study approach therefore is its ability to capture the dynamic nature of health care provision. For example, sometimes the aims and characteristics of a service are ill defined, at least at the outset,

**Table 12.1** Major approaches to evaluation: framework of evaluation literature

| Philosophical framework | Ideological framework | Principal audiences | Methods | Evaluation questions |
|---|---|---|---|---|
| Positivism | Measurement Causal knowledge Outcomes Efficiency Summative | Senior policy decision makers | Quantitative: RCT, experiments, cost-benefit analysis, quasi-experiments | Is this service/programme efficient and cost effective? |
| Post-positivism | Measurement Correlation | Senior policy makers | Surveys Document reviews | How efficient is the service/programme? How do different programmes/services compare? |
| Pragmatism, eclecticism and utility | Quality assurance, utility, practicality Formative evaluation | Middle managers/decision makers | Eclectic: surveys, structured and unstructured interviews, observation, document review | Which parts of the service work well and which need improvement? |
| Interpretivism | Pluralism, understanding diversity | Service staff at 'grass root' | Qualitative: case studies, document review, observation, ethnography, in-depth interviews | How is the service experienced by stakeholders and users? |

Source: adapted from Ingleton.[46]

and so cannot easily be identified. Even where the aims are well defined, a complex mix of changes, both external and internal, may occur over the time span of the evaluation. This is a particularly pervasive problem in the health care arena, which is frequently experiencing widespread upheaval. Case study research allows these changes to be examined over time and the implications for various stakeholders can then be explored.

The attraction of case studies to health service researchers is often the opportunity they afford for triangulation. Using this technique, detailed analysis of a single case from a variety of perspectives can allow data drawn from any of the available methods to be focused on a common issue or research question. Moreover, this will be done in ways which will allow the particular case to be understood in its wider context.

Krishnasamy[24] used a multiple case study design to explore the nature and impact of fatigue as experienced by patients, relatives and health care workers involved with their care. She justified her choice of method as follows:

> A case study approach was selected since it allows the researcher to focus intensive observation on a single subject. A case study enabled the researchers to focus on understanding the particular (the fatigue of advanced cancer) in addition to the general (the lived experiences of patients, relatives and professionals). Throughout the case study, the unit of analysis was the experience of fatigue, and a case was defined as incorporating a patient, a relative or friend of choice, and a health care professional involved with their care.

She conducted in-depth, tape recorded semi-structured interviews, reviewed medical and nursing notes and asked patients to complete self-rating questionnaires.

## Triangulation

Triangulation has its origins in navigational, military or surveying contexts where it refers to the use of two known and fixed points in order to locate the position of a third. Conceptually the approach dates back to Campbell and Fiske[25] who argued the need to measure a single concept in a number of different ways. This early application lodged triangulation firmly within the positivist paradigm of measurement. This is somewhat paradoxical given that the entire spectrum of qualitative approaches is now defined, at least in part, in terms of triangulation. There is general agreement that triangulation can take a variety of forms. However, most writers follow the framework developed by Denzin[26] which encompasses four types of approach: data, method, investigator and theoretical triangulation. Data triangulation is based on the use of different data sources to explore the same phenomenon. Methodological triangulation involves employing different methods within a single study.

Investigator triangulation, as the name suggests, involves the use of different researchers in the same study. Theoretical triangulation involves the use of several different frames of reference or perspectives in the analysis. Similarly, and of relevance particularly in palliative care evaluation, Janesick[27] suggests a fifth category of triangulation which she terms 'interdisciplinary'. This may best be described as an extension of theoretical triangulation in which theories or perspectives from a range of disciplines are brought to bear on the topic of inquiry.

Although many writers extol the virtues of triangulation, it is not without challenges. First, difficulties may arise at the 'paradigm' level: researchers often adopt different and mutually exclusive positions and reject the merits of approaches other than their own. However, it appears that most of the literature supports the view that it is possible to mix qualitative and quantitative methods. Perhaps the most challenging task in triangulation is the attempt to integrate data. This is seldom a straightforward process because, given the arguments in the early chapters of this book about the kind of questions that particularly lend themselves to qualitative methods, it is likely that quantitative and qualitative methods will eventually answer different questions that do not easily come together to provide a single, well-integrated picture of the situation. The question perhaps which is still to be debated is that if different methodological approaches lead to contradictory outcomes, which information should be considered most valid. Ingleton and Seymour[28] report how they used triangulation not as a method for checking the 'truth' of one method or source against another, but as a way of achieving 'completeness' or depth. Seymour discusses how this worked in practice, in relation to her doctoral work:

> The interviews undertaken after the observational phase of the field work provided an opportunity to incorporate the views of the research participants into my early analysis of the observational data. This approach allowed for clarification of complex and confusing issues that had emerged during observation and added depth to the analysis.[28]

A further challenge in applying triangulation techniques within evaluation studies is that it is resource intensive, and attracting funding is often difficult. Mixed methods may produce large volumes of data which can become unfocused, thus impacting upon the ease of analysis and interpretation. The use of participatory research methods, whereby the focus and methods of the evaluation are negotiated with the research 'subjects', may overcome such difficulties. The use of participatory methods is the focus of the next section.

## Participatory and action research

Both action research and participatory research (also sometimes known as cooperative inquiry) can be seen as part of a 'new paradigm' of evaluative research.

This new paradigm supports the notion that the advancement of science and the improvement of human welfare are best achieved by research strategies that closely link research and action.[29] Both action research and participatory research are best seen as 'styles' of research rather than specific methods. Reported action research studies tend to involve practitioners whereas participatory research more often seeks to involve service users. Both approaches attempt to involve participants in the creative thinking that goes into designing a research project; involve participants as co-researchers; educate participants, either explicitly or implicitly; and change people's behaviour/experiences.

As a consequence of these broad goals, both action research and participatory research approaches are unpredictable and demand flexibility on the part of all participants. In this context, the distinction between researcher and participants becomes blurred, leading at least one commentator to suggest that these terms are irrelevant within the context of participatory and action research.[30]

## Participatory research

Participatory research methods challenge traditional dichotomies between researcher and researched, and between lay and professional knowledge.[31] They highlight the importance of alliances or partnerships between different stakeholders, in order to promote understanding across traditional boundaries. In effect, participatory approaches turn the traditional research model on its head, advocating that, rather than a researcher deciding at the outset of a study how they will solve a particular problem on behalf of service users, problems are actively constructed or shaped, at an early stage in the research, in a reflexive way between users and researchers. Within the context of health care, participatory research methods aim to ensure that the actual process of research has a therapeutic potential for users of health care services.[32]

There are well-documented examples of research that has effectively involved users of palliative care services as research collaborators. Krishnasamy and Plant,[32] for example, describe how they attempted three projects: a multicentre study to evaluate a nurse-led clinic for breathlessness in patients with advanced lung cancer; a study to explore the experiences of the families of patients newly diagnosed with cancer; and an exploration of the nature and impact of fatigue in patients with advanced cancer.

These studies used different designs but what they have in common is a commitment to the development of knowledge which fosters new ways of working with patients.[32] These new ways of working involve reciprocity and flexibility within the research relationship. In doing so, the studies acknowledge the expertise of participants rather than treating them as passive providers of information.

**Table 12.2** Alternative criteria for assessing the quality of participatory research

| Original criteria | Renamed |
| --- | --- |
| Fairness | *E*qual *A*ccess |
| Ontological authenticity | *E*nhanced *A*wareness of the position/views of self/own group |
| Educative authenticity | *E*nhanced *A*wareness of the position/views of others |
| Catalytic authenticity | *E*ncouraging *A*ction by providing a rationale or impetus for change |
| Tactical authenticity | *E*nabling *A*ction by providing the means to achieve, or at least begin to achieve, change |

Source: Nolan *et al.*[47]

Swantz[33] proposes four different degrees of participation and control in the evaluation process which depends on the extent to which people participate in the different phases of the project. The critical criterion, she concludes, is not the extent to which people are enabled to participate, but the degree to which the research contributes to an individual's ability to articulate their experiences in a way which can be heard and appreciated. This suggests that the traditional criteria of validity and reliability that are used to assess the quality of a research product are inappropriate within the context of participatory research. Indeed, Lincoln and Guba have identified an alternative set of criteria, which Nolan *et al.*[34] have recently attempted to render more accessible (Table 12.2).

Participatory research is not without its critics. In particular, it has been suggested that the ideal of participation often amounts to little more than tokenism. Priorities for research are often identified in a 'top-down' rather than 'bottom-up' approach. Furthermore, there are costs to service users associated with the approach. These may include the need for unanticipated levels of commitment and input, a high demand on personal resources and frustration at lack of impact.[31] These issues may be particularly relevant to users of palliative care services who are likely to have a range of competing demands on their time and whose personal resources may be diminished. It may therefore be more appropriate to involve family carers and staff in participatory approaches and to attempt to minimize the demands for patients.

An important component of participatory research within the context of health and social care is hearing the voices of service users. This will now be explored in more detail.

## User involvement in research

Although user involvement in health services research and development has been almost universally adopted as a 'good thing',[35] engaging patients and service users in evaluation and research is not an easy task. Mental health services, intellectual disability services and social care have long advocated more explicit involvement of people who use services in the monitoring of care, and palliative care researchers could learn much from their work. In the field of disability research, writers provide examples of the ways in which people with intellectual disabilities have extended their roles within the research process in terms of: helping to shape the research agenda, advising and assisting in research, doing research themselves and being involved in research dissemination.[36] However, most of the discussions about the participation of people with intellectual disabilities in the research process have been reported by academics, and largely in academic journals. In seeking to set the research agenda, Ward[36] points out that funding bodies, such as The Joseph Rowntree Foundation and Community Fund, in the UK have set the requirements for voluntary organizations to submit proposals in collaboration with academic researchers.

Active involvement in the research process can take place in any or all of the stages, from setting the research agenda and reviewing grant proposals, through commissioning and undertaking research, to disseminating results.[9] In reality, however, most users play a nominal role in the research process, and the priorities, ideas, design and data remain firmly in the hands of professionals and academics. Crawford et al.[37] conducted a systematic review to examine the effects of involving patients in the planning and development of health care. The findings from this review suggest that papers often described changes to services that were attributed to involving patients, including attempts to make services more accessible and producing information leaflets for patients. However, an evidence base for the effects on use of services, quality of care, satisfaction or health of patients does not exist.

In the context of palliative care, there are a number of specific obstacles to involving people near the end of their life and their families in research. It cannot be assumed, for example, that patients or carers will wish to spend time (which is a precious commodity) engaged in activities which are unlikely to benefit them directly. Moreover, they may feel too tired, too distressed or too overwhelmed by their day-to-day experiences to have the desire or the energy to participate in the completion of questionnaires and interviews or travel long distances to attend meetings. A desire not to think about disease progression may also mitigate against membership of groups, as this is likely to involve mixing with people at different disease stages. Characteristically, research paradigms in palliative care have cast patients and carers in a passive and reactive role, and their involvement has mainly been confined to responding to questionnaires and measures of quality of life. Furthermore, Payne[17] suggests that a single 'user' is relatively powerless in an academic setting where his/her presence merely enables researchers to claim that user involvement requirements have been fulfilled. Cynically, it could be argued that academic researchers rationalize their research as worthwhile simply on the grounds that users have been 'involved'. In posing the question, how can we help patients and carers feel comfortable and valued in these roles, Payne[17] suggests that a radical re-think is necessary in order for the rhetoric of user involvement to become reality, where researchers work in partnership with their 'subjects' or even are led or directed by them. Another evaluative research design that explicitly seeks to develop partnerships between researchers and those they are studying is action research.

## Action research

Action research does not focus exclusively on user and carer involvement, although this is often an important aspect of the work. Rather, it may involve working with practitioners to develop their practice. Indeed, action research is often seen as a way of addressing the research–practice gap by involving practitioners as collaborators in the research process. Action research is seen by many as a way of improving the quality of health care by narrowing the gap between 'researching' and 'doing', and consequently between theory and practice.[38,39] Waterman et al.[40] provide the following helpful definition:

> Action research is a period of inquiry that describes, interprets and explains social situations while executing a change intervention aimed at improvement and involvement. It is problem-focused, context-specific and future-oriented.

Action research most commonly focuses on a local issue and attempts to problem-solve within a local context. It is cyclical in nature, with methods evolving as the research progresses, normally in response to feedback from participants.[41] However, most action research projects include the following stages: the problem to be studied is identified: problem concepts are investigated and related literature is studied; baseline measures are taken; the plan of action to solve the problem is designed; the plan is put into action and its workings observed and monitored; a second set of measures are taken; and a reflective stage follows where changes and modifications to the solutions can be made.

This cycle of events may be repeated until practical considerations such as time and resources terminate the study.

Challenges and pitfalls of this approach have been described. For example, Meyer[39] describes the difficulty of introducing change in areas with a constantly changing workforce. Furthermore, lack of precision in relation to definitions and models of action research may result in confusion about roles and responsibilities.[42] Action research also poses a number of ethical challenges, particularly in relation to protecting the confidentiality and anonymity of participants.[43,44] Since action research can have political consequences, the potential for the research to result in harm for participants also needs to be carefully considered. Moreover, introducing a change in practice is always difficult, and it has been suggested that action research should not be judged only on the extent to which change is achieved, but also in relation to what has been learned from the experience.[39]

## Challenges of evaluation research

Whichever approach is used, researchers are likely to face a number of challenges in attempting to evaluate a health care programme or intervention. Negotiating access may prove difficult as practitioners can often feel threatened by a project which specifically sets out to evaluate their practice, particularly if they hold a firm belief that their particular practice works! Identifying the aims and objectives of a programme or intervention can also prove difficult. Often an intervention has multiple objectives which may be difficult to prioritize.

Many of the approaches to evaluation described within this chapter are relatively new, and much remains to be done to refine and test these methods and to determine their impact upon, and consequences for, all participants, particularly within the context of palliative care. In particular, many researchers are experimenting with approaches to involving service users in research, without being fully aware of the potential benefits, pitfalls and consequences. A participatory conference held in Sheffield in 2003 explored these issues with older people and family carers who had experienced direct involvement in research. While participants identified a range of benefits, a number of challenges were described including:[26] accessing the views of 'hard to reach' groups, such as older people living in care homes and those with dementia; coordinating input so that everyone's voice is heard; ensuring that older people do not feel they have been exploited; minimizing distress caused by research on sensitive topics; ensuring that participants do not feel let down and abandoned when the project ends; and raising people's expectations when often there are insufficient resources to change services or not enough action to follow through proposed changes. Although these issues were identified on the basis of discussions with older people and their families, similar issues are likely to apply in conducting research with people with palliative care needs.

## Selecting an approach to evaluation

Different evaluation approaches do tend to draw on specific research strategies, but crucially the evaluation question itself will determine the appropriate strategy or combination of strategies to use. The good evaluator is one who is able to select a technique or combination of techniques that are appropriate to the given situation, in full understanding of the aims of the evaluation and any theoretical perspective which has been adopted.[5] Moreover, it is important to bear in mind that since evaluation research almost always takes place within a political arena and is often fed into a policy making process, key stakeholders (such as supporters and opponents of a particular programme or intervention) are likely to have a vested interest in influencing the focus and methods of any evaluation.

Since evaluation itself is a fiercely contested terrain with many distinct and competing views as to what form an evaluation should take and how it should be conducted, Beattie[45] proposes a new paradigm evaluation in which a key starting point is to ask questions about participants' power and ownership by focusing on:

- Who has a stake in the project and its evaluation?
- Whose interests are likely to be affected by it?
- Who has the authority in resource allocation and decision making in the project?
- How close to the project are such stakeholders?
- In what way does the evaluation strategy for a project engage or marginalize different stakeholders?

The importance of acknowledging and accepting stakeholders as partners in the process encourages ownership of evaluation findings, with the resultant greater likelihood of their use for reflection and action.

## Conclusion

Within this chapter, we have tried to show how mixed approaches to evaluation research are likely to produce the most comprehensive picture of the effects of an intervention or service. This involves incorporating a combination of qualitative and quantitative research methods, and accessing the views of a range of stakeholders. We have suggested that involving service users is an essential feature of all evaluation research, independent of the research strategy used. However, this does pose particular challenges within palliative care research. In addition to pursuing the development of knowledge that will inform service delivery and practice in palliative care, there is an urgent need to explore the impact of methods used in evaluation research in order to identify the most sensitive, acceptable and appropriate strategies for conducting rigorous and ethical research in this field.

# References

1. St Leger AS (1992) *Evaluating Health Services Effectiveness*. Milton Keynes: Open University Press.
2. Clarke A (2001) Evaluation research in nursing and health care. *Nurse Researcher* **8**: 4–14.
3. Clark D, Ferguson C, Nelson C (2000) Macmillan schemes in England: results of a multicentre evaluation. *Palliative Medicine* **14**: 129–39.
4. Addington-Hall JM, MacDonald LD, Anderson HR, Chamberlain J, Freeling P, Bland JM, Raftery J (1992) Randomised controlled trial of effects of coordinating care for terminally ill cancer patients. *British Medical Journal* **305**: 1317–22.
5. Robbins M (1998) *Evaluating Palliative Care: Establishing the Evidence Base*. Oxford: Oxford University Press.
6. Tolson D (1999) Practice innovation: a methodological maze. *Journal of Advanced Nursing* **30**: 381–90.
7. Donabedian A (1980) Criteria, norms and standards for quality assessment and monitoring. *Quality Review Bulletin* **12**: 99–108.
8. Ingleton C, Field D, Clark D (1997) Multi-disciplinary care study as an approach to the evaluation of palliative care services: two examples. *International Journal of Palliative Nursing* **3**: 335–9.
9. Small N, Rhodes P (2000) *Too Ill to Talk: User Involvement in Palliative Care*. London: Routledge.
10. Bredin M, Corner J, Krishnasamay M, Plant H, Bailey C, A'Hern R (2001) Multicentre randomised controlled trial of nursing intervention for breathlessness in patients with lung cancer. In: Field D, Clark D, Corner J, Davis C, (ed.) *Researching Palliative Care*. Buckingham: Open University Press, pp. 119–27.
11. Corner J, Plant H, Warner L (1995) Developing a nursing approach to managing dyspnoea in lung cancer. *International Journal of Palliative Nursing* **1**: 5–10.
12. Redfern S, Norman I (1990) Measuring the quality of nursing care: a consideration of different approaches. *Journal of Advanced Nursing* **15**: 260–71.
13. Pawson R, Tilley N (1997) *Realistic Evaluation*. London: Sage.
14. Bond S (1989) The experimental design. In: Cormack D, (ed.) *The Research Process in Nursing*. Oxford: Blackwell Scientific Publications.
15. Corner J, Clark D, Normand C (2002) Evaluating the work of clinical nurse specialists. *Palliative Medicine* **16**: 275–7.
16. Ingleton C, Hughes P, Noble B, Gray H, Clark D (2003) An evaluation of a Macmillan GP clinical facilitator project: the post holder perspective. *Primary Health Care Research and Development* **4**: 177–86.
17. Payne S (2002) Are we using the users? (Guest Editorial). *International Journal of Palliative Nursing* **8**: 212.
18. Patton M (1990) *Qualitative Evaluation and Research Methods*, 2nd edn. Newbury Park, CA: Sage.
19. Smith G, Cantley C (1991) Pluralistic evaluation. In: *Evaluation: Research Highlights in Social Work 8*. London: Jessica Kingsley Publishers.
20. Parlett M, Hamilton D (1987) *Evaluation as Illumination: A New Approach to Study of Innovatory Programmes, Occasional Paper 9*. University of Edinburgh: Centre for Research in Educational Science.

21. Guba E, Lincoln Y (1989) *Fourth Generation Evaluation.* Newbury Park, CA: Sage.

22. Yin R (1994) *Case Study Research.* Thousand Oaks, CA: Sage.

23. Ingleton C, Field D, Clark D, Carradice M, Crowther T (1995) *King's Mill Hospice: Three Years on (1991–94). Occasional Paper 16.* Sheffield: Trent Palliative Care Centre.

24. Krishnasamy M (2000) Fatigue in advanced cancer: meaning before measurement. *International Journal of Palliative Nursing* 5: 401–14.

25. Campbell DT, Fiske DW (1959) Convergent and discriminant validation by multi-trait multi-dimensional matrix. *Psychological Bulletin* 56: 81–105.

26. Denzin NK (1970) *The Research Art in Sociology. A Theoretical Introduction to Sociological Methods.* London: Butterworths.

27. Janesick V (1994) The dance of qualitative research design. In: Denzin NK, Lincoln Y, (ed.) *A Handbook of Qualitative Research.* Thousand Oaks, CA: Sage, pp. 209–19.

28. Ingleton C, Seymour J (2001) Methods of analysing qualitative research: two examples from studies in palliative care. *International Journal of Palliative Nursing* 7: 227–34.

29. Meyer J (1995) Stages in the process: a personal account. *Nurse Researcher* 2: 24–37.

30. Lincoln Y (2002) Engaging sympathies: relationships between action research and social constructivism. In: Reason P, Bradbury H, (ed.) *Handbook of Action Research: Participative Inquiry and Practice.* London: Sage.

31. Parry O, Gnich W, Platt S (2001) Principles in practice: reflections on a 'post-positivist' approach to evaluation research. *Health Education Research* 16: 215–26.

32. Krishnasamy M, Plant H (1998) Developing nursing research with people. *International Journal of Nursing Studies* 35: 79–84.

33. Swantz ML (1995) *Milk, Blood and Death: Body Symbols and the Power of Regeneration Among the Zamaro of Tanzania.* Westport, CT: Bergin & Garvey.

34. Nolan M, Grant G (1993) Service evaluation: time to open both eyes. *Journal of Advanced Nursing* 18: 1434–42.

35. Gott M (2004) User involvement and palliative care: rhetoric or reality? In: Payne S, Seymour J, Ingleton C, (ed.) *Palliative Care Nursing: Principles and Evidence for Practice.* Buckingham: Open University Press.

36. Ward L (1998) Practising partnerships: involving people with learning difficulties in research. *British Journal of Learning Disability* 26: 128–37.

37. Crawford MJ, Rutter D, Manley C, Weaver T, Bhui K, Fulop N, Tyrer P (2002) Systematic review of involving patients in the planning and development of health care. *British Medical Journal* 325: 1263–5.

38. Hart E (1996) Action research as a professionalizing strategy: issues and dilemmas. *Journal of Advanced Nursing* 23: 54–61.

39. Meyer J (2000) Using qualitative methods in health related action research. *British Medical Journal* 320: 178–81.

40. Waterman H, Tillen D, Dickson R, de Koning K (2001) Action research: a systematic review and guidance for assessment. Health Technology Assessment 5 (On-line) Available at, http://www.hta.nhsweb.nhs.uk/fullmono/mon523.pdf

41. Hart E, Bond M (1995) *Action Research for Health and Social Care. A Guide to Practice.* Buckingham: Open University Press.

42. Titchen A, Binnie A (1993) Research partnerships: collaborative action research in nursing. *Journal of Advanced Nursing* 18: 858–65.

43. Coghlan D, Brannick T (2001) *Doing Action Research in Your Own Organisation.* London: Sage.

44. Williamson GR, Prosser S (2002) Action research; politics, ethics and participation. *Journal of Advanced Nursing* **40**: 587–93.

45. Beattie A (2003) Dialogical evaluation and health projects: a discourse of change. In: Siddell M, Jones L, Peberdy A, Douglas J, (ed.) *Debates and Dilemmas in Promoting Health: A Reader,* 2nd edn. London: Macmillan/Open University, pp. 239–56.

46. Ingleton C (1996) Multi-disciplinary evaluation of two hospice units. PhD Thesis, University of Sheffield.

47. Nolan M, Hanson E, Magnusson L, Anderson B (2003) Gauging quality in constructivist research: the Äldre Väst Sjuhärad model revisited. *Quality in Ageing* **4**: 22–7.

# Chapter 13

# Ethnography

Jane Seymour

## Introduction

A great deal of our knowledge about palliative care, especially in relation to the experience of pain and suffering, understandings of death and dying, and the processes and organization of clinical care, communication and interaction, stems from a relatively small collection of ethnographic studies. In these, the researcher became involved in the daily lives of a particular group of patients or caregivers, recorded aspects of these lives in a detailed way, and subsequently made analytical interpretations that allow us, as readers, to consider the broader implications of these for our own work and for palliative care as a whole. Ethnographers provide an in-depth understanding of sensitive issues that are difficult to address using other research approaches. For these reasons, ethnography has been described as opening the 'black box'.[1]

Although not classically considered to be 'ethnographers', Cicely Saunders and Elisabeth Kubler-Ross made use of many ethnographic techniques: they focused on the patient's point of view, they set patients' accounts within a broader context and they used a range of resources to shed new interpretive light on what was the wider message communicated by the stories they recorded. Perhaps best known of the more formal ethnographies are those of hospitals in 1960s America by Sudnow,[2] Glaser and Strauss,[3] and Quint.[4] From these have come our understandings of 'social death', 'awareness contexts' and the paradoxes that threaten the nurse's role in caring for dying people. Since these classic studies, the ethnographic method has been used in cancer wards and clinics,[5–7] hospices,[8,9] in the community and in the general hospital,[10–13] and even in 'high tech' areas such as intensive care where patients with palliative care needs often predominate.[14] Some authors have used the approach to study several settings.[11,15] More recently, the approach has been applied in a focused and time-limited way to produce 'mini-ethnographies' of clinical areas.[16] In all these ethnographies, the stories of patients, carers and staff are interwoven, giving a rich sense of the complexities and challenges that make up palliative care. This chapter explores what is ethnography, its complex history and how it may be used by researchers in palliative care.

## What is ethnography?

The term ethnography refers to a social scientific description of a community and their culture, drawing on the Greek word 'ethnos' meaning people, race or cultural group.[17] The emphasis on description is important, with what has been termed as 'thick description'[18] seen as the hallmark of those ethnographies which give us a sense of privileged insight into an otherwise hidden world. Seale explains elegantly the differences between 'thin' and 'thick' description by drawing on the anthropologist Clifford Geertz's ethnographic description of Balinese cockfights.[19] He explains how Geertz rejected simplistic interpretations of the cockfights as expressions of Balinese men's masculinity and how instead, through careful description of a wide variety of events, Geertz showed that they symbolized a range of religious and cultural issues in Balinese society. Such description has an explanatory power since it allows and encourages theoretical thinking about social phenomena and enables inferences to be made that have a wider applicability beyond the context of the study at hand.[20]

In a widely accepted characterization, Hammersley and Atkinson[21] outline the following features of modern ethnographic research: people's behaviour is studied in everyday contexts; data are gathered from a range of sources, with observation and informal conversation being the main sources; there is an unstructured approach to data collection; the research focus is usually a single setting or group; and analysis involves interpretation of the meanings and functions of human action.

Hammersley and Atkinson's emphasis here is on the procedures for gathering and handling data that are associated with ethnography. However, ethnography is much more than a collection of particular methods for gathering data: it also implies a particular methodological perspective, i.e. the philosophical and theoretical stance that the researcher takes when conducting any research study.[22] The methodological perspectives associated with ethnography have changed over time, making the task of pinning down exactly the meaning of ethnographic research rather difficult. Like all other forms of qualitative research, ethnography has been caught up in ontological and epistemological debates. Without wishing to get too distracted by disputes that are essentially irreconcilable, it is important to raise awareness of how they have contributed to shaping the character of ethnographic research studies, and to recognize their salience to the decisions that are made in the design, conduct and reporting of ethnographic research. In the few paragraphs of the next section, I outline the major methodological shifts that have taken place in relation to ethnographic research. As Denzin and Lincoln[23] note, these shifts have been marked by the relative weight accorded to the interpretation of the researcher; the extent to which the researcher attempts to 'share' power with the researched; and the extent to which it is assumed that there is an absolute reality that can be 'captured' by the researcher.

## A brief methodological history of ethnography

Ethnography has varied antecedents: historical, anthropological and sociological. The field trips of early twentieth century anthropologists, who were predominantly British, are often seen as particularly important. The work of Malinowski, who lived among the New Guinea and Trobriand Islanders between 1914 and 1915 and 1917 and 1918[23] (p. 13), is among the most well known. Later, techniques of observational fieldwork were developed in the field of sociology and applied to the study of a wide range of issues in our own society. Key players here were sociologists in the USA at the University of Chicago in the 1920s (known as the Chicago School and led by Robert Park). Collectively, they produced some famous studies of small town America; of inner city life in Chicago; and later of crime and deviance, medicine and education. They relied on a combination of observation, informal interviewing and study of personal documents in undertaking their work.

While at first sight different, the orientations of the anthropologists studying 'foreign' cultures and early ethnographers of 'home' society share many characteristics. In their discussion of historical shifts in qualitative research, Denzin and Lincoln[23] identify that both were characterized by three principles: objectivism, looking at 'strange' people as 'other'; imperialism, assuming a position of superiority; and monumentalism and timelessness, attempting to create an enduring work of art by 'capturing' a culture.

Researchers at the Chicago school introduced 'slice of life' and narrative techniques which reported the language and meanings of the people in the social contexts under study. They adopted a 'naturalist' stance to social research that has had a major influence on ethnographic research. In this, three major assumptions can be discerned: (1) the social world is not reducible to that which can be externally observed, but is something created, recreated, perceived and interpreted by people themselves; (2) knowledge of the social world must give access to actors' own accounts of it; and (3) people live in a bounded social context, and are best studied in their natural setting (adapted from Brewer[22] pp. 34–5).

While being in the vanguard of the naturalist tradition, researchers from the Chicago school tended to maintain the 'outsider' stance of the British social anthropologists. Moreover, they were equally preoccupied with ascertaining

some 'real truths' about their subjects, making attempts to portray a 'true picture' of them. In their attempts to bring their research subjects to life, they
tended to romanticize them and turn them into the equivalents of what has
been called the 'sociological version of a screen hero'[23] (p. 13). Moreover, the
voices of the researchers were not manifest, except insofar as they tried faith-
fully to recount the 'tales of the field'.[24]

The naturalist and realist influences of the Chicago school persisted into the
post-Second World War period of 1950–1970. It was during this period that
efforts to formalize and 'scientize' the ethnographic method reached their
peak. Grounded theory, with its step by step approach to producing theory
from data that have been systematically collected, was produced during this
time, and became overwhelmingly popular because it appeared to offer a clear
and relatively straightforward recipe for reaching 'external truths' as long as
particular procedures were followed.

The end of this period saw the beginnings of recognition that qualitative
research was not, and arguably should not be, politically neutral and that
achieving one 'true' account was not the only goal of such research. During the
1970s and 1980s, critical theory and feminist perspectives emerged and were
used by ethnographers to argue for the importance of recognizing that interpretation without critique risked reproducing and perpetuating a societal status
quo that often oppressed and disempowered the people studied. Feminist
ethnographers called for recognition of the risk that researchers merely reproduced relations of power and domination vis a vis their research and subjects.
Anne Oakley's famous text 'Interviewing women'[25] is perhaps the best example of advocacy for ethnographic research that is accessible, usable and related
to issues of critical concern in the lives of the persons studied. The moral value
of taking a participatory stance to ethnographic research for which Oakley
and others argued so eloquently and in which a deliberate attempt is made to
equalize power between researchers and researched has become widely accepted.
From these influences, ethnographic research and writing became more
reflexive, and how issues of gender, class and race were dealt with became central to the researcher's task. The researcher's voice thus became central to the
ethnographic account.[23]

Such radical stances represented one strand of a rapidly developing broader
anti-realist, or postmodern, attack on the 'naïve realism' of previous traditions mobilized in the fields of sociology and cultural anthropology.[22] This
attack sought to establish the idea that ethnographies produce accounts that are
only one of a number of multiple, and potentially equally valid, accounts of a
social world that are possible. The critiques of classical ethnography brought
with them a renewed crisis in arguments about what were, and indeed whether

it was even possible to establish, criteria for the evaluation of ethnographic research. Recently, there have been some pragmatic attempts to resolve this crisis. Before leaving this discussion to focus on some practical aspects of ethnographic research, I want briefly to look at one that I personally have found valuable in resolving some of the methodological problems outlined above. Researchers at the National Centre for Social Research in the UK[26] were commissioned to produce a framework for assessing or appraising evaluative research evidence for the Government Chief Social Researcher's Office. In so doing, they presented an elegant and detailed analysis of the issues outlined above. Before setting out their framework of assessment, they argued that while we must accept that qualitative research contains many different paradigms and is based on diverse assumptions, it is possible to specify a range of philosophical and methodological assumptions which allow one to engage practically in qualitative research and to set out meaningful criteria for its evaluation. These are that: reality is mediated through shared human constructions; the world is affected by the researcher; neutrality is not attainable, but is a guiding ideal; subjective perspectives should be articulated and documented; claims to knowledge are desirable but must be seen as provisional; and there are no valid or invalid methods: they should be used appropriately and flexibly to fit the aims of particular research projects (summarized from Spencer *et al.*[26]).

The appraisal questions that form the basis of the framework of assessment for research developed by Spencer *et al.*[26] (p. vi) flow logically from the assumptions they outline: those that are relevant to ethnographic research are presented below (each of these is complemented by a series of aspects that could be considered in making this judgement; see Spencer *et al.*[26] for further details).

- How credible are the findings?
- How has knowledge been extended by the research?
- How well was the data collection carried out?
- How well defended are the target selection of cases/documents?
- How well has the approach to and formulation of analysis been conveyed?
- How well are the contexts of data sources retained and portrayed?
- How well has diversity of perspective and content been explored?
- How well has detail, depth and complexity (i.e. richness) of the data been conveyed?
- How clear are the links between data, interpretation and conclusions?
- How clear and coherent is the reporting?
- How clear are the assumptions/theoretical perspectives/values?

- ◆ What evidence is there of attention to ethical issues?
- ◆ How adequately has the research process been documented?

These helpful questions, which are an amalgam of those found in many famous methodological texts with which readers may be familiar, concentrate on the practical aspects of the research process in ethnography, reminding us that any piece of ethnographic research can only be judged by: (1) the goodness of 'fit' between the research objectives outlined and strategic choices during the study—these are issues of research design; (2) the extent to which the account given of fieldwork is defensible, detailed and transparent; and (3) the quality of the manner in which it is reported (i.e. 'thick' rather than 'thin' description). I turn now to look at these practical aspects in some detail.

## Issues of research design and process in ethnography

Research design means setting out a strategic plan for a research study: it addresses issues of suitability of the overall approach selected to the research problem identified, selection of study site(s) and negotiation of access, sampling of 'cases' and identification of the units of analysis in the study (e.g. whether these are individuals or groups of individuals); selection of data collection methods and consideration of ethical issues; mapping out of the time scale and costs of the study; and developing a plan for analysing and reporting the data. These issues are, of course, of relevance to any research study and are addressed at various points throughout this text. For the purpose of ethnographic research, some design issues are arguably particularly critical, namely the specification of research objectives that are appropriate for this sort of approach; the negotiation of access to selected sites for study; and the management of the participant observation and interactional interview techniques that characterize data collection in ethnography.

### Developing research objectives

The first step in ethnographic research design entails a critical consideration of whether your study objectives and philosophical stance to research are best addressed by this type of approach. This means analysing whether the objectives you compose and the assumptions that you hold are best suited to an approach that involves: an evolving and flexible design; the presentation of a mediated reality; seeing the researcher as an instrument of data collection; and focusing closely on research participants' views and the contexts within which these are expressed.

In my own PhD study,[14,27] objectives, which were framed as questions, focused on gaining an understanding of how death and the withdrawal of active treatment was managed in intensive care units. I realized, after some thought in the early months of developing the proposal for the study, that only a time-consuming ethnographic approach could come close to allowing me to address these. A proposal was thus developed in which participant observation, documentary analysis and semi-structured interviewing were embedded within a multiple case study design. Each 'case' consisted of the interactions and perceptions of those involved with selected critically ill individuals from two general adult intensive care units. Within each case study, there were two stages of data collection: (1) observations of care and treatment given to the selected patients and the surrounding interaction; and (2) a series of semi-structured interviews with the ill person's companions, and with key members of the health care team. Setting out my ideas logically in the proposal was invaluable in helping me to keep the study within a manageable framework and also in presenting it clearly to those who were responsible for deciding whether or not I could conduct the fieldwork.

## Getting in: managing access and social relationships in ethnography

The success or failure of ethnographic research clearly hangs on the ability to gain access to the places that you need to study: no access, no study! This can be difficult and extremely time consuming. There is a tendency to think that access involves mainly jumping through the hurdle of research ethics committee approval and governance requirements, but in ethnographic research this is only one aspect of a complex process of becoming, hopefully, an accepted part of your study environment. The way in which access is gained fashions the way in which research participants see you, and thus shapes all the possibilities surrounding your study.

Gaining access entails gentle but persistent persuasion, confident (but not overly confident) demonstration that your study is worthwhile and will give something back to those with whom you are trying to engage and, most importantly, manifestation of your trustworthiness as a person and as a researcher. It is perhaps obvious that in studies which touch on issues related to palliative care, these factors are likely to be magnified since patients and their carers may be regarded as potentially vulnerable and at risk of harm. These may give rise to a sense of 'potentially impenetrable obstacles' to negotiate[9] (p. 26). The process of negotiating access is not, however, only a practical process. It can also shed light on aspects of the research setting and culture that you hope to study. To this extent, gaining access becomes part of the data collection process in ethnography.

Perhaps the best way of thinking about and considering the issues that may be faced in this process is to learn from other people's accounts of how they negotiated access in their studies. Revealingly, however, in some of the most widely cited and classic studies related to palliative care, little is said about access.[3] This undoubtedly is a reflection of the vastly different circumstances in which research is now conducted, in particular the greater scrutiny applied to studies conducted in clinical settings. In the mid 1990s, Atkinson[28] was concerned to study the way in which haematologists and pathologists in the UK and USA defined and categorized disease during their interactions with each other. Atkinson is an eminent sociologist, with a longstanding record of research in the sociological study of medicine. He writes:

> The pathologists who I approached were, at best, lukewarm and at worst chose not to respond to any overtures I made. Even the senior pathologist in the American hospital—who had apparently agreed to my research in general terms—proved unwilling or unable to go so far as to set up any practical access to his colleagues. The reception offered by the haematologists, on the other hand, was entirely accommodating. Not only were the respective Chiefs of Service sympathetic to my proposed research, but they were able to indicate just how I could establish a practical presence with some of their colleagues and so observe their daily work[28] (p. 3).

Atkinson went on to complete his study in two American haematology units. He was able to attach himself to the clinical fellows as they went about their everyday work, but did this selectively to suit his purposes at hand. He attended the early morning 'rounds' when new patients were discussed, and also the main weekly haematology–oncology conference at which patients were more formally presented, as well as engaging in some more general participant observation.

One of the most stressful experiences for the ethnographer is going into the 'field' for the first time. Once this has been done, then relationships have to be sustained through the process of developing and nurturing rapport with research participants. Atkinson[28] reports how, on the whole, the process of early participant observation in his study went well, although he recounts vividly one critical incident in which one doctor became unhappy about his presence and suspicious of his motives. This arose in the context of a difficult exchange this doctor had had with a patient who complained about the treatment he was receiving. The doctor in question complained to his senior and Atkinson subsequently had to send out a memo to all the doctors with whom he came into contact explaining that 'I had no intention of evaluating and criticizing their work, nor of intruding on it'[29] (p. 16). He reflected candidly that he had fallen foul of a common error: relying on goodwill of senior figures and not adequately corresponding with, or talking to, the rest of the key personnel.

In my own study, I was able to draw on Atkinson's experience to good effect. In negotiating access to two intensive care units and all the relevant staff, I found that I had to write upwards of 40 letters at each site and held two or three preliminary meetings in each unit to meet staff and talk about aspects of the study. I found that this 'set up' process was invaluable, since once I started participant observation people had, at the very least, heard of me and at best perceived accurately that they had contributed something important to the way in which the study was conducted. Indeed, it was through these meetings that a practical and ethically appropriate way of addressing the problem of consent to observation in a context where patients were not conscious was developed.[14] These early meetings smoothed my path, and perhaps made it possible to sustain the relationships necessary to nurture participant observation in an environment which can, at times, be stressful and demanding.

Julia Lawton in her study of a hospice reports similar meetings[9] (pp. 26–28) and was able, through these, to work out an observational identity or role that she could assume once the study started. She writes in relation to the first period of observation in day care:

> As we all agreed, I needed to be in a role that would give me a legitimate reason to spend large amounts of time within day care, without my presence necessarily having to affect the internal dynamics there. A decision was thus reached that I should work in a volunteer capacity as this would allow me considerable contact with patients'[9] (p. 27).

While it is impossible to set out 'rules' of engagement for participant observers, some transferable principles can be outlined which are likely to increase the chances of success in sustaining social relationships in the field. Bogdewic[29] recommends the following, most of which are common sense:

- ◆ Be unobtrusive: at the beginning, be more observer than participant, and try not to draw attention to yourself too much. Pay careful attention to what you wear and how you behave. Your goal should be to 'fit' in.

- ◆ Be honest: deal with queries about your presence directly and honestly without overwhelming people with too much detail.

- ◆ Be unassuming: you may know a lot about the setting under study, but play this down. You may be perceived as a threat to the research participants otherwise.

- ◆ Be a reflective listener: by doing this you can better understand the culture you have entered.

- ◆ Be self-revealing: a willingness to discuss common interests or to give away some information about yourself can lead to a sense of reciprocity which helps the relationship between you and your research participants to develop.

## Anything you say may be taken down as data:[30] participant observation in ethnography

Participant observation, usually complemented by more or less informal interviewing, and by the collection and analysis of relevant documents, is the hallmark of ethnography. It is rooted in the tradition of symbolic interactionism which focuses on how individuals are engaged in a constant process of interpretation and definition as they move from one situation to another. For example, Perakyla[31] demonstrates how varieties of 'hope work' are manifest in the exchanges between hospital staff who care for individuals dying in hospital environments. 'Hope work' is employed differently by the various staff members, but, through their interactions with one another, they achieve a shared interpretative view where 'hope' for a medical cure is dismantled and the dying individual is given up to 'nature'.[31] For Perakyla, developing such sophisticated and nuanced understandings meant taking part in the everyday life of the hospital staff: watching them, listening to them, being with them while they worked, and talking to them to discover and reflect on how they made sense of the challenges they faced in caring for dying people. This involves active involvement and interaction on the part of the researcher: it cannot be gained by any 'arm's length' stance to those under observation. However, nor can it be gained by entering too completely into the world under study and losing the ability to reflect in an analytical, critical and theoretically sensitive manner. A delicate balance has to be reached between being an 'insider' and an 'outsider'. There has been, over the years, much debate about different forms of participant observation: one famous and oft cited typology posits a continuum between complete observer and complete participant.[32] Junker's[33] classic paper on roles for social observation remains a useful resource for thought in relation to this. The complete participant's research activities are likely to be concealed from those in the study setting, meaning that the researcher must record data covertly. The ethical and methodological problems to which such a position gives rise make this an unlikely role for any contemporary ethnographer in health care. At the other end of the continuum, the complete observer could hide behind a one-way mirror, or could watch activities 'on camera', but would take no part in talking to or interacting with participants. Again, given contemporary understandings of the importance of accessing participants' meanings, this is an unlikely stance for ethnographers to adopt. Rather, most ethnographers will move in and around the middle territories of these opposite poles during their research study and will be known to be working as an ethnographer by the study participants. Moreover, the researcher's very presence in a social setting means that she will be perceived as a participant, even if her chosen role involves little 'action'.

Anne-Mei The's ethnography 'Palliative Care and Communication: Experiences in the Clinic'[7] portrays a demanding and time-consuming ethnographic study of people with lung cancer. Unusually for the modern ethnographer, The spent 5 years monitoring the illness process of patients from the time of receiving their diagnosis to their death. She incorporates a variety of perspectives: her own powerful narrative descriptions, patients themselves, their families and relatives, doctors and nurses. Her reflections on the process of observation are very revealing of the difficulties that can be encountered in trying to maintain the balance between insider and outsider, and in trying to 'manage' compassionately the relationships that she made with patients and their families in a context in which they developed certain expectations of her:

> I had to admit to myself that sheer neutral observation was not possible. As time went by I acquired a role. ...one day at the hospital I received a direct appeal. It started with Mrs Dekker paging me through Dr Liem during an outpatient consultation in order to ask her big question, 'Have they given him up?' Following my suggestion she made an appointment to see the doctor. During that meeting she kept looking at me, imploring help, each time she asked a question. I nodded encouragingly. She cried, at first of anger, later due to grief. Whether I liked it or not, I had become a player in what I was studying[7] (p. 233).

The further reflects that because of her research role she was with patients and their relatives for prolonged periods: she listened to them, had time, was always there. She became a known and friendly face within the hospital to which people could relate during a time of stress and fear. Patients, and subsequently doctors and nurses, gave her feedback that her involvement was perceived positively. Many appeared to forget that she was a researcher, or saw that as merely incidental to the fact that she was a helpful and supportive presence. Candidly, however, she reflects that she felt that it must be acknowledged that she had an ulterior motive in maintaining these relationships:

> Even though I provided support to patients and to their relatives, I still 'used' them. I did not only listen with a sympathetic ear, I listened and observed as a researcher. This still sometimes made me uneasy. Another problem was ending the relationship with relatives after the patient had died. The job was done, but the affection that had developed through the sharing of intimate moments was still there. I visited the bereaved families at home and attended most funerals. But then, perhaps when the bereaved families needed the most support, I distanced myself. This sometimes clashed with what I felt I should be doing, but it was practically impossible for me to maintain contact[7] (p. 234).

As The reveals, working as an ethnographer in a palliative care environment means becoming fully aware of one's own mortality and entails sharing in the lives and feelings of others as they face loss, grief and suffering. Acknowledging this and preparing for it is essential, but has been somewhat underemphasized in the literature. To some extent, these issues can be addressed by the ethnographers themselves, perhaps through careful reflection and thought before entry into the field. The supervisor relationship (where it exists) is another important venue for examining issues such as these. There may also be a need to consider engaging external supervision to enable issues which lie beyond the purely academic to be addressed in a confidential and safe environment.[34]

While the above has outlined some general methodological considerations that the ethnographer needs to consider when preparing to conduct observational fieldwork, a major practical challenge is how data will be recorded and how choices will be made about exactly what to observe and what to record. Observation involves trying to document systematically, and thus to some extent interpret immediately, what it is that is happening around you, and where it is of relevance to your research focus. It must necessarily be a selective process, and is time consuming. It can involve hundreds of hours, over many months and, in some cases, years. The process is not that of 'smash and grab',[22] (p. 61) but that of slow acclimatization and acculturation. In deciding what to focus on, it is important to think back at this point to your research objectives. These will, to a greater or lesser extent, define your observational scope, ruling some issues in and others out. Developing a role in the research setting, perhaps based on early conversations that you have with your participants before you enter the field, will also assist by defining what it is possible to observe. Field, in his ethnography of nurses caring for dying people, gives a helpful definition of the research process in ethnography:

> Both participant observation and the unstructured interview attempt to be nondirective and responsive to new and unexpected information, although the latter inevitably has a narrower focus of concern and cannot draw on the direct experience of the researcher. In both, the researcher asks questions to test leads and hunches derived from previous research contacts, and both attempt to gather detailed descriptive material on the ways in which individuals make sense of their lives without imposing the researcher's concepts or categories upon them[10] (p. 152).

Field describes here the process of 'theoretical sampling' whereby methodological choices are made as the study unfolds about what to observe and of whom to ask questions or engage in conversation. This iterative process follows and complements the careful design of study objectives which directed the observational focus in the first instance.

Documentation of observational data usually takes place through the making of field notes, although it may on occasion also involve the use of film making, study of documents, voice recordings, etc. These field notes may be complemented by a fieldwork diary that is kept by the researcher or by analytical notes in the margin of the field notes. The following example of field notes is taken from my own work; they are drawn from a study of older adults' understandings of technologies used in end of life care.[35]

> We positively looked forward to meeting this group again and found the Church easily. We had been told to park in a 'permit only' space, and then walk into the main body of the Church. This was, however, deserted except for one person praying. We went out again and walked around the building, which was large, imposing but modern, until we could see signs of activity. We came upon a large room with trestle

tables set up for lunch, and a kitchen/bar area set to one side. Quite a few people were there, among them Susan and Penny, both of whom greeted us warmly. Penny explained that she had set one table aside for our group and showed us where it was. Barbara was already there, and was joined fairly rapidly by Edith, and Peter. All three looked very well—particularly Peter, who told me that since his wife had died he had been able to take several holidays and trips to visit children and grand children. Edith also looked very well, and told me that, at 87 in January, she was now a member of Weight Watchers! I asked her what advice was for a long life, and she reported: 'a good sense of humour' and 'I can see the funny side even when I shouldn't you know; it's got me into trouble sometimes!!' It was clear that all three wanted to have intimate conversations with either of us, which was actually a bit difficult to manage. I was acutely aware of trying to be even handed in the degree of conversational attention directed to each. Barbara caused slight difficulties with another member of the lunch club who came over to say hello to her. She told this person quite firmly that 'We are with people from the University; I can't talk to you now' and gestured the woman away, who retorted 'I've only come to say hello' before retreating in an obvious huff with Barbara. (Extract from field notes taken following a follow-up meeting with focus group participants who were members of a church lunch group for older people. All names have been changed.)

Spradley[36] provides a helpful and practical guide to the process of making field notes, recommending that three principles are adhered to:

1. The language identification principle: is this your interpretation, or something which reflects the terms used in the setting? Try to reflect the various ways in which language is used.

2. The verbatim principle: try, wherever possible, to write down verbatim what is said. Make this clear by the use of quotation marks, and identify the speaker.

3. The concrete principle: when describing your observations, use concrete language, not academic terms. Give as much specific detail as possible.

Spradley[36] also recommends that in order to make observation manageable, it is a good idea to make condensed notes, which can be expanded as soon as one has time; preferably as soon as that period of observation has ended. Choosing what to condense is crucial: there may be some verbatim data that must be recorded at the time of fieldwork, otherwise it will be distorted or forgotten. Developing a system that works for you is important, and getting into the habit of noting the date, time and other basic details is valuable. The recording of field notes in the research setting, even in a condensed form, may make you feel uncomfortable and may raise concerns among your research participants. Personally, I feel that it is not an option to try to record data covertly, and that, if asked, you should be willing to share your notes with the research participants: far from 'cramping one's style', this focuses the mind on trying to develop the accurate, and critical yet compassionate account that is the foundation of good ethnographic writing. Moreover, participants should be aware when you are recording things: this gives them the chance to say if they do not wish something to be noted down, or to move out of your earshot if they wish. Researchers should also exercise some judgement in deciding whether to record data: people will often be encouraged by your listening stance to disclose things that they may later regret. The need to maintain one's common sense and moral integrity in this process is obvious. However, while staff and carers may be able to distance themselves from the ethnographer, many patients in palliative care settings are a relatively 'captive audience' in the research situation, especially where their condition is deteriorating. Being aware of this and thinking about ways of addressing it sensitively is essential. As Lawton reports in her discussion of the observational process in an in-patient hospice:

> The practical and ethical difficulties I experienced whilst conducting fieldwork in the hospice were, in many respects, considerably more complex than those experienced in day care. One of my major and repeated concerns centred upon the issue of informed consent: I became acutely aware that, just because patients had given consent to be included in my research on their admission to the hospice, such consent could not necessarily be taken for granted in my later encounters with them. It is precisely because patients experienced a loss of self as their diseases progressed that I could not necessarily assume that a patient that I observed in the final stages approaching death was necessarily the same person who had originally given their consent[9] (p. 33).

These issues are discussed in more depth in Chapter 10 and should be read in conjunction with this chapter.

A final issue that ethnographers in health care need to think about relates to the possibility that you may be planning to conduct work in your own culture, or somewhere in which you are a very familiar figure. In my own work in intensive care, I had years of prior clinical work in the setting—my task was to use that familiarity actively in developing a 'thick' description of intensive care. In so doing, I made some aspects of the setting visible, but others invisible, precisely because of my familiarity. There is a literature on this in the nursing literature,[10,16,37,38] which highlights the complexity of the methodological and ethical issues that have to be negotiated when working in familiar cultures. For example, Goodwin,[37] a nurse, reports the everyday dilemmas that she encountered in an ethnographic study which involved her following anaesthetists during their daily work, and how her dual identity as researcher/nurse was sometimes enabling, but sometimes disabling to her project. Manias and Street[16] highlight the vital importance of reflexivity in ethnographic work in familiar cultures, meaning that the researchers must constantly critically examine their interactions within the research setting and consider candidly how their taken for granted values and views may have shaped what is seen and what is written in the final ethnographic account.

## Conclusion

Ethnography offers the potential for providing a subtle understanding of issues and problems that are poorly addressed by other research approaches, but is both complex and contested.[39] Conducting ethnography well takes considerable time, is therefore costly and requires the researcher to sustain critical engagement with a topic of study that is often familiar to them, while effectively becoming incorporated into the culture of the chosen research site. Ethnographers thus need highly developed research skills, a sound sense of their position in methodological debates related to ethnography and other qualitative methods, and good supervision if they are to succeed.[40] In palliative care, one of the biggest challenges to the ethnographer is to address issues of informed consent to participant observation, and to sustain a discrete yet compassionate role in observation that does not overly interfere in the dynamics of clinical care or make participants feel threatened or criticized. The changing environment of research governance and ethics committee approval in the UK means that these issues are under particular scrutiny at the moment. However, in spite of these difficulties, it has been recognized that ethnography, carefully and ethically conducted, can shed light on critical questions facing palliative care. Clark,[41] in an editorial about patient-centred death published in the *British Medical Journal* in 2003, called for greater use of ethnography and what she called 'other novel qualitative approaches' to address the following:

> We know little about the needs and desires of people from non western cultures, patients with dementias and non-malignant conditions, and dying children ...what does it 'mean' for patients to say that they want to die with dignity, or quietly or suddenly? What is the meaning of the desire for death? Does suffering have any meaning? How do these notions vary across cultures, space and time?[40] (p. 174).

Of course, ethnographic methods should only be seen as part of the palliative care researchers' 'kit box', but they are important and hitherto relatively underused: this chapter has tried to provide the means by which readers can think about issues involved in using them.

## References

1. Pope C, Mays N (1996) Opening the black box: an encounter in the corridors of health services research. In: Mays N, Pope C, (ed.) *Qualitative Research in Health Care.* London: BMJ Publishing Group, pp. 68–75.

2. Sudnow D (1967) *Passing On: The Social Organization of Dying.* Englewood Cliffs, NJ: Prentice Hall.

3. Glaser BG, Strauss A (1965) *Awareness of Dying.* Chicago: Aldine.

4. Quint JC (1967) *The Nurse and the Dying Patient.* New York: Macmillan.

5. McIntosh J (1977) *Communication and Awareness in a Cancer Ward.* London: Croom Helm.

6. Schou K, Hewison J (1999) *Experiencing Cancer: Quality of Life in Treatment.* Buckingham: Open University Press.

7. The AM (2002) *Palliative Care and Communication. Experiences in the Clinic.* Buckingham: Open University Press.

8. James N (1986) Care and work in nursing the dying: a participant observation study of a continuing care unit. Unpublished PhD thesis. Aberdeen University.

9. Lawton J (2000) *The Dying Process. Patients' Experiences of Palliative Care.* London: Routledge.

10. Field D (1989) *Nursing the Dying.* London: Tavistock/Routledge.

11. Hockey J (1990) *Experiences of Death. An Anthropological Account.* Edinburgh: Edinburgh University Press.

12. Young M, Cullen L (1996) *A Good Death. Conversations with East Londoners.* London: Routledge.

13. Riches G, Dawson P (2000) *An Intimate Loneliness.* Buckingham: Open University Press.

14. Seymour JE (2001) *Critical Moments: Death and Dying in Intensive Care.* Buckingham: Open University Press.

15. McNamara B (2001) *Fragile Lives. Death, Dying and Care.* Buckingham: Open University Press.

16. Manias E, Street A (2001) Rethinking ethnography: reconstructing relationships. *Journal of Advanced Nursing* 33: 234–242.

17. Vidich AJ, Lyman SM (2000) Qualitative methods: their history in sociology and anthroplogoy. In: Denzin NK, Lincoln YS, (ed.) *Handbook of Qualitative Research.* Thousand Oaks, CA: Sage, pp. 37–84.

18. Geertz C (1993) *The Interpretation of Cultures.* London: Fontana.

19. Seale C (1999) *The Quality of Qualitative Research.* London: Sage.

20. Hammersley M (1990) *Reading Ethnographic Research: A Critical Guide.* London: Longmans.

21. Hammersley M, Atkinson P (1983) *Ethnography: Principles in Practice.* London: Tavistock.

22. Brewer JD (2000) *Ethnography.* Buckingham: Open University Press.

23. Denzin NK, Lincoln YS (2000) *Handbook of Qualitative Research.* Thousand Oaks, CA: Sage.

24. Van Maanen J (1988) *Tales of the Field: On Writing Ethnography.* London: Sage.

25. Oakley A (1981) Interviewing women: a contradiction in terms? In: Roberts H, (ed.) *Doing Feminist Research.* London: Routledge, pp. 30–61.

26. Spencer L, Ritchie J, Lewis J, Dillon L (2003) *Quality in Qualitative Evaluation: A Framework for Assessing Evidence.* London: Government Chief Social Researcher's Office.

27. **Seymour JE** (1997) Caring for critically ill people: a study of death and dying in intensive care. Unpublished PhD thesis, The University of Sheffield.

28. **Atkinson P** (1995) *Medical Talk and Medical Work: The Liturgy of the Clinic.* London: Sage.

29. **Bogdewic SP** (1992) Participant observation. In: Crabtree BF, Miller WL, (ed.) *Doing Qualitative Research.* London: Sage, pp. 45–69.

30. **Bell C, Newby H** (1977) *Doing Sociological Research.* London: Allen and Unwin.

31. **Perakyla A** (1991) Hope work in the care of seriously ill patients. *Qualitative Health Research* 1: 407–33.

32. **Gold R** (1958) Roles in sociological field observation. *Social Forces* **36**: 217–33.

33. **Junker BH** (2004) The fieldwork situation. Social roles for observation. In: Seale C, (ed.) *Social Research Methods. A Reader.* London: Routledge.

34. **Clark D, Ingleton C, Seymour JE** (2000) Support and supervision in palliative care research. *Palliative Medicine* **14**: 441–6.

35. **Seymour JE, Gott M, Bellamy G, Clark D, Ahmedzai S** (2004) Planning for the end of life: the views of older people about advance statements. *Social Science and Medicine* **59**: 57–68.

36. **Spradley J** (1980) *Participant Observation.* Fort Worth: Harcourt Brace, Jovanovich College Publishers.

37. **Goodwin D, Pope C, Mort M, Smith A** (2003) Ethics and ethnography: an experiential account. *Qualitative Research,* **13**: 567–577

38. **Allen D** (2004) Ethnomethodological insights into insider–outsider relationships in nursing ethnographies of healthcare settings. *Nursing Inquiry* **11**: 14–24.

39. **Savage J** (1995) *Nursing Intimacy: An Ethnographic Approach to Nurse–Patient Interaction.* London: Scutari Press.

40. **Savage J** (2000) Ethnography and health care. *British Medical Journal* **321**: 1400–2.

41. **Clark J** (2003) Patient centred death. *British Medical Journal* **327**: 174–5.

Chapter 14

# Documentary analysis and policy

Margaret O'Connor

## Introduction

Palliative care services in most Western countries have substantially developed, first through community lobbying and pressure groups, and then through government funding. Overt policy has not played a large role.[1] Nonetheless, significant policy documentation now exists, and this body of work can show important trends in the emergence of the discipline and its practice.

In understanding the development of a comparatively new discipline such as palliative care, there is much to be learned from the analysis of policy documentation, and understanding its part in how the discipline has developed as well as the connections between policy and practice. Because palliative care is a developing discipline, there is a 'closeness' to the written documentation; there are also not a lot of documents, particularly in seeking a historical perspective. It is possible, however, to analyse the emphasis given to palliative care and related issues such as the rights of the dying, through an analysis of documents such as the daily newspapers, the academic literature and annual reports, as well as more formal government and agency policy documents.

While analysis of language and its structure has been a part of traditional language studies for a long time, social and political connections with the written word are more recent developments, which may assist understanding of the place of policy and its connections in establishing or reflecting changes in society.[2] There is now firm recognition of the role of language in the social fabric, in particular its centrality in social change processes.[3] Policy is obviously structured from language and, because language is never neutral, one can analyse and interpret meanings, community values and directions from such documentation. Critical and interpretative documentary analysis may cover a wide range of areas: social and political sciences, education, law, psychological and health sciences. The material viewed can be almost any written document: formal policies, legal rulings, speeches, letters, media and other publicity material, and historical documents.[4]

Perhaps the importance of understanding policy in relation to palliative care is best illustrated by the dearth of policy that exists in most countries. This is mainly because, reflecting the death-denying character of many societies, the issues of dying and death do not feature in health policy in an obvious way.[1] This chapter seeks to get behind that hidden-ness to discuss the role of analysing policy, as well as utilizing the method of discourse analysis. An example of how to undertake such an analysis using palliative care documentation is included, drawing primarily on the Australian setting and on reflections of palliative care policy in that country.

## Policy

Numerous definitions of policy exist;[5,6] however, the dictionary suggests that policy is:

> a course of action adopted and pursued by a government party, ruler, statesman, etcetera; or any course of action adopted as advantageous or expedient.[7]

For the purposes of this chapter, in describing a broad sweep of documentary analysis, Gardner and Barraclough[5] use all-encompassing approaches which delineate a field of activity, an expression indicating a general purpose or areas of specific content. Policy may take several forms: clear organizational directions, a programme or material that focuses on government output and outcomes[5] (p. 7). Hennessy and Spurgeon[6] state that policies are neither: 'conceived consciously nor logically developed', but are 'the strategies and courses of action adopted as being advantageous and expedient to provide within the resources available from a health system that at least maintains and preferably improves, health'[6] (p. 6). There are competing opinions and views inherent within this definition. Policies may also be regarded as:

> management tools aimed at describing the preferred organisational responses for particular circumstances. They may be seen as either facilitative or inhibitive depending on the degree of restraint built into a particular policy[8] (p. 131).

While policies on a particular issue may shape political agendas, they are by no means the only way that direction on an issue is shaped. In all democratic countries, policy development will have idiosyncratic political development pathways. In democratic countries such as Australia, where there are regular elections of government, the associated political processes work towards shaping policy. During the lead up to an election in particular, policy formation may involve compromise between opposing views either within or between political parties; views gained from voters, from workers and users of a particular programme such as health or welfare; the media; the community's preconceived opinions and attitudes; and the general philosophical stance of a particular political party. Given divergent interpretations and understandings of policy, which are contextual to the political particularities within each country and its place within the fabric of democratic processes, this very complexity provides rich material for undertaking analysis.[2]

Policy development is a process that occurs at a number of levels and may involve politicians and public servants, community lobby groups, other loosely organized issue and interest groups, unions, corporations and individual institutions. In any policy development, it is important to understand which of these parties are involved, their vested interests and the role they play.

Policy may also develop from three different, but compatible sources:

- As an *authoritative* voice, responding to a public issue or problem—the intention to pursue specific directions; making decisions, identifying the steps in the chosen direction and testing the outcomes. Decision making involves identifying key people, the resources required and the implementation process; it is political in that it expresses one choice over others, thus making the authority of the choice visible.[2]

- As a *hypothesis*—policies develop in response to particular world-views, with inherent assumptions about human behaviour, to bias one behaviour against another (e.g. taxes and evasion). Policy (particularly public policy) is made in an uncertain environment, so good policy making incorporates evaluation as an inherent part of the policy cycle.[2]

- As an *objective of government action*—particular policy development is about achieving the objectives; they are the means to the end. Thus the goal to be achieved will always be explicit in good policy; if not, then policies may lack direction and outcomes will be diffuse.[2]

It is also recognized that consistent policy making will occur within a continuous cycle.[2] The process begins with *identifying the issue*, which may emerge in a variety of formal or informal ways—the corridor, conversations, lobby groups, meetings, pressure groups, a political activity, lobbying and pressuring.

A policy analysis should then be undertaken; the interest group or groups such as analysts specifically employed by the public service will undertake this process as a focused activity. Such written documents as briefing papers may emerge at this stage. The *policy instruments* used in the analysis need to be appropriate to the issue. Some will require a community discussion paper, others will require legislative change.

Appropriate *consultation* needs to occur in order to ensure that stakeholders are informed and involved, which should result in better and more relevant policy, with more chance of eventual acceptance of the proposed policy changes. Part of the consultation process is *coordination*, to ensure that differences between groups are resolved. These may be most apparent at different levels within the issue, e.g. consumers and funders, the community and government.

Following these processes, a *decision* is required at some level. The information feeds into the final information given to decision makers, which should be at an appropriate level, as too much information may result in a decision being held up, and too little information may result in an ill-informed decision.[2]

*Implementation* is an important stage in the cycle, requiring a 'selling' of the policy and subsequent acceptance. An effective process, and one which closes the cycle, is an *evaluation stage*, that gauges effect and makes allowances for adjustment as appropriate. Then the cycle starts again.

## Policy analysis

There is little methodological/definitional agreement about how one analyses texts such as policy,[3] being dependent on various theoretical and disciplinary standpoints taken. Policy research is also a relatively recent method of research, in terms of its contribution to the political process.[9,10] Both Majchrzak[10] and Quade[11] emphasize the importance of understanding the social setting in definitions of analysis, with Majchrzak suggesting that analysis is: 'the process of conducting research on, or analysis of a fundamental social problem…it begins with a social problem …'[10] (p. 15).

Quade[11] says that in endeavouring to understand a social problem, policy analysis assists, but it is a form of research that is as much about the process, and not just the end product[11] (p. 13).

Policy analysis focuses on the dimensions of a particular social problem and its outcomes. In providing an overview of this issue, many possible actions may be addressed. Policy analysts are also typically interested in the processes behind the adoption of policies, and their effects once adopted. To capture this complexity, a broad sweep of many kinds of literature associated with a particular issue is often required. Pragmatic policy analysts would also say that:

> policy is virtually synonymous with decisions; … patterns of decisions over time or decisions in the context of other decisions … these are taken by political actors … and are about both means and ends. They are contingent in that they refer to and depend on a specified situation. Policy is restricted to that which can be achieved, over which the State has authority and to what actions/results are actually feasible[12] (p. 3).

Identifying connections between policy and practice requires taking a broad view of the social issue as expressed in policy, raising awareness and questions for the practitioner, in relation to a particular area of clinical practice. There may be no definitive end-point reached however, because, in a Foucauldian sense, there is no one true view of what is 'truth'.[13] It is:

> ...not a battle 'on behalf' of the truth, but a battle about the status of truth and the economic and political role it plays[13] (p. 132).

So a need for open questioning is the required approach to analysis, which may support the model of a dynamic cyclic continuum already described—starting with the social issue, examining the policies, and funding which influences strategic directions and models of care. In the light of this analysis, policy may change, evidenced by changes in practice. The social issue may then require further anayisis with the process reciprocated, stimulated by the dynamics of policy changes arising from previous policy changes.

Thus Majchrzak[10] (p. 20) claims policy analysis to be 'a challenging endeavour', suggesting that much that is defined as policy research is only a small part of the required continuum between an experienced researcher, an open and attentive policy maker and the policy-making environment.

> The researcher must be able to consider all aspects of the multidimensional social problem, identify and maintain a focus on the most malleable variables, study the social problem without imposing a predefined theory, consider the effects of both past and future trends on the present, explicitly incorporate values into the research process and be responsive to study users despite their numerous and sometimes conflicting demands[10] (p. 20).

## Discourse and discourse analysis

Discourse is defined in language as to: 'talk, converse; hold forth in speech or writing on a subject; give forth'.[7]

In linguistic understanding, discourse contributes to the construction of community by establishing identity, in particular attention to language usage and its place in providing shared patterns of meaning.

Discourse analysis is a valuable research tool in providing a critical research perspective that examines phenomena across the human and social sciences, building on insights from linguistics, philosophy and social theory. Discourse analysis produces meaning from talk or texts, revealing aspects of cultural understandings, which may have been hidden. Fairclough[3] sees its use:

> in social theory and analysis, ... to refer to different ways of structuring areas of knowledge and social practice ... Discourses ... are manifested in particular ways of using language and other symbolic forms such as visual images ... Discourses do not just reflect or represent social entities & relations, they construct or 'constitute' them[3] (p. 3).

Discourse analysis is part of the larger body of social and cultural research that produces meaning through examination of words and texts. Like other qualitative methods, discourse analysis challenges the dominant knowledge about a particular issue or phenomenon, and seeks to disrupt easy assumptions about the meanings and organization of social life. Discourse analysis does not aim to give a definitive and representative overview of public attitudes towards a particular issue; rather it seeks to examine how: 'public attitudes ... are shaped, reproduced and legitimised through the use of language[4] (p. 253).

If society is symbolized by the words that are used to describe it, then language is an important part of that society's social construction. Fairclough argues that something becomes a social reality only in its linguistic representation and the use of language.[3] He makes a two-layered distinction in the construction of discourse; it is influenced from the outside by such things as culture, context and political theories, as well as from the inside by the textual meaning that is applied. A social theory of discourse becomes clearer and more distinctive through the process of political debate, comment, writing and referencing[3] (p. 5). Texts utilized in discourse analysis provide insight into societal changes[14] and, in tracing the discourse of a particular policy over time, one can consider the influence of policy issues over a continuum—past, present and planned direction in the future.[15]

Thus discourse is not only socially shaped, but also contributes to shaping society—systems of communication, social relations and differing knowledges or 'truths' arise from discourse. The analysis of discourse is concerned with the connections between meanings, power and knowledge; about how social and cultural constructions are shaped, giving particular groupings a common ground of communication and understanding.

Within the framework of analysing discourse is a basic recognition that language is socially and culturally situated, as well as being inherent in the values contained in words themselves, and the content and setting of groups of words that comprise a discourse. Besides being used by those with interests in pure linguistics, discourse has been used by both analysts and theorists in helping to construct social relationships, and contributing to systems of knowledge and belief, thus assisting us to understand each other. Discourse can connect meanings through the way in which it brings together both individuality and sameness—we are at once free individuals, but in particular cultures we speak the same language, with agreed meanings; we have similar values and know the same truth.[9] For example, if our collective language about ageing and dying is negative—old people are a societal burden, because they cost money and contribute little to the economic life of society—this may lead to the devaluing and disempowerment of older, dying people within that society.

Language is an important area of reflection in all aspects of life, because changes in common language usage may represent changes in communal attitudes. The analysis of particular discourse involves a broad critique of language usage, which may be drawn from many sources. These sources may include:

> official documents, legal statutes, political debates and speeches, media reports, policy papers, maps, pictorial and exhibition materials, expert analyses, publicity literature and press statements, historical documents, tourist guides, interviews, diaries and oral histories[4] (p. 245).

Discourse analysis may take many forms. It assists the researcher to view beyond the words, as more than tools for communication, and to examine the context of their usage, the meanings understood; what is symbolized within the community, and implied values. Language is highly symbolic, rarely politically neutral, and illustrates the world-view of the user to the listener, thus language is never just descriptive, but often shapes the way the community views an issue or a phenomenon. An example in Australia is the media's shying away from usage of the word 'dying' and increasingly favouring phrases such as 'passed away' or 'passed'; this is perhaps suggestive of a communal discomfort and hidden-ness about issues to do with death.[16]

Discourse analysis may be a way of moving beyond the actual words to draw a rich picture of an issue within a particular setting and the emphasis it is given within a group or community. It is also important to consider that discourse may take the form of delineating an 'expert' language that belongs to a particular group and serves to define membership of that group.[4] This kind of discourse also carries an authority with it, so that those who know the language can communicate with each other, excluding those who do not. Another consideration of discourse analysis is the relationship between a particular knowledge of a group and the inherent power that is created in relation to those who do not have that knowledge. Medical terminology is the most common example of this kind of exclusive discourse.[3] This understanding of discourse is particularly pertinent for palliative care services, and will be discussed further.

Through thematic development, different discourses about an issue develop from different perspectives—the many 'truths' of the issue. As stated, the method is reflective, open-ended in the questioning of text, rather than seeking solutions or developing a particular dominant view. In a contemporary sense, discourse analysis has provided a legitimate way of balancing many perspectives of one issue, without needing to establish the correctness of any one perspective. Issues often develop through the push and pull of conflicting discourses, communicated to the community in different ways, raising awareness of an issue and forcing political debate.

## Foucault's understanding of discourse

A word should be said about the post-structural understandings of discourse, mainly under the influence of Michel Foucault, who expanded the strictly linguistic understandings of discourse to incorporate the concept of a discipline in relation to a particular body of knowledge, its connection to politics and the power that 'exclusive' knowledge carries. A post-structural view of discourse is one where social reality arises from language and which may balance different or competing views of the one reality. In contrast, the opposite view holds that social reality is reflected in language and is a fixed identity. Foucault[13] argues that there are terms identified by a set of particular rules, which carry with them a sense of control and therefore power. Medical language is commonly noted as an example of this[13] (p. 112 ff).

Foucault's work on discourse encompasses a political view, bringing together

> Linguistically-oriented discourse analysis and social and political thought relevant to discourse and language, in the form of a framework which will be suitable for use in social science research, and specifically in the study of social change[17] (p. 62).

In his work, there are connections in the relationship of discourse to power, and of discourse to social change.[18]

> Language partakes in the world-wide dissemination of similitudes and signatures. It must, therefore, be studied itself as a thing in nature ... Language itself stands halfway between the visible forms of nature and the secret conveniences of esoteric discourses[18] (p. 35)

Discourse is not only about the words themselves, but also the meanings behind them, the power they symbolize and what they say about their author. Foucault's early example of a changed (or discontinuous) historical discourse was that of mental illness or 'madness', moving from being regarded as a moral lack in the eighteenth century, to a psychopathology (illness) in the nineteenth century[19] and a social inconvenience in the late twentieth century. Perhaps the historical discourse about dying could be viewed in a similar way as a discontinuous discourse: once a shared communal family activity and regarded as part of human beginnings and endings, it is now not only separate and hidden from the community gaze and family involvement, but has become a medical event in the hands of those who have made care of the dying their specialty, with its own particular language.

The analysis of power in discourse assists in understanding the way that power impacts and shapes issues within a community or group. Foucault redefined understandings of power as not necessarily negative, but as something that can provide energy to issues; developing not from outside or above, but from within. It is evident in the way it is exercised through knowledge, in particular with knowledge and power being mutually interdependent. The generation of knowledge generates power; power cannot be exercised without knowledge. Power is implicit within all aspects of everyday life, but is masked behind the practices and discourses of a society. Power in Foucault's eyes[20] is not necessarily regarded as 'power over' another; power is not to be 'had' by a person or persons—rather it is everywhere: '"power" is primarily a matter of the administration of "life"'[20] (p. 143).

Power is a mechanism, a system of particular relations, whereby the parts of a society are shaped, particularly as it is articulated in institutional life, and can empower or become a mode of surveillance or regulation.

Foucault's work reveals that in any institution there is a discourse hierarchy, based on power, that is applied to particular groups within that institution. Foucault's interest is not discourses in general, but the power of their construction within specific disciplines such as medicine.[21]

> We must cease once and for all to describe the effects of power in negative terms: it 'excludes', it 'represses', it 'censors', it 'abstracts', it 'masks', it 'conceals'. In fact power produces; it produces reality; it produces domains of objects and rituals of truth[21] (p. 194).

Change occurs through struggle/resistance, in particular with the power relations inherent in all discourses. Macdonnell notes that it is:

> through the possibilities of being pinned down and defined through opposites, in these struggles that discourses find their meanings[9] (p. 10).

In this process, the dominant discourse then becomes the 'truth', which Foucault argues is a constantly changing construct. We understand truth through power:

> ... and we cannot exercise power except through the production of truth ... we must speak the truth ... power never ceases its interrogation, its inquisition, its registration of truth[13] (p. 93).

Meanings are created through the language used, not vice versa. In a social sense then, the analysis of a particular discourse will articulate and inform community values and opinions. Thus the discourse on death, for example, is not just composed of the words that describe people's experiences; it also involves the rituals, the practices and the settings surrounding the words, making discourse and practice inseparable.

As stated, the organization of language within a specific discipline, the language of that discipline and the use of power inherent in particular language are important in understanding the relationship of power and knowledge to discourse. Using this mode of thinking, for example, the conversation between two doctors, compared with a lay person seeking an opinion from a doctor, would be quite different and according to a hierarchy. Particular words are used for particular groups when relating to others. Language has inherent power, especially if, as noted, it is used to define membership of particular groupings. Forms of societal power—legal, economic, administrative and others—underpin society, contributing to the 'truth' of that society, transmitting and producing power:

> it reinforces it but also undermines and exposes it, renders it fragile and makes it possible to thwart it. In like manner, silence and secrecy are a shelter for power, anchoring its prohibitions, but they also loosen its hold and provide for relatively obscure areas of tolerance[22] (p. 107).

## Undertaking discourse analysis

Even though discourse analysis is not regarded as an exact science,[11] it is nevertheless a legitimate qualitative research method, thus requiring consistency, a lack of bias and ethical standards in the methods used, that are defendable to the observer. Additionally, although this kind of analysis does not use a particular method, there are still common techniques that can be gathered.[14] These include highlighting key words, variations and themes within and between texts; and reading documentation looking for emphasis, missing texts and detail. Vague but difficult to challenge language and descriptions such as 'the good death' or 'the team' may also be noted.[4] What follows is an example of discourse analysis that was undertaken to examine aged care policy in Australia in relation to discourses on care of the dying.

Before commencing analysis, objective questions that may set the scene for more detailed questioning of the text itself include:

- ◆ What is the status of the text?
- ◆ Is the text part of a wider text? For example, is it part of a series of policies, a series of special newspaper articles on an issue?
- ◆ Who is the author of the text?
- ◆ Who is the intended audience?
- ◆ Are there stakeholders in what has been written?
- ◆ Who are the people with the power to make decisions and how are they using their power?
- ◆ Are there hidden agendas/biases, hidden issues or aspects of a bigger issue?
- ◆ What sort of authority has been given to the document?
- ◆ What sorts of decisions have been made, with what level of authority and influence?

## Ways of selecting and approaching the data

As with all research, the starting point is often a vague interest in a particular issue and involves a process of clarifying the question: like other qualitative methods, it requires an open-ended question that is not seeking answers as much as seeking the meanings that contribute to a particular view (Chapter 9). My research question (above) was generated from a clinical situation, whereby I became aware of the disadvantaged dying who live in residential aged care, compared with those who are fortunate to die in a palliative care service. There are visible inequities in access to expertise, environment, staffing levels and funding, even though it could be argued that the clientele have much in common. I was interested in why this situation existed and from where these differences arose; hence the decision to look at policy, not practice.

Then begins a process of collection of written documentation about the issues; as stated elsewhere, this does not require collection of *everything* written, but a more measured approach in weighing up what is pertinent to exploring aspects of the issue. There is no 'correct' way to collect documents, no number of documents that are regarded as sufficient and no incorrect type of documents. It depends on the individual design of the research, and working out what will be the most appropriate sort of documentation that will provide material relevant to the research question. For my study, I chose a variety of documents, but wanted to concentrate on formal policy at the highest level I could access, thus only examining the Australian Government documents. Then a strategic decision was made, based on time limits and the volume of documentation, to limit documentation to a particular time period, and a contrast created within the design, by examining documentation in the daily newspapers, providing a lay view of a topical issue. Ultimately one is seeking data that will add insight to the question or issue being addressed.

The design will necessarily combine a number of research methods to strengthen the picture and give insight from a range of perspectives. My research included a statistical analysis of deaths in an aged care setting, thematic analysis of recent academic literature, and examining commonalities and differences in and between discourses in formalized policies as well as informal sources such as the daily newspapers. An understanding of the social setting of the issue was also required, informed mostly from the daily newspapers.

The analysis methodology needs to make sense in consideration of the issue and (for me anyway) needed to be outcomes focused and relevant to practice. So for my study, an interaction with the practice area of aged care and an understanding of the issues of dying in that setting and from that perspective was vital, in order for the picture that emerged to be grounded in the reality.

Many methodologies could have been chosen for this question, but a multilayered thematic analysis was chosen to encompass the complexity of the picture gleaned, as well as to provide structure to varied information gained from many different sources.

## Sorting, coding and analysing the data

Seale[4] notes that discourse analysis is a method that is perfected by the doing and by working with someone else who understands the process. The process of 'doing' the analysis is what enables the researcher to get a 'feel' for the question or issue and, as familiarity increases, may often be the way that a researcher sorts through the relevance of particular documentation. Supervision or other ways of working with another person can be helpful in the process, in seeking other perspectives of the issue. It is also sometimes helpful at this stage to find other examples of discourse analysis in order to ascertain previous use of discourse analysis methods.

As with many other qualitative methods, one needs to suspend one's own particular view of an issue, otherwise they may find themselves seeking out particular views to support their own biased view. In my design, I utilized two expert aged care practitioners to oversee and read my data.

A commencement of seeking out themes, words, approaches and emphases begins. This may be slow at first, but an open-minded reading and re-reading of a number of the texts chosen will soon provide the basis for common thematic beginnings. This does not mean that these themes will remain but, at the beginning, it is important to start with something and to build the analysis from there. For example, I began my analysis by reading the Australian Government aged care policy documents, expecting that I would find much material of care of the dying there. During the time period chosen, the International Year of the Older Person was celebrated, which saw an overemphasis on images of healthy ageing as the dominant discourse, with a discounting of issues of frailty, vulnerability and dying; thus, I needed to expand my study design, both to incorporate this emphasis and to find documents on care of the dying elsewhere.

Like other qualitative methods that analyse words, key themes or words may then emerge from the materials being examined. There is no one way to organize this, and one may need to sift and change the material in order to organize it in a way that will respond to the original question. As noted, my study issue turned out to be more hidden in the literature that I viewed than I had originally anticipated, so I utilized the symbolism of a 'veil' to show this.

There may be commonalities and consistencies, differences or plain contradictions both within and between texts. These all need to be captured in a thematic design. Variations in texts are important to highlight, demonstrating that there is not universal agreement on an issue and illustrating the political nature of discourse analysis particularly when examining contemporary or contentious issues. For example, during the time period chosen, the International Year of Older People was lauding the achievements of older people, while the daily newspapers exposed the scandals of levels of care in aged care facilities. If language is found that is difficult to understand (words used without explanation, or where common understanding is assumed), these require highlighting and comment. An example is the word 'team'. Further examples of this are seen below.

## Presenting the analysis

The emphasis of discourse analysis is on the meaning of text, and meaning is open to different interpretation. This is acceptable, however, since, as has been stated, the end-point is not to seek a definitive truth, rather critically to interpret text and to offer ways in which this impinges on policy and political processes.

The chosen design needs to reflect the socio-political environment by interacting with the study and by predicting changes as a result of the study. As noted, for me, the implications of this research for the practice environment were an important consideration. This requires a level of sophistication in showing the hidden discourses, power relations and contextual considerations in order to make such predictions. I experienced sometimes defensive reactions, when I presented my study in aged care facilities, as opposed to a more open listening when I presented it to palliative care services.

The data should be ordered, understandable and accessible to the reader. The researcher needs to be able to justify their chosen design and to defend criticism. In this kind of research, there will always be other views of the issue (particularly if it is contentious), so the researcher needs to be prepared for challenges and to stand confidently by their methodology, design and outcomes, and to engage in constructive defence.

## An analysis of palliative care discourse

'Expert' or exclusive language serves a 3-fold purpose for those who share the discourse:[23]

- It defines an area of knowledge, which immediately denotes 'membership' of a group and defines an area of expertise. For example, for a person who does not understand the rules of cricket, what do the terms 'out for a duck' or 'bowl the maiden over' mean? More seriously, as will be seen below, those who work in palliative care have a particular understanding of the terms used and even of those that are not necessarily exclusive—'multidisciplinary team' for example.

◆ The use of particular language creates a discourse that allows those who belong to communicate with each other, to the exclusion of others. The cricket example applies readily here, but one only needs to recall conversations with doctors who use medical language that may not always be understood by the sick layperson.

◆ A distinctive language gives authority to the speaker. So the former cricket player makes the best cricket commentator. The listener may not understand, may be intimidated or (in the case of the medical practitioner) may feel consoled that someone knows more than they and so understands his or her medical problem.

The commonly used definition for palliative care in Australia is:

> Palliative care is specialised health care of dying people which aims to maximise quality of life and assist families and carers after death.[24]

To ask some of the objective questions listed above of this question, the author of the statement is Palliative Care Australia, and the intended audience is the Australian public. Agreed during the 1990s and utilized until very recently, the brevity of the definition was purposeful, to assist with gaining media attention, as well as attempting to be a plain language statement for the general public. The authority of the document is that it comes from a body which represents and speaks on behalf of services throughout Australia. The stakeholders in what has been written are those who deliver or who are responsible for the delivery of palliative care services. It is interesting to note, however, that many services choose not to use this definition, preferring the World Health Organization, Canadian or their own local definitions, which all have subtle language differences.[16] Thus the authority achieved by the national body speaking with one voice is discounted by those who make these individual organizational choices.

What does this definition mean to the uninitiated or uninformed? Does a person need to be dying in order to get this specialized care and what is 'special' about it? Unless a person has experienced palliative care within their social structure, it is still not uncommon for someone to have never heard of palliative care or, even if they have, not to know what it is, or be confused about the aims of care (e.g. 'it's what you get in that place you don't come out of'). The term 'palliative care' is not in common language usage and it is misunderstood even in health care circles (e.g. the care plan suggested in an aged care facility: 'he's on palliative care; we don't need to *do* anything there'[25]).

Using the word 'dying' in the definition may be confrontational within a death-denying society. How this word is interpreted would vary along a continuum, depending on the experience of the audience—from understanding dying as a trajectory, occurring over a period of time, to understanding dying as an instant action. When the short Australian definition was written, there was spirited but ambivalent discussion about inclusion of the word 'dying' in the definition, some preferring 'care of those with a life-threatening/limiting illness' or those whose 'disease is not responsive to curative treatment'. This euphemistic language has also been noted in many definitions used by local services, perhaps in an attempt not to offend the community.[16]

However, these phrases are difficult to access and intimate a denial of the real work of palliative care, and, if used by staff, need to be questioned as avoidance. Language about dying will always disaffect some people—some people not 'dying' will need care—thus avoidance defeats the purpose of endeavouring not to offend. Like Seale's description of 'expert' language[23] (p. 20), there appears to be a contradiction that 'palliative care language', so commonly used and understood as the dominant discourse within the discipline, may be a barrier that confuses and separates people from understanding the reality of palliative care service.

Exclusive language may serve to make palliative care mysterious and thus disempower the very people that the discipline claims to empower. Even though there is a sense of moving away from the use of excluding medical terminology (which denotes the power of one group over another), the above language has been demonstrated as difficult to interpret. In bringing Foucault's discourse hierarchy framework to bear in this reflection on language,[13] the dominant discourse in traditional health care settings is medical language. Palliative care language is quite different, as seen above, and indeed has been overtly developed to be different from medical terminology. In placing palliative care language against traditional medical language, it can be seen that they do not readily mix. Another level of discourse hierarchy is seen and perhaps may account for the resistance to palliative care in some health care settings. Without even considering the separation from everyday language, do other health professionals, who work side by side with palliative carers, actually understand the language and the care that is implied?

Thus does this language usage risk being misunderstood not only by the community, but also by health professionals. This language is now in such common usage among palliative care practitioners that they are too close to its usage to comprehend the power that is created in being a language shared among one group, but not universal. Exclusive language is a discourse that serves to communicate power and control.[13]

Mellor says[26] that this special care of the dying has distinctive, individualistic meanings and language that remove it from the gaze of the community. The above demonstrates a power relationship, in that some have the knowledge and some do not. For those who do not have the knowledge, palliative care remains mysterious. Seale[27] notes that because of excluding language, there are certain forms of knowledge that are privileged, certain modes of argument that are persuasive and therefore certain speakers will be heard as authoritative. This kind of expert language serves to define the membership of a discipline, marking out a particular body of knowledge, and is by definition exclusive[27] (p. 248).This demonstration of power in language is worthy of reflection on the part of those who work in palliative care, even if it is not conscious or purposeful, because of the centrality of the value of empowerment of those in their care.

## Conclusion

An understanding of analysing policy in palliative care has been demonstrated in this chapter. This kind of analysis is important simply because of the relative lack of policy in this area, reflecting the death-denying character of many societies. Discourse analysis has provided a suitable overall critical research tool for removing the hidden-ness that surrounds care of the dying.[3,4,17,22,28] Foucault's work[13,18–21] has demonstrated the more philosophical understandings of discourse in shaping and constructing community values; of particular relevance is his work addressing the symbolism and truth of particular discourses, and the continuous or discontinuous historical path. The process of analysing discourse illustrates the place of an issue in the community fabric, and the role of power in relation to the voices present or hidden. This chapter has demonstrated that the use of discourse analysis of policy is possible at many levels, in a way that can more overtly make care of the dying more accessible to the community and health professionals.

## References

1. Smith M (2000) Death, health policy and palliative care. In: Kellehear A, (ed.) *Death and Dying in Australia*. Melbourne: Oxford University Press.

2. Bridgman P, David G (2004) *The Australian Policy Handbook*, 3rd edn. Crows Nest, Australia: Allen and Unwin.

3. Fairclough N (1992) *Discourse and Social Change*. Cambridge: Polity Press.

4. Seale C, (ed.) (1998) *Researching Society and Culture*. London: Sage Publications.

5. Gardner H, Barraclough S (1992) *Health Policy Development, Implementation and Evaluation in Australia*. Melbourne: Churchill Livingstone.

6. Hennessy D, Spurgeon P (2000) *Health Policy and Nursing: Influences, Development and Impact*. Basingstoke: Macmillan.

7. *Concise Oxford Dictionary* (1964) 5th edn. London: Oxford University Press.

8. Barnum M, Kerfoot K (1995) *The Nurse as Executive*. Gaithersburg, MD: Aspen.

9. Macdonnell D (1986) *Theories of Discourse*. London: Blackwell Press.

10. Majchrzak A (1984) *Methods for Policy Research.* Thousand Oaks, CA: Sage Publications.

11. Quade ES (1989) *Analysis for Public Decisions.* New York: Elsevier.

12. Hill M, Bramley G (1986) *Analysing Social Policy.* Oxford: Basil Blackwell.

13. Foucault M, Gordon C, (ed.) (1980) *Power and Knowledge—Selected Interviews and Other Writings 1972–77.* New York: Pantheon Books.

14. Lupton D, McLean J (1998) Representing doctors: discourses and images in the Australian press. *Social Science and Medicine* **46**: 947–58.

15. O'Connor M, Pearson A (2004) Ageing in place, dying in place: competing discourses for care of the dying in aged care policy *Australian Journal of Advanced Nursing* **22**, 31–7.

16. O'Connor M (2005) Mission statements: an example of exclusive language in palliative care? *International Journal of Palliative Nursing* **11**: 190–6.

17. Fairclough N, (ed.) (1992) *Critical Language Awareness.* London: Longman Group.

18. Foucault M (1970) *The Order of Things: An Archeology of the Human Sciences.* New York: Pantheon Books.

19. Foucault M (1965) *Madness and Civilization: A History of Insanity in the Age of Reason.* London: Tavistock Publications.

20. Foucault M (1978) *The Archeology of Knowledge.* London: Tavistock Publications.

21. Foucault M (1977) *Discipline and Punish: The Birth of the Prison.* Harmondsworth: Penguin.

22. Weedon C (1997) *Feminist Practice and Poststructuralist Theory.* Oxford: Blackwell Publishers.

23. Seale C (1998) *Constructing Death: The Sociology of Dying and Bereavement.* Cambridge: Cambridge University Press.

24. Palliative Care Australia (1999) *Palliative Care Australia Standards for Palliative Care Provision*, 3rd edn. Canberra: Palliative Care Australia.

25. Commonwealth Department of Health and Aged Care (2003) *Community Attitudes to Palliative Care Issues—Quantitative Report.* Canberra: Commonwealth Department of Health and Aged Care; Publication No: 3281(JN7665).

26. Mellor P (1993) Death in high modernity: the contemporary presence and absence of death. In: Clark D, (ed.) *The Sociology of Death: Theory, Culture, Practice.* Oxford: Blackwell Publishers.

27. Seale C (1999) *The Quality of Qualitative Research.* London: Sage Publications.

28. Seale C (1995) Dying alone. *Sociology of Health and Illness* **17**: 376–92.

## Section 5

# How to …

Chapter 15

# How to develop a research question

Laura Kelly and Patrick Stone

## Introduction

This chapter addresses the first and most basic aspect of study design—namely the formulation and development of a research question. Surprisingly, this aspect of study design often receives scant attention from prospective researchers. There is sometimes a temptation to decide upon a broad area of investigation and then to leap into a detailed consideration of the research methodology without ever clarifying the precise research question that is being addressed. The perils of this approach are well illustrated by Douglas Adams in the '*Hitchhiker's Guide to the Galaxy*'. He relates the story of a race of 'hyper-intelligent pan-dimensional beings' who design a supercomputer to calculate the answer to the ultimate question of 'life the universe and everything'. After many generations the computer is ready with its answer, but the programmers are not pleased.

> 'Forty-two!' yelled Loonquawl. 'Is that all you've got to show for seven and a half million years' work?'
> 'I checked it very thoroughly' said the computer, 'and that quite definitely is the answer. I think the problem, to be quite honest with you, is that you've never actually known what the question is'[1] (p.152).

This chapter will serve to emphasize the importance of having a clearly defined research question before embarking on a research project, and will provide the reader with advice on transforming an abstract 'research idea' into a concrete 'research aim'.

## The importance of defining a clear research aim

Researchers are usually eager to start the process of writing the study protocol, submitting ethics committee applications and then collecting data for their project. However, time spent early on, in the planning and framing of a suitably robust research question, will usually pay dividends as the study progresses. The benefits include the following.

## Informing the choice about appropriate study methodology

Researchers often agonize over the relative merits and drawbacks of different types of research methodology. In broad terms, researchers may choose to answer a question using quantitative or qualitative methodologies. Qualitative research:

> explores and describes social phenomena. It interprets and describes these phenomena in terms of their meaning and helps to make sense of these meanings.[2]

In contrast, quantitative research addresses biomedical questions and: 'tests hypothesised causal relations between variables'.[2]

Each methodological approach has its own proponents and detractors.[3,4] However, to a large extent, the debate about which research methodology or paradigm is most 'valid' is misplaced. Different approaches are needed to answer different types of question. If the research question is 'In patients with prostate cancer and incident pain from bony metastases, does sublingual fentanyl provide quicker pain relief and have fewer side effects than oral morphine?', then a quantitative approach (e.g. a randomized controlled trial) is probably the methodology of choice (Chapter 2). If, however, the research question is 'What is the impact that incident pain has on the lifestyle of patients with metastatic prostatic cancer?', then a qualitative methodology (perhaps using purposive sampling and in-depth interviews) would be the most appropriate approach[5] (Chapter 9). In a *British Medical Journal* editorial, Sackett and Wennberg[6] made a plea for investigators to stop arguing about different methodological approaches and return their focus to the research question:

> Our thesis is short—The question being asked determines the appropriate research architecture, strategy and tactics to be used—not tradition, authority, experts, paradigms or schools of thought'[6] (p. 1636).

## Guiding the data analysis and guarding against 'data dredging'

The data analysis must be based on the research question. In the absence of a clear research question, the study is likely to produce a wealth of data but no clear results. This can lead to the researcher looking for meaning in the data collected rather than looking to answer the question posed.

As an example, consider a hypothetical study that sets out to 'explore the effects of exercise on patients with cancer'. The hapless researchers do not clarify the aims of their study but decide to use a combination of assessment methods 'for completeness'. Quantitative data are collected on health-related quality of life, fatigue, anxiety and depression. Patients complete some blood tests and a subset also undergo in-depth interviews about their experience. In the absence of a clear research aim, the study will almost certainly 'discover' a variety of statistically significant findings. After all, the potential number of hypotheses that could be tested in this cohort of patients is legion—and by chance some of them will be found to be statistically significant. It is crucial, therefore, that the study has *one* primary aim (and no more than two or three secondary aims) that can be tested. The researchers should guard against excessive sub-group analyses (unless pre-planned) or exploration of alternative hypotheses not covered within the original aims (Chapter 2).

## To improve the chances of being successfully published

Once a research study has been completed, the results should be written up for publication in a peer-reviewed journal. The presentation of such papers follows a standard format, part of which includes a statement of the aims and objectives of the study[7] (Chapter 19). Checklists for appraising the quality of research papers invariably include 'clearly stated aims' as an important indicator of the quality of the research. In his guide to the critical appraisal of research papers, Crombie writes:

> Clearly stated and tightly focused aims suggest that the research hypothesis has been specified in advance, resulting in a well-planned study. In contrast, wide-ranging and woolly aims suggest many different issues were being pursued to see what popped up'[8] (p. 23).

Thus, if one wishes to have one's paper positively evaluated by one's peers (and editorial boards of journals), then it is important that the aims are clear and unambiguous.

# Generating the research idea

Individuals are sometimes deterred from embarking on a research project because they do not have an *original idea* to investigate. This concern arises from a misapprehension about the day-to-day business of science. New ideas or discoveries are few and far between. Most research is more mundane and involves a clarification and/or an extension of existing ideas rather than the development of anything truly original. How then should a prospective investigator identify a suitable area to research?

## Personal areas of interest and clinical practice

It is likely that undertaking a research study will take a number of years. Therefore, it is helpful for the topic to be an area of personal interest to the investigator. Many studies are conceived or started, but relatively few are completed and published. Personal interest in the project is likely to lead to a higher completion rate.

One fruitful source of research ideas is from clinical practice. Palliative medicine is a relatively new specialty and accepted practice is often based on very little evidence. Consider the use of a double dose of morphine at night as an alternative to a strict 4-hourly regimen. This is an area of clinical practice that is largely influenced by expert opinion and consensus; however, the evidence to support such practice is lacking. A recent study compared the 'traditional' double-dose approach with an alternative regimen and found the traditional approach wanting.[9] The details of the study and the validity of its conclusions are not the relevant issue. The importance of this study lies in the way that it posed a novel research question based soundly on a day-to-day clinical practice that most other practitioners had taken for granted.

## Reading the literature

The medical literature is a fruitful source of research ideas. Most academic papers conclude with a list of research questions that still need to be answered. Indeed, it sometimes seems that studies pose more questions than they answer. Although browsing journals for articles of interest is a good way to generate ideas, ultimately a more systematic review of the literature will need to be undertaken (Chapter 8).[10]

## Consulting patients

The National Institute for Health and Clinical Excellence (NICE) *Guidance on Cancer Services Improving Supportive and Palliative Care for Adults with Cancer* states that:

> peoples whose lives are affected by cancer can be viewed as experts on living with its consequences.[11]

If this is true, then involvement of patients should be an invaluable tool for generating and refining research questions. Users may add a different perspective on the research problem. For example, a patient who has previously been involved in a clinical trial may be able to advise researchers on the aspects of the study that deterred them from participating or improved their compliance. Users can also provide insight about the aspects of clinical care that they perceive to be most important to them, and thus ought to be considered as research priorities. It is increasingly likely that ethics committees and funders will expect researchers to have consulted users in the design of their study. Despite the attractions of involving patients in study design, there can be practical problems particularly in recruiting appropriate individuals for palliative care studies. However, many specialist palliative care units now have user representatives and there is a National Cancer Research Network initiative on consumer involvement in research activity.[12]

## Priorities highlighted by professional bodies or funders

Since most studies require at least some degree of financial support, it is prudent to know what are the research priorities of the relevant funding bodies. The NICE *Guidance on Cancer Services Improving Supportive and Palliative Care for Adults with Cancer* has made a number of suggestions on the priorities for palliative care research. These include research looking at determining effective solutions rather than re-assessing needs, longitudinal studies of patient and carer experiences, and evaluative research to determine which interventions are most effective.[11] The National Cancer Research Institute Palliative Care Clinical Studies Development Group have also identified a need for research in several areas including symptom control and access to services.[12]

## Prioritizing the research ideas

After generating a number of research ideas, it can sometimes be difficult to choose between them. In these situations, it is useful to have a scheme for identifying which ideas should be properly worked up into a research protocol. One method for doing this is to consider how urgent and/or important it is to find the answer to the research question. Ideas can then be categorized into four groups:[13] very urgent but of low importance; very urgent and very important; very important but not urgent; neither urgent nor important.

The importance of a question is obviously a rather subjective matter, but in terms of clinical research it is useful to think about the potential impact that the study could have on patients' care. The questions which are felt to be both urgent and important would then be identified as the top priority for research.

Other factors will also influence the priority that an individual will place upon undertaking a particular study. It is important to consider the practicalities of undertaking the research. Who will collect the data? Will the patients be able to complete all of the assessments? Can I reliably measure my chosen outcome? (Chapter 3). It is also important to consider the ethical aspects of the study. Studies which are too onerous for patients are unlikely to be sanctioned by research ethics committees, and even if they are approved they are likely to struggle to recruit sufficient patients.

## Turning the idea into a research question

Sackett and colleagues[14] have suggested that a well-structured research question should be made up of four components and be contained within a single sentence. These four components are: a problem; an intervention; a comparison; and an outcome.

This process of framing a research question can be summarized by remembering the acronym PICO—Problem, Intervention, Comparison, Outcome.[13] As an example, consider a study concerned with the use of gabapentin for the management of neuropathic pain in cancer patients. One suitable research question might be: (Problem) for patients with malignancy who have neuropathic pain; (Intervention) does gabapentin; (Comparison) when compared with amitriptyline; (Outcome) result in better pain control.

Framing the question in this way should prompt the investigator to think very hard about several aspects of the study (see below). This should result in the research question being refined so that the study does indeed answer the question that the researcher is interested in.

## A problem

A problem is defined as the patient, population or condition that is being dealt with. There are difficulties associated with either defining too narrow or too broad a population. For example, consider a study comparing erythropoietin and blood transfusion for the management of fatigue in cancer patients. If the chosen population is narrowly defined as 'fatigued, anaemic, in-patients with advanced breast cancer on a palliative care unit with an expected prognosis of greater than 6 months' then the study will benefit from having a relatively homogenous population. However, the study may suffer from difficulties recruiting sufficient numbers of patients. Furthermore, the results may be difficult to generalize to clinical practice because they have been obtained from such a highly selected population (i.e. will the treatment help fatigued *out-patients*? Or patients with advanced *prostate* cancer? Or patients with an expected prognosis of *less than* 6 months?). Alternatively, if the chosen population is broadly defined as 'fatigued patients with advanced cancer', then there ought not to be any difficulty recruiting sufficient patients to the study. However, the enormous variability in the population is likely to make any treatment effect difficult to detect above all the 'noise' from uncontrolled extraneous factors.

Clinical studies should be undertaken in a population that is as similar as possible to the population within which the intervention is likely to be used. In palliative care practice, the patient population often has multiple symptoms, the nature of which is continuously changing. Furthermore, the patients have multiple diagnoses, unpredictable prognoses and are undergoing (or have recently undergone) multiple medical interventions. All of these factors make the population difficult to define.[15] So what does constitute a palliative care population for the purposes of a research study? A pragmatic answer might be that a palliative care population consists of all patients referred to a palliative care service. However, there is a wide variation in which kinds of patients are referred to palliative care services across the country (and even more so if one considers international variations). Referrals may be influenced by factors such as the accessibility and resources of the local specialist palliative care service or the ability of funders to purchase such services. Even within an individual specialist palliative care service, there is a wide variety of patients within the so-called palliative care 'population'. Patients may be referred to the service for psychological support at the time of diagnosis, symptom control, respite, terminal care or bereavement support. Patients may have cancer, heart disease, respiratory failure or AIDS. There is currently no consensus on which patients should be considered to be 'palliative' for the purposes of research. This means that investigators need to be explicit about which patients they intend to include in their particular study.

## An intervention

The term 'intervention' is a very broad one. It includes treatments, diagnostic tests, prognostic factors or exposures to risk factors. It is usual for the intervention to be kept as simple as possible and for extraneous variables to be minimized. However, this is not always possible, and some studies explicitly set out to investigate the effectiveness or otherwise of 'complex' interventions. For example, consider the hypothesis that a multidisciplinary clinic 'intervention' alleviates fatigue in breast cancer survivors. One could attempt to test this hypothesis by breaking the intervention down into its component parts (e.g. counselling, optimization of medical therapy, physiotherapy) and testing each of these individually. However, this assumes that there is no synergy between the different components and that the sum is no greater than the parts. Alternatively, one could take the intervention as a whole and test whether or not it has any effect. The drawback of this approach is that it will not be clear which part of the intervention is the 'active' part and which other parts could safely be omitted.

## A comparison

A comparator is defined as an alternative intervention with which to compare the intervention of interest. Comparisons are usually with an accepted or standard therapy. To give a patient a placebo would be unethical when there is a proven treatment available. Thus, a new anti-emetic should be tested against the best available treatment rather than 'no treatment' or placebo. If there is no accepted treatment for a condition, then comparison against placebo is recommended. However, this is not always a straightforward matter. Consider designing a study to investigate the use of phenothiazines for the management of excessive sweating in patients with cancer. What would be a suitable comparator? If an inactive placebo is used, then it is likely to be spotted by both patients and investigators. It may be that the placebo needs to contain a sedating agent in order to keep the study blinded[4] (Chapters 2 and 3).

## An outcome

An outcome is a measurable study end-point. In some studies, this may be relatively straightforward to define. Thus in a study investigating the ability of clinicians to predict survival of patients newly admitted to a hospice, the outcomes will be 'clinician estimate of survival' and 'actual survival'. Both of these are relatively easy and accurate to measure. However, in other studies, the endpoint may be much more difficult to define. How, for instance, does one measure fatigue, breathlessness or quality of life? Even more awkwardly, how does one measure quality of death, existential distress or terminal restlessness? These questions obviously assume greater importance when one comes to the process of deciding upon the details of the study methodology. Nonetheless, it is important to consider these questions at an early stage. There is no point in choosing a research question that is 'unanswerable' because there is no valid method to measure the outcome (Chapter 7).

## Conclusion

Writing a clearly defined research question is the first and possibly the most important aspect of study design. If the question is ambiguous, then the answer will be too. It is definitely worth investing time and energy on getting the question right before embarking on a detailed consideration of study design or statistical methods. The practice of defining a clear Problem, Intervention, Comparison and Outcome for each research question is a useful technique for improving the quality of a study's aims.

## References

1. **Adams D** (1979) *The Hitchhiker's Guide To The Galaxy. A Trilogy in Five Parts*. London: Pan Macmillan. Reproduced with permission from Pan Macmillan.
2. **Gaicomini MK** (2001) The rocky road: qualitative research as evidence. *Evidence Based Medicine* **6**: 4–6.
3. **Clark D** (1997) What is qualitative research and what can it contribute to palliative care? *Palliative Medicine* **11**: 159–66.
4. **Mazzocato C, Sweeney C, Bruera E** (2001) Clinical research in palliative care: choice of trial design. *Palliative Medicine* **15**: 261–4.
5. **Stone PC** (2002). Issues in research: deciding upon and refining a research question. *Palliative Medicine* **16**: 265–7.

6. Sackett DL, Wennberg JE (1997) Choosing the best research design for each question. *British Medical Journal* **315**: 1636.

7. British Medical Journal (1997) Getting published in the BMJ. *British Medical Journal* **314**: 668.

8. Crombie IK (1996) *The Pocket Guide to Critical Appraisal*. London: BMJ Publishing Group.

9. Todd J, Rees E, Gwilliam B, Davies A (2002) An assessment of the efficacy and tolerability of a 'double dose' morphine sulphate at bedtime. *Palliative Medicine* **16**: 507–12.

10. Murray DM (1998) Planning the trial. In: *Design and Analysis of Group Randomized Trials. Monographs in Epidemiology and Biostatistics*, Vol. 27. Oxford: Oxford University Press, pp. 19–20.

11. NICE (2004) *Guidance on Cancer Services Improving Supportive and Palliative Care for Adults with Cancer*: Oxford, NICE.

12. http://www.ncrn.org.uk/csg/index.htm Accessed on 14 May 2004.

13. NHS-Executive-Anglia-and-Oxford (1999) Asking the question: finding the evidence. In: *Evidence-based Health Care—An Open Learning Resource for Heath-care Practitioners*, Vol. 2. Luton: Chiltern Press, pp. 3–16.

14. Sackett DL, Strauss SE, Richardson WS, Rosenberg W, Haynes RB (2000) *Evidence Based Medicine: How to Practice and Teach Evidence Based Medicine*, 2nd edn. Edinburgh: Churchill Livingstone.

15. Mazzocato C, Sweeney C, Bruera E (2001) Clinical research in palliative care: patient populations, symptoms, interventions and endpoints. *Palliative Medicine* **15**: 163–8.

Chapter 16

# Writing a research proposal

Chris Todd

## Introduction

In this chapter I intend to give some top tips on navigating your way towards funding for a research proposal. Before we go any further, the first thing you must have is a good research idea. Only if you have a decent research idea are you likely to obtain funding. However, just because you have a good research idea does not guarantee funding.

Most new researchers will be looking for relatively modest funding to support a specific project. As such, neophytes are likely to be applying to a charity or a government grant-giving body such as, in the UK, the Medical Research Council, the Economic and Social Research Council or the Department of Health, or, in the USA, the National Institutes of Health. Most charities and government agencies have numerous forms of funding arrangements. You should ensure that you are applying for a form of grant which fits the sort of study you intend to do and reflects your own level of research experience. As a beginning researcher, schemes for small 'responsive' projects or training fellowships might be the right sort of scheme. It is very important to ensure you are applying for a scheme for which you are eligible. Thus read the regulations for the scheme before you do anything else. Probably the best way to find out about sources of funding is through the Internet. The process is then normally to make a written submission (or online application) to the funding agency: most funding agencies have a form which has to be completed outlining the nature of your research and explaining who you are and why they should fund you. Most agencies have specific closing dates for research applications so that the process can be run as a competition for funds that are available in any one year. It is *very important* to make sure that you know the dates when specific funding agencies close their call for applications. Identifying the funding agency can be difficult, but you must try to identify the right agency for your proposal. Many universities, hospitals, hospices and professional organizations (e.g. The Royal College of Nurses in the UK) have a research office who can help you identify the right funder and sources of funding.

## How are applications appraised?

Whilst individual funders and funding schemes will differ, in general, the sorts of criteria that are likely to be used by funding agencies when deciding whether or not to fund an application are outlined below.

### Importance of the issue

This can be expressed in terms of the burden of disease. Burden may be to do with the scale of the problem, i.e. the epidemiology. For example, dying from cancer is very common and therefore important. Another component of burden may be the impact of the disease process on individuals, for example the patient and his or her family or the community at large. One could justify research into an uncommon problem because whilst it is uncommon it causes a lot of suffering, distress and difficulties for a small number of people. A third issue considered in terms of the burden of disease is the potential for health gain. Is your research likely to bring about change to ameliorate the suffering of a group of individuals or society at large?

Another way of thinking about the importance of the issue is what are the resource implications. How much does caring for patients cost the health service, social services or the individuals themselves or health insurance agencies? Is there a real opportunity for change which would make the provision of services more efficient and more cost-effective so that the same amount of resource provides a greater amount of care?

A further way of identifying importance is to relate to priorities set by the funding agency. For example, at any one time, the NHS will have prioritized specific areas for development. The publication of the Cancer Plan and the creation of the National Cancer Research Institute has set up a series of priorities for research in cancer including palliative care in the UK, during the early part of the twenty-first century. Many charities relating to medical and health research are disease-specific charities. Nonetheless, they will prioritize certain areas of research relating to their disease, and it is worth checking to see if their priorities match your research ideas. It is normally very important at the beginning of your research proposal to make it very clear why your proposal is important using one or more of the above criteria.

### Impact of research findings

In health-related research, it is quite clear that we are undertaking essentially applied research. Thus any funder is going to appraise the degree to which the results of your research are likely to make a difference in terms of prevention, treatment, management or care provided. Very often in palliative care research, the decisions are likely to relate to the nature and method of service delivery and organization. Are you going to be in a position to demonstrate that organizing care in a different way has an important benefit to patients, their families or the service?

## Originality

You will need to demonstrate convincing evidence that your work is original. Thus you will need to review the literature to show that what you intend to do will add to knowledge, and that the question you are asking has not been answered previously. This is probably most effectively undertaken by providing a systematic review of the literature[1] (Chapter 8). However, very often a systematic review in itself requires funding because it is a rigorous and time-consuming procedure. Beware, however, because many new writers of research proposals spend far too much of the few pages allowed in the application reviewing the literature and too little time describing what they themselves intend to do. Your review must be focused and appropriate to demonstrate the importance of your intended work. If a similar study has been done before, you will need to provide clear arguments as to why you need to do this study again. The obvious reasons may be that: (1) you will do it better; (2) you will correct some methodological flaw in the original study; (3) you will undertake a bigger study with greater generalizability; or (4) the original study may have become outdated. All of these are valid reasons for undertaking work which is similar to previous studies, but you need to argue this clearly and cogently.

## Timeliness

Timeliness is particularly important for health technology assessment and for service delivery research. If a new service is being introduced which is different from what has gone on before, it may be very timely to undertake a study of the new service. In a year's time, the opportunity to evaluate the new service will have been lost. The same thing goes for new health technologies. If a new technology is being introduced, there will be a window of opportunity for rigorous evaluation before the health technology becomes widely implemented. So evaluation needs to be undertaken when uncertainty is at its peak because, once a service or technology has been widely adopted, it is much more difficult to persuade clinicians and patients to accept evaluation or randomization to different treatment arms, especially if that means they do not get the most 'up to date treatment' (Chapter 3).

## Design and methods

This is probably the most important part of a proposal. You need to describe the design of your study and the methods that you intend to undertake in order to answer the question you have posed. You must ensure that the design that you propose is appropriate for the question. You will also need to ensure that your design is rigorous and scientifically sound. However, as well as simply ensuring that you are undertaking good science, you will have to make sure that the study has an acceptable design. There is no point in designing the 'perfect study' if nobody would be willing to take part in it, if no clinicians would be willing to refer patients or if an ethics committee would not be willing to let you undertake the study. The issue of ethical acceptability is difficult to define since standards do change with time. It is quite clear that some studies would never be acceptable, whereas others may be acceptable because they really offer a future advantage to patients. You will need to ensure that you comply with the ethical requirements of the funder as well as regulatory requirements. Another very important issue to consider when designing your study is the appropriateness of measures. The rest of this book is about study design, and hence I will not cover these issues in this chapter. However, it is all important that you design a rigorous, clearly thought out study and that you make your intentions very clear and *explicit* in your application. You should not assume knowledge by your readers—and it is useful to discuss your project with colleagues at an early stage.

## Feasibility of methods

A relatively common failing amongst new researchers is not to consider the feasibility of their design and methods when writing their research proposal. For example, are the participants that you want to recruit into your study actually available in the numbers that you will require? How long will it take you to recruit your sample of, for example, 100 patients? Does the clinic in which you work or in which you are basing your study see one patient a year of the sort you wish to recruit or 100 or 1000? If you are using clinical records, will you be able to access those records? If you are using biological samples, will you be able to access or collect the samples in the amounts required? Also, you have to think through not only the numbers but how long and the time frame required for your study to be undertaken. It is very important to be realistic here and perhaps even more important to realize that whilst you are being optimistic as you write your research proposal, it may be more realistic to be pessimistic about the numbers. It is almost a truism in research that the supply of patients who are suitable to take part in the study almost always dries up as soon as you start your study.

Once you have identified your methods and clearly indicated how you can undertake the study, it is going to be important to identify what resources you will require to undertake the work. New researchers seem to make two diametrically opposite mistakes here. Very often they will ask for too few resources to allow the work to be undertaken. It is not unknown to see a proposal in which when you think it through the researcher will have to work 18 h a day, 7 days a week for 2 years in order to collect the data. On the other hand, asking for too many resources can also be the 'death' of a proposal. So it is important to estimate realistically what resources in terms of personnel, equipment, consumables and the like are required to make the study feasible. It is important to commit sufficient time for preparation prior to the study starting and sufficient time after completion of the data collection for analysis, writing up and dissemination of results. Prior to the study starting, it is important to ensure there is enough time for any pilot studies to be undertaken and to arrange for access to the study site, the study population and the like. Do not forget that if you are using a questionnaire you will have to have the questionnaire printed and you will have to obtain permission to use questionnaires designed by other people, etc. Another important issue to consider is how much time it will take to set up the study so that it is acceptable within research governance regulations. Thus you have to allow time for your study to be considered by an ethics committee and for permission to be given for you to undertake your study. You also have to ensure that the health care facility in which any study is being undertaken has given permission and has put in place research governance mechanisms to ensure that your study is properly undertaken. Such research governance issues can take many months and must be sorted out in advance of the study starting. Most funders want to see the research they have funded appearing in the public domain, so time to write up is important.

## Value for money

You have to ensure that your proposal provides good value for money and you will need to undertake a careful and comprehensive costing. Many institutions have research finance officers who can assist you in undertaking your costing. You also need to provide a detailed justification of the support requested. It is no good just saying you will need a research assistant for 2 years. You have to clearly justify what the research assistant will do and why it will take 2 years. Thus it is very useful to sit down and work out a timetable and a clear schedule for recruitment and follow-up, etc. and the resources you need.

## Research team

As a new researcher, is it often very important to ensure that you have the support of other people. Very often a multidisciplinary team, including clinicians (e.g. doctors and nurses), will have to have help from statisticians, psychologists, economists or other health research disciplines to undertake research.

A very thorny issue for the new researcher is that whilst you may have a good idea and you may have actually thought through the issues quite carefully, many research bodies are loathe to fund researchers who do not have a track record. You will not be able to build up a track record without funds, you will not be able to get funds without the track record. The best solution is probably to find an experienced researcher, to act as a supervisor to assist you in your first studies.

## Overview

When considering your first research proposal you must think in terms of:

- What? The title, the question, the hypothesis.
- Why? The timeliness, the relevance, the impact and the burden of the disease.
- How? The design, the methods, the time scale and the deliverability.
- How much? Detailed costings and value for money.
- Why you? The track record of yourself and collaborators, the team and any pilot work that has gone before.
- So what? What will the impact of the study be, what will the outcomes of the research imply, what can it lead to and how it will be disseminated.

# Making the application

Most funding applications will use a standard form. The first thing to do of course is get your hands on the form, and to read it and any guidelines or guidance that are available on how to complete the form and the rules related to applying. Do not forget to check that *you* are eligible or that the study that you want to undertake is likely to be of interest to this particular funder. Check the closing date for applications and give yourself plenty of time to make the application. Even if there is no form from the funder, it is useful to structure your application using, for example, the UK MRC application structure. Some application procedures invite applicants to submit an outline bid or expression of interest bid first, and then shortlist bids to invite those successful at the first hurdle to submit full proposals. Probably the most successful strategy for these sorts of bids is essentially to write the full application (or at least do most of the intellectual work) prior to writing a precise expression of interest. Writing a 'back of an envelope' outline bid is unlikely to be successful.

The first thing that you are likely to have to give information about is the title of your study. This is important since the title must describe your project is but must do so in a way that makes it interesting. You will then need to write a summary of your proposal. Again this must be interesting and should normally be written for a non-specialist audience. Some funders actually ask for two summaries, one for a specialist audience and one for a lay audience. It is imperative that you make sure that your study is described in ways that non-specialist or lay audiences can understand. Remember, the review team may include people who are very specialized in your area, but will probably include generalists and user representatives as well. You must persuade them just as much as the specialist. First impressions count, and the first impression that you will be giving is your brief summary on the front page of your proposal.

## Contributions

You will then often be asked to identify what contribution each member of the study team is making to the overall study in terms of design, analysis, data collection, etc.

## Background

Most proposal forms then ask you to describe your study in terms of background or introduction, the aims of the study and the plan of investigation. In the background or introduction, you must provide a review of the literature which indicates why your study is needed and why it is important. Most proposal forms have a word limit or a page limit. Do not make the mistake of using two-thirds of the available space describing the background to your study. At the very most, you should be aiming for 20 per cent of your application being background, probably less. Outline the aims of your study clearly. Think in terms of bullet points and list the central aims of your study. Do not list too many aims but clearly identify what it is you intend to find out. If you are proposing a hypothesis-testing study, now is the time to outline and list your hypothesis. Do ensure that you list your hypothesis and the null hypothesis.

## Plan of investigation

The plan of investigation is the core of your research proposal. You need at this point to explain exactly what you are going to do and how you are going to do it. You may well wish to give an overview and then go into specific detail of how your study is to be conducted. You must ensure that you identify very clearly the participants or the sample, where they will be identified from (the sampling frame), how you will approach them, indicating how this approach will be made and by whom (yourself, a research nurse, the clinical staff?) and whether the approach will be on admission or at some other point during their disease career. You must also clearly identify the size of your sample and demonstrate that it is feasible for you to collect this sample size. You need to make sure that you identify your participants clearly, specify any inclusion or exclusion criteria and how sampling will be undertaken. Clarify your recruitment plans and, if you are assigning participants to groups, quite how you intend to assign to different study groups. It is not enough simply to say that patients will be allocated at random to two groups; make it very clear using CONSORT criteria how you will do this.[2] You will also need to justify your sample size. If it is a quantitative study, you will need to seek statistical advice so as to calculate a sample size sufficient for your hypothesis testing (Chapter 18). You should ensure that how you derive your sample size is clearly indicated in your application. This is equally important for qualitative studies. How participants will be recruited and how many participants will be recruited need to be made clear and justified. If you are, for example, using purposive sampling techniques, you may wish to indicate how many people you think you will need to recruit before, for example, saturation is achieved. You could only do this perhaps on the basis of previous work, but you have to provide an estimate so that reviewers can decide if this is sensible. You should also outline your data analysis approach in relation to these sample size considerations.

When identifying your sample and sampling frame, not only do you have to make sure to identify the numbers available and the inclusion and exclusion criteria, but you have to give very specific plans on how you will approach potential participants, how study contacts will be organized, who will contact the person, where, when and how. It is necessary to explain clearly that you will, for example, write to the participants at their home address or that you will approach them as they come to the clinic. You must not forget that in the UK, as in all other countries, there are clear guidelines and ethical considerations to be taken into account into how you are allowed to approach potential participants. Ensure that your recruitment plans are acceptable within the ethical constraints and the research governance arrangements in which you intend to work. The other thing you need to remember is how will any researchers who are working with you be trained or how will you ensure that you are adequately trained to undertake the study. You must ensure clear plans for training so that competent interviewers or researchers are used.

You will also need to think carefully through how you will follow patients up, if there is to be more than a single data collection point. This is particularly important in community-based studies or in longitudinal studies where the participant may move. However, it is equally important in an in-patient study since you will need to ensure that the time that you may want to return to see the participant is going to be suitable as part of their clinical or personal routine. When considering the sample size, you must also ensure that you allow large enough numbers of participants for your study to take into account the effect of people dropping out of the study and people refusing to take part in the study in the first place. Attrition is a major problem for all studies, but is especially important in palliative care since patients are often deteriorating rapidly and may not be well enough within 24 h of an initial contact to continue. Perhaps the most useful tip for ensuring that adequate numbers of participants can be recruited is to point out that if you undertake pilot work with exactly the same population that you intend to study, you will gain a good idea as to the nature of the problems involved in recruitment and retention of participants.

## Interventions

If you are planning to undertake an intervention study, you will need to describe your study interventions in considerable detail. As well as the data collection, you need to ensure that you describe the nature of the intervention and the control treatments in some detail. Make sure that you make it clear how the intervention and control treatments will differ in those areas which you are specifically testing. It is vital that you clarify the difference between your intervention and control treatments and that you make it clear how the interventions are delivered by the service. Ensure that you give precise details about how participants are to be allocated to groups if you are doing this kind of study (Chapters 2 and 6).

## Data collection

You need to describe exactly what measures are to be collected from participants and you should also justify them. Think carefully about which variables you are going to collect, in terms of structure, process and outcome variables[3] (Chapter 7). Ensure that you consider not only outcomes, but variables which may be confounders, and how you will collect this information to permit statistical analysis at a later date to unravel any causal relationships that may occur. Whilst on the one hand you need to be fairly abstract and conceptual in your thinking, on the other hand you need to be very concrete when describing the method of data collection to be undertaken. Exactly what measures will be used? It is not enough to say, for example, quality of life (QoL) measures will be undertaken. You have to specify exactly which QoL scales you intend to use and when, how and by whom they will be administered. It is also important that you justify the use of any measure for your particular study. It is important not only to think of the scientific principles (e.g. reliability and validity) but also to ensure that the instruments that you intend to use are practical and acceptable (Chapter 7). You also need to describe in detail the procedures for administration of any data collection instruments. This is important because unless you have given considerable thought to how you will operationalize your study, it is likely that you will run into problems when you come to try to undertake your study.

Once you have described how you intend to do the study, you must also describe the analysis that you expect to undertake on the data. It is often useful to involve a statistician at a very early stage of thinking about your study, if you do not have these skills yourself (Chapter 18). You should also consider talking to experts in qualitative methods or other methods who may be able to help (Chapter 9).

Once you have written your full plan of investigation, you will need to think through the timetable. Most application forms request that you outline the timetable for your work. Ensure that you leave enough time for each part of the project, but do also think about how parts of the project may overlap in time (e.g. you could be undertaking transcription or data entry before all of the data have been collected). You will also need to write a clear justification for any resources you are requesting. This needs only to be a few lines if it is obvious why you would need, for example, a Research Assistant to help you undertake the study, but may need to be considerably more detailed if your requests are less obvious.

## Costing

While preparing your research proposal, you will need to consider a number of areas of costing. Most grant-making bodies will make it very clear in the application forms what you are allowed to apply for and what you may not apply for. Make sure you read the forms carefully and only apply for things that are permissible under the scheme. You will also need to ensure that you get exact costings rather than just pull 'numbers out of a hat'. You should discuss costing issues with your institution's financial office or accountant to ensure that the costings are reasonable. Your project may justifiably require secretarial or technical support or other research staff, and you will need to include other costs such as travel and subsistence, consumables and equipment. You will need to seek advice to ensure you estimate the full costs of your study. You also have to think very carefully about the effects your research will have on the provision of services and what costs your research imply for service provision. These costs also have to be estimated, and you will have to ensure that there are adequate arrangements in place to cover the costs that your study will have for the provider of services. You should look at the Department of Health website in the UK to view the most up-to-date guidelines in this area, or check local arrangements for service costs.

## Benefits of your study

Many application forms ask you to explain what are the potential benefits of your study, and you should write a brief paragraph describing not only the purpose but the potential outcomes for your study. What good will it do for human kind to fund this piece of research? Unless you can justify the research in terms of potential benefits, it would be unlikely that most funding agencies will be terribly interested.

## Dissemination plans

Many funding agencies require applicants to outline how they will disseminate the findings of their study. It is very useful to specify your plans for publishing in peer-reviewed and professional journals, your intentions to present at conferences, and so on. You should include the costs of this in your budget plans. Do you intend to write a report and make this available? Do you intend to run a workshop for local clinicians so that you can tell them about the findings of your study? All of these sorts of plans may also have cost requirements which you should think about.

## Curricula vitae

Most funding agencies will also ask for applicants to supply a brief curriculum vitae (CV), and these are often on a standard form and can be as brief as one page. It will be your responsibility to ensure that not only is your own CV is up to date and in the correct form but also the CVs of any co-applicants. So do not forget to ensure that you tell everyone who is a co-applicant that you will need their CV in good time.

## Ethics and permissions

Many funding agencies will require that even if you do not yet have ethical approval, you have at least thought about the ethical issues and you are in the process of making applications to the right ethical committees. The rules here differ between funding agencies and change over time. Currently the practice in the UK and many other countries is that ethics committees will only consider studies for which funding is agreed, and funders will only release funds after ethical approval has been obtained. Thus it is important to ensure that you prepare your ethical application as soon after you have made your application for funding as possible if you are to ensure that you can start on time. However, check the regulations of the funding agency. You will also need permission from the health or social care organisation where you intend to undertake the study. You should ensure that you have letters from the relevant officers supporting your application. You will also need to make an application at an early stage through the research governance mechanisms which are administered by the health care provider. Check carefully what permissions you need and from whom.

## Common failings

There are a number of common failings to be found in applications made to research funding committees. Perhaps one of the saddest is a failure by the applicant to read the forms and the guidance of the funding committee properly. Careful reading of the guidelines and the forms will reveal, for example, whether or not you are eligible to apply. It is a terrible waste of time to make an application for which you are not eligible. Careful reading of the guidelines will also indicate whether your area of research is a priority and thus whether it is likely to be funded. Another very common failing amongst applications which are not funded is that it is an uninspiring project. Remember you are trying to inspire a group of reviewers and a funding committee as to why this is an interesting issue. Therefore, you need to ensure that you get across to them why anyone would want to research this issue. Another problem is that people write rambling descriptions where they have not structured their application carefully. Think carefully about ensuring that there is a logical and clearly organized description and justification of your project. Make sure you get the balance between the amount of text describing the background to your project and the amount of text describing what you actually intend to do. Another common failing is that the methods are poorly developed or unclear. Ensure that you think through the methods very carefully and describe them in detail. It may be very useful to undertake a pilot study prior to making your application to try out your ideas to see if they work. Occasionally funding committees see studies which are just poor science. Make sure that the method that you intend to use is appropriate to answer the questions that you pose. Make sure that the science that you are undertaking is rigorous and well thought out.

The funding requested can itself be a reason for failing to be funded. Sometimes people ask for excessive amounts of money for a study. It is perhaps less common but equally problematic to ask for less funding than is required. You must ensure that you adequately justify the funding and that you do not just, for example, say 'wouldn't it be nice to have a couple more laptops' and throw those in. Most funding committees will notice this kind of thing and mark you down for it. Again read the forms and the guidance from the funding agency. There is no point in asking for a quarter of a million if the top amount awarded is one hundred thousand!

Another common failing amongst applications is the amount of detail provided for what they intend to do. Paradoxically some applications fail because they give too little detail, whilst others can fail because they give too much extraneous detail. You have to ensure that you are giving sufficient detail for people to understand what you are doing and why within the constraints of the application form. It is probably better to give too much rather than too little detail, but you do not want to bore your reader.

Unfortunately for people who are new to research, a not uncommon failing is that the research funding committee will think that there is insufficient expertise in the research team. Ensure that you team up with people who have the right expertise and a track record if you possibly can. Remember that there may be a trade-off between the perceived risk that the committee may be willing to take in funding a relatively inexperienced researcher and the amount of money they would be willing to provide. It is one thing to offer £10 000 to an inexperienced researcher to undertake a study, it is quite another thing to offer £100 000 to an inexperienced researcher without a track record.

Sometimes applications fail because they have clearly been cobbled together from a series of previous presumably failed applications, and obviously so. Do ensure when you are writing an application that it is coherent in itself.

A very common failing for projects is the problem of being conditional. By this, I mean one should never in a project grant put forward a project which is conditional on some findings which you have not yet got. Funders are very loath to commit money to studies which depend upon the results of other work which is not yet complete.

Finally, plan your study with care and give yourself time to work up the proposal and discuss it with colleagues. At the end, carefully proofread the application prior to submission. You do not need to make your reviewers think you are sloppy by submitting a poorly formatted application, or one with lots of typographical errors. So check your application carefully before you post it off!

## Six top tips for success

1. *Allow time.* This is perhaps one of the most difficult things to do. Ensure that you have plenty of time to write your proposal. Keep a look out and identify as soon as possible the closing dates of funders so that you can ensure that you have as much time as possible to write your application. Begin writing as early as possible. You will be surprised at how difficult it is cogently to describe your ideas in a few thousand words even if you think you have worked it all out in your head.

2. *Select funder and programme.* Think about your study and see if you can target your work to a specific funder who is interested in this area. Look out for potential funding programmes that may be announced from time to time in the press or on websites. Many universities and professional organizations have services which alert researchers to potential funding calls. Once you have identified a potential funder to whom you are going

to target your study, check your eligibility and possibly even ring them up and talk to someone in the funding office as to whether they think the committee might be interested in your ideas. A telephone call at an early stage could save many hours of work.

3. *Read and follow the instructions.* Check what are the terms of reference, what is required in the funding application. As a reviewer, it is a great shame to see that somebody has put hours of work into what is perhaps a nice, competently written research proposal but which is completely ineligible because the applicant has not read the terms of reference of the funding call. There is no point in applying for a Post-doctoral Award, for example, if you have not already got a PhD (believe me, it happens).

4. *Begin writing.* Writing a research proposal for the first time can be a salutary experience. It may be very easy to discuss your ideas with your colleagues, but it is often surprising how difficult it is to write those ideas down. Write clearly and concisely, and beware of the use of jargon. Remember you are writing for an intelligent layperson or a non-specialist. Avoid too many complex sentences and avoid sentences that go on forever. Lay your work out clearly and structure it using headings and subheadings. Try to write in *plain English*. You are aiming for clarity more than anything else. It is also useful to write for reviewers or readers. Can you think of two or three people who might be the readers of your research proposal, for example two people who are the leaders in the field. Try to write an application which they will find interesting. Remember that reviewers and committee members have day jobs, and that for the most part they provide their services as reviewers or members of funding committees on top of everything else they do. So whilst you may have spent 6 weeks working on your research proposal, the reviewer and the research committee considering your application may have a pile of 50 applications to look at prior to the meeting. They will need to squeeze that work in over weekends or in the evenings, so you must write in such a way that it is accessible and clear. You need to grab and maintain the attention of the reviewers. You need to do this by clearly explaining the issue and why it is important; clearly explaining why you will succeed especially if others have failed in the past.

5. *Seek advice at an early stage.* You need to turn to people who can provide you with statistical or other methodological advice and who can help you with costing if this is not something that you are familiar with. You need to build your team early; find people who can help you and bring expertise which perhaps you do not possess to your study. Think of building a multidisciplinary team: statisticians, clinicians, psychologists, health economists, etc.

The earlier you do this, the more likely you are to put together a good and helpful team. Think about the layout of your study and the way you present it. Try to make it easy for reviewers and committee members to follow by using headings and subheadings, bullet points and to number points in the text so that it is obvious that you are making a series of different points. Aim for a well written and well laid out professional application. Pay attention to detail. However brilliant your research plans may be, if your application is full of typographical and spelling errors, this will reflect badly on you because it will suggest that you have little ability to attend to detail. That would suggest that you may be a bad bet in terms of the science as well as the writing. So carefully reread and check, and possibly get other people to read and check your application before sending it off.

6. *Be tenacious.* Whilst Homer Simpson said 'if at first you don't succeed, it's too hard', this is not really the best advice. If at first you do not succeed, try again, but use the feedback that is provided by the funding committee to whom you have applied to improve your application. Show it to a colleague and discuss it with other people to see if you can improve on your application.

## References

1. Chalmers I, Altman D, (ed.) (1995) *Systematic Reviews*. London: BMJ Publishing.
2. Moher D, Shulz KF, Altman D for the Consort Group (2001) Revised recommendations for improving the quality of reports of parallel group randomised trials. *Lancet* **357**: 1191–4.
3. Donabedian A (1966) Evaluating the quality of medical care. *Millbank Memorial Fund Quarterly* **44**: 166–203.

# Chapter 17

# How to gain research ethics approval

Peter Speck

## Introduction

Every institution or organization undertaking research which uses human participants should have in place a system of ethical scrutiny of each proposed study. The way in which that scrutiny takes place will vary from country to country, but should at least conform to the Declaration of Helsinki where Principle 5 states:

> In medical research on human subjects, considerations related to the well-being of the human subject should take precedence over the interests of science and society.[1]

Ethical review is designed to protect the human participant and ensure that he/she is able to make informed choices about any trials and investigations they are invited to enter.

Within the UK, Research Ethics Committees (RECs) came into being in 1968 and have undergone several revisions since then. The most recent of these has been the establishment of the Central Office for Research Ethics Committees (COREC)[2] which now scrutinizes all research undertaken within the NHS and requires researchers to submit proposals to the appropriate Local Research Ethics Committee (LREC) or a Multicentre Committee (MREC) depending on the nature and scope of the project. In 2001, new Department of Health guidance was issued which placed RECs within the new Research Governance Framework of the NHS. This guidance[3] now imposes time constraints on RECs in order to address a common complaint that decisions often took too long and were affecting grant applications. Decisions should be reached and communicated to research applicants within 60 calendar days of submission. Requests for further information should be limited to one occasion, and the running period is suspended until a satisfactory response has been received from the researcher. For amendments to research projects already commenced, a request for approval of the amendment should be answered within 35 days. With these time constraints in place, researchers need to ensure that their application forms are completed correctly, the accompanying documentation is provided in the required format, and they have addressed any likely ethical issues arising from their research project in the documentation or covering letter. For projects undertaken by students, their supervisors need to be vigilant since delays in obtaining approval can lead to students running out of time to undertake their project. It is important that researchers and their supervisors adopt a 'check-list' approach to ensure that everything is present and complete before submission for review if approval is to be gained. This includes ensuring that the correct signatures have been obtained, use of appropriate headed notepaper, licences have been obtained if appropriate, and that participant information and consent forms in user-friendly language are included. Incomplete application forms are no longer accepted by the committee for review.

While there is no legal requirement for research undertaken outside of the NHS to be subject to REC approval, it would still be deemed good practice for such approval to be sought. Many non-NHS bodies and universities have also established their own ethics committees to advise on ethical issues relating to research undertaken in their name.

The ethics committee exists to facilitate and not prevent research. Many of the major journals and grant-awarding bodies now require evidence that the proposed or completed project received appropriate ethical approval. However, some researchers may feel the process is obstructive if their proposal is turned down, or sent back for modification. A tension can develop between a research team and the REC. This tension can be creative if they are able to cooperate with each other throughout the process of study design, submission and progress reports of studies which have stopped, or been completed and published.

## What steps can researchers take to facilitate ethics approval? (Table 17.1)

### Ensure scientific validity of the study

The Declaration of Helsinki (Principle 11) states

> Medical research involving human subjects must conform to generally accepted scientific principles, be based on a thorough knowledge of the scientific literature, other relevant sources of information, and on adequate laboratory and, where appropriate, animal experimentation.[1]

Does the study have scientific validity and are there any potential benefits from the question being answered? This should have been addressed, prior to any submission to the ethics committee, by a process of scientific review, usually by peers. This review should look at the aims of the research, ascertain whether there is duplication of previous work and, if so, what is the justification for

**Table 17.1** Aspects involved in process of obtaining ethical approval

1. The scientific validity of the study (already peer reviewed)
2. User involvement in research design (especially pertinent in palliative care)
3. Does the researcher/research team have the necessary skills?
4. Does the research ethics committee have the necessary skills?
5. Recruitment of participants
6. Consent: information + consent forms
7. Confidentiality and data protection
8. Community considerations—relevance of any results to concerned community

repeating the study. Is there a justification for the selection of scales, tests and assessment tools that will be used, and are there better, more appropriate, ones? Have the necessary safety precautions been incorporated into the design (e.g. radiation hazard, exposure to toxicity) and has a risk/benefit analysis been undertaken, and the relevant licences obtained? Is the method to be employed appropriate for the stated aims and is the method statistically sound? Within the UK, have the requirements of the R&D Department of Clinical Governance within the NHS been met? This might include consideration of any cost implication for an NHS Trust of additional clinical investigations undertaken because of the research. Are there clear criteria for terminating the research or early withdrawal of research participants? Finally, is there clear discussion of the manner in which the findings will be published and reported?

## User involvement in research design

With the current focus on user involvement in the planning and delivery of health care, committees may also look to see if users have been involved in the planning and design stage of the proposal. This can be especially important in studies that REC members may deem to be intrusive or requiring the recruitment of 'vulnerable' people. The inclusion within a proposal of evidence that a study is deemed acceptable to potential participants can help alleviate anxieties that a particular study would be 'too distressing' to participants. This is especially relevant in the field of palliative care research. Where a research team wishes to commence a series of studies, which an REC believe to be intrusive or distressing, it can be beneficial for the lead researcher to meet with one or more members of the REC to discuss the methodology and any evidence of acceptability to participants. This evidence may be gained by quoting peer-reviewed published work, which may not be known to the REC, or by incorporating an 'exit-audit' into a pilot study to show acceptability. This can be especially important for studies of a more psychological nature, or those that use a qualitative methodology which may not be familiar to members of the REC who may be more medically orientated.

## Does the researcher/team have the necessary skills?

The REC may decide that the project design and aims are acceptable but have concerns about the researcher's ability to undertake the work. This may be because the research project lies outside the normal range of activities of the team or, in the case of a more psychological study, the researcher does not appear to have the necessary interviewing or counselling support skills deemed to be required. The prime concern of the REC in all of these situations is the protection of vulnerable people involved in end-of-life care or bereavement research. Specific attention to any limitations within the research team, and their provision of access to appropriate help and support if required, can often lower the likelihood of a rejection of approval.

## Does the REC have the necessary skills?

Some studies have indicated that there may be case for research ethics committees to receive some training in the variety of study methods used in end-of-life research, in particular those of a qualitative nature. Stevens *et al.*[4] interviewed the Chair and Vice-Chair of the multicentre RECs within the UK to ascertain their attitudes to palliative care research. Respondents stated that they reviewed only a small number of studies and felt less skilled to review those utilizing a qualitative approach. Some of the themes that emerged from the interviews included concerns that the study design should explicitly take into account the potential difficulties of recruiting research participants due to their poor clinical condition, high attrition rates and the importance of obtaining informed consent. They also had concerns about the impact of the research on the participant, the influence of the researcher, and the existence of adequate support mechanisms. There was special mention of identified groups receiving palliative care who might be especially vulnerable, such as children, older people, bereaved families and those from ethnic groupings.

Lee and Kristjanson[5] also highlight, in an Australian setting, three major issues related to ethical approval in palliative care research: denial of ethical approval because of a view that the palliative care patient is dying and should not be troubled by research; lack of understanding of the methods needed to conduct ethically sound research with palliative care populations; and an unbalanced approach that is weighted primarily toward a negative stance of 'preventing unethical research' without careful regard for potential benefits that may arise from conducting the study.

Bereavement research is another area where the REC may have difficulties in approving studies unless the researcher has clearly addressed the methodological and ethical issues. Stroebe *et al.*,[6] writing from The Netherlands, emphasize the importance of methodological sophistication to ensure that the research is 'good' research. They highlight the need to consider recruitment criteria carefully and the ability of people to say 'no' without embarrassment. They also discuss issues of timing of the research approach and the problems associated with evaluation of services.

It is difficult for an REC to be skilled in all these areas and aspects of work. While a committee can seek confidential external expert opinion, this can add to the time scale of obtaining approval. It is far better for the researcher to be aware of ethical discussion of issues relating to their specialist area and ensure that these are addressed in the documentation they submit to the REC. In this way, they can perhaps pre-empt some of the questions that might arise in committee and also extend the knowledge base of the members in respect of this line of research.

## Recruitment issues

The characteristics of the population from which the participants will be recruited and the means by which initial contact and recruitment will be conducted must be addressed. Statistical issues may also be a feature. Similarly, there must be discussion of how information will be conveyed to potential participants and the inclusion/exclusion criteria that will be used. In many instances, a committee would not wish the researcher to approach possible participants directly but via a third party. Thus staff in an out-patient clinic might give literature relating to a study to 'suitable' patients who could then express an interest or throw the leaflet away without embarrassment. This can be especially important if the research is being led by a clinician to whom the patient may feel a sense of obligation to 'help' because of their gratitude for care received so far. These issues are closely linked to those of consent as they help to mitigate against any feeling of coercion to participate.

## Consent

For consent to be valid, the participant must be competent to give consent, based on adequate and understandable information, in the absence of any coercion or inducement. Therefore, researchers should ensure that people receive an information sheet which is sufficiently complete and understandable to the research participant of whatever age is to be recruited. This information should be written in plain English, or translated into the participant's own language if appropriate, and include:

- *The title in simple terms*: what the research aims are, the method to be employed and confirmation that a research ethics committee has approved the study.
- *An invitation paragraph*: stating that this is research and why the person is being invited, together with the legal rights and safeguards.
- *Do I have to take part?* Explaining the voluntary nature and the ability to withdraw without prejudice to any current or future treatment and care.
- *What will happen to me if I take part?* What is required of the participant, any likely inconvenience, and effects of randomization if appropriate. Details of any lifestyle restrictions should also be given and the offer of travel expenses if required to attend hospital or clinic more frequently.
- *What is the drug or procedure to be tested, what are the alternative treatments, possible side effects of taking part?* For non-drug/treatment trials, details of interviews, questionnaires or activities to be undertaken should be given.
- *Disadvantages and risks associated with taking part.* These might be clinical risks or risk of psychological distress. If future insurance status may be affected by participation, this should be clearly stated. There should also be details of what will happen if other health needs are revealed in the course of the study. The participant's rights in the event of something going wrong and details of compensation arrangements should also be discussed.
- *Possible benefits of taking part.* If there is no intended clinical benefit, this should be clearly stated. However, possible benefits should not be exaggerated. If new information becomes available during the study, the participant should be informed and the options reviewed.
- *At the end of the study.* Will the drug or treatment continue to be available is a key issue for many and should be addressed.
- *Confidentiality.* Permission to access medical records and the protection of privacy and confidentiality should also be clearly stated, together with the method of storing personal information, as well as the anonymity of participants in any publications or presentations of results. Access to the results of the study and who is funding of the research may also be of interest to many participants.
- *Who has reviewed the study and how to contact the Committee in the event of ethical concerns.*
- *A contact person for further information if required.*

Many proposals become problematic at the REC stage when researchers have not given sufficient time and thought to the participant information sheet. It is helpful, sometimes, to give the sheet to a non-research colleague or family member and invite them to comment on its readability and comprehensibility. If you are very close to a particular area of work, it is easy to assume certain phrases and procedures are non-frightening or easily understood. It is on the basis of this information, and any subsequent discussion, that consent is obtained.

The consent form is an essential document for valid research and must be signed by a competent person: one who is capable of making reasonable decisions, of understanding the information given, and assessing rationally the 'pros' and 'cons' of a particular procedure. Researchers should be aware of issues relating to 'capacity' and be able to address these in the proposal if they are likely to be recruiting people whose 'capacity' may be questionable or likely to be compromised by drugs, pain, etc. (Chapter 3). Methods to assess competence should be described where children or non-competent adults are to be part of the study.

In the event of research involving the collection and storage of human tissue (as defined within the Human Tissue Act[7] and eventual Human Tissue Authority UK), the consent form may need to be staged[9] to enable the participant to specify any restrictions on the use of donated and stored tissue and organs.[8] For example, there may be concerns about the tissue being used for genetic studies now or in the future. The REC would expect this to be set out clearly within the information sheet and in the consent form.

## Confidentiality

Each REC will consider who will have access to personal data and other information about participants, how the data will be kept secure, how long any samples will be kept and whether they are likely to be sent elsewhere for analysis. Within the UK, compliance with the Data Protection Act is also a requirement. Anonymization is an issue if samples or the results of data analysis can be linked back to the donor. The results of some studies could have consequences for family members of the participant. This possibility should be anticipated if at all likely, and the implications of a sample being anonymized in a linked or unlinked way discussed with the participant. The possible use of data or samples for studies other than the one currently being recruited for should also be discussed.

## Community considerations

This is a new area of concern for RECs and requires some consideration of the effect of the research findings upon and relevance to the local community and the concerned communities from which the participants are drawn. As mentioned earlier in relation to 'user involvement', the community aspect requires researchers to explain the extent, and ways, in which they have consulted with concerned communities in the design stages of the study. Other significant factors include the extent to which the research contributes to the building of capacity within local health care provision and its ability to respond to public health needs. The availability and affordability to concerned communities of any product or approach recommended as a result of the study should be detailed, together with a clear description of how the research results will be made known.

This requirement links closely with the requirement by many funding bodies for researchers to outline the extent to which they believe their work will shape policy relating to social and health care provision.

## Conclusion

> The primary task of an ethics committee lies in the review of research proposals and their supporting documents with special attention given to the informed consent process, documentation, and the suitability and feasibility of the protocol[9] (section 6.2, p. 19).

If researchers are to obtain approval for their research proposals, then they must bring the same attention to detail to the preparation of their protocol that they will ultimately bring to the analysis of data and the publication of their findings. The time spent in preparing the protocol prior to submission should then be rewarded by a much smoother passage through the REC.

## References

1. World Medical Association (2000) *Declaration of Helsinki: Ethical Principles for Medical Research Involving Human Subjects.* Edinburgh: World Medical Association.
2. www.corec.org.uk See especially, guidance notes for applicants.
3. Department of Health (2001) *Guidance Arrangements for NHS Research Ethics Committees.* London: Department of Health. www.dh.gov.uk
4. Stevens T, Wilde D, Paz S, Ahmedzai SH, Rawson A, Wragg D (2003) Palliative care research protocols: a special case for ethical review? *Palliative Medicine* 17: 482–90.
5. Lee S, Kristjanson L (2003) Human research ethics committees: issues in palliative care research. *International Journal of Palliative Nursing* 9: 13–8.
6. Stroebe M, Stroebe W, Schut H (2003) Bereavement research: methodological issues and ethical concerns. *Palliative Medicine* 17: 235–40.
7. Human Tissue Act (2004). See www.hta.gov.uk
8. Medical Research Council (2001) Human Tissue and Biological Samples used in Research. www.mrc.ac.uk
9. World Health Organization (2000) Operational Guidelines for Ethics Committees that Review Biomedical Research. www.who.int/home-page

# Chapter 18

# How to use a statistician

## Malcolm Campbell

A statistician can help you at different stages of the research process, from designing a quantitative study through to writing it up. This will not be a lesson in Statistics, although several textbook and online references are included to help you find out more about the subject. Instead, the aim is to show you how a statistician may be able to help you with your research, how you can help the statistician help you and how you can benefit from the contact.

## Statistics and statisticians

Statistics has been described as 'the essential skill required for the collection, analysis and evaluation of numerical data', and the 'core science of evidence-based practice'[1] (p. 1), as it allows quantitative evidence to be rigorously assessed.

Statisticians range from the highly applied to the highly theoretical. They may seem to be precise, even pedantic, in their terminology, and you may feel that they think and talk in a different language. Statistics involves complicated terms and concepts as it has a mathematical underpinning, and the language has to convey exact meanings but, like most languages, you only need to learn a little to get by. It is well worth finding a statistician who can also speak in layman's terms (and some do!), but remember that you must speak to him or her in layman's terms too. Perhaps most importantly, a statistician may see your research from an entirely different point of view, providing you with a second opinion from another perspective.

One of the key roles of a statistician is to teach statistics. From conversations with researchers and students, however, Medical Statistics seems to me to be poorly taught at times, often pitched at a mathematical level beyond the comprehension of health care students and practitioners. Given its importance, this is a pity as the basic principles are not difficult to grasp, especially if presented in an easy to understand format with illustrative graphics targeted at the level of the student.[2]

## How a statistician can help with your research

Once you have formulated your quantitative research questions, a statistician can help you with designing a quantitative study to help answer the research questions; estimating a sample size for the study, if required; choosing appropriate software for data management and analysis; collecting data for the study and entering them on a computer; analysing data for the study; and with writing up the study in research papers, dissertations or theses.

The stage where a statistician may be of little use is that very first stage when you put the research questions together, although that has not stopped researchers asking my opinion....

## Designing a quantitative study

You should discuss the design of your quantitative study at an early stage. It may be descriptive, comparative or equivalence based, and investigate either cause-and-effect or association. There are a number of standard research designs,[1,3] which can be broken down into *deliberate intervention studies* or *controlled trials* (e.g. parallel design, crossover design or cluster-randomized trial) (Chapter 2) and *observational studies* (e.g. cross-sectional survey, prospective or cohort study, or case–control study) (Chapter 6). A statistician may ask whether you are using an appropriate design for your research question, whether you are collecting the right data and whether your proposed outcome measures are adequate (Chapter 7).

The statistician may discuss whether there may be any *bias* due to the selection of subjects in the study[1] (pp. 16–21, 32–64). This may occur if the participants differ systematically from non-participants, if groups in a non-randomized design differ, when subjects recall information differently in a retrospective study or when subjects are lost to follow-up in a prospective study. The statistician may also discuss whether *confounding* may be present due to the relationship between an outcome measure and explanatory variables being distorted by other variables (e.g. age, sex, severity of illness)[4] (pp. 177–80).

Intervention studies require allocation of subjects to groups (*randomization*) (Chapter 2); surveys may require *probabilistic sampling* to help guarantee that the data are representative (Chapter 4). A statistician can suggest how these techniques can be performed in practice.

Once the above have been taken into account, the statistician can advise on implications for the statistical analysis. There may be potential problems with missing values in the data, or it may be possible to adjust the analysis using regression techniques to allow for confounding[4] (pp. 98–106, 208–13). Analysis may be straightforward, or the study may require advanced statistical methods and software, which may raise the question of who should perform the complicated analysis.

A statistician can also help in the writing of the research proposal for a study, covering the type of design, estimation of the sample size and the wording of any statistical text in the proposal. Funding bodies often want to know where your statistical advice will come from, so it is important to include a statistician as a consultant or even a co-applicant. As a minimum, a statistician can act as a sounding board: as a reviewer with a different perspective, he or she may spot problems in the proposal.

The Research Methods Knowledge Base[5] and STATS—STeve's Attempts to Teach Statistics[6] give good general advice on study design online, while the Statistics Guide for Research Grant Applicants[7] is an indispensable guide to designing and submitting a quantitative research proposal.

In an informal rather than systematic review to see what kind of designs were used in palliative care research, I searched the public access BMJ website[8] for suitable studies, looking for those with the word 'palliative' in the title or abstract and at those in their 'Palliative Medicine' collected resource. Papers were included if they were published online between 1 January 1994 (the earliest online starting date) and 31 December 2003. Papers found may reflect the types accepted by a general medical journal, and may differ from those in specialist palliative care journals.

I only came across 20 quantitative papers in my search (there were six qualitative papers). Their details were analysed descriptively using SPSS® 11.5.2.1.[9] Not surprisingly, the most commonly used study designs (Table 18.1) were cross-sectional surveys, randomized controlled trials, and cohort studies where patients are followed-up repeatedly, an obvious design for palliative care research.

## Estimating the sample size

Apart from some pilot studies, research proposals generally require sample size calculations. A study needs just enough cases, allowing for potential attrition, to detect a clinically meaningful result. Incidentally, the definition of 'clinically meaningful' is your responsibility, not the statistician's! If too few subjects are recruited, their time, effort and goodwill may be wasted as the study may not be large enough to demonstrate the desired effect. If too many are recruited, some will have been needlessly given interventions or questionnaires. Clearly either eventuality has serious implications in palliative care research, where recruitment is likely to prove particularly difficult and ethically worrying.

Sample size calculation is based on the expected behaviour of one or more primary outcome variables in the study, depending on the research question

**Table 18.1** Study designs and statistical methods used in quantitative palliative care research in BMJ database (1 January 1994 to 31 December 2003)

| Study design | Main methods of statistical analysis[1] | None | Descriptive | Basic inferential | Confidence intervals + basic inferential[2] | Advanced methods | Meta-analysis | Total |
|---|---|---|---|---|---|---|---|---|
| Randomized controlled trial | Parallel pilot | 1 | | | | | | 1 |
| | Parallel | | | 2 | 1 | 1[3] | | 4 |
| | Crossover | | | | | 1[4] | | 1 |
| Cross-sectional survey | Individual | | 4 | | | 1[5] | | 5 |
| | Clustered | | | | | 2[6] | | 2 |
| Cohort study | Prospective | | | | 2 | 2[7] | | 4 |
| | Retrospective | | | | | 1[8] | | 1 |
| Systematic review | | 1 | | | | | 1 | 2 |
| Total | | 2 | 4 | 2 | 3 | 8 | 1 | 20 |

[1] Software reported included: SPSS (2), MLwiN (2), SPSS + Statistica (1), SAS (1), SAS + SUDAAN (1), EpiInfo (1), Metaview (1) and Stata (1).
[2] For example, $\chi^2$ tests, $t$-tests, ANOVA.
[3] Survival analysis.
[4] Analyses for crossover designs.
[5] Time trade-off analysis.
[6] Multilevel modelling, ANCOVA with clustering.
[7] Repeated measures ANOVA, multinomial logistic regression.
[8] Multilevel modelling.

and how such variables will be analysed. A statistician should have access to the relevant formulae, a look-up table or a software package to suggest answers. You should find out what he or she needs to know about your data in order to perform the calculations. This is usually in the form of meaningful ranges of values or differences you would like to detect. I give a range of alternative sample sizes for different clinically meaningful results, as the final decision on sample size is usually pragmatic.

Details on the most commonly encountered examples are given in good introductory textbooks on medical statistics[1] (pp. 335–47). Advice on how to adjust the sample size to allow for different sized groups, loss to follow-up, confounding variables, detecting interactions and clustered designs is also available[4] (pp. 413–28). There is also good advice online.[7,10]

The more common sample size calculations are supported by general purpose statistical software such as SAS[11], Stata[12] and StatsDirect,[13] while nQuery Advisor[14] is a specialized package covering a wider range of designs. There are some sample size calculators freely available on the Internet.[15]

## Choosing software for data management and analysis

The statistical software you use for data management and analysis will depend on the complexity of the data, and the nature of the required analysis, and you! For example, StatsDirect can be used for small data files and basic calculations using the latest methods; SPSS is suitable for large data files and simple designs such as parallel interventions and surveys; while Stata is required for complex designs such as cluster-randomized trials and surveys with stratification and clustering. The choice may also depend on your experience and expertise, and what is available at your site.

The *British Medical Journal* does not require the software used for data analysis to be reported. Although not a requirement of the CONSORT statement[16] for randomized controlled trials, naming the software lets readers know what is required in case they wish to run the reported analyses on their own data. Even commercial statistical software may use different algorithms, so results may vary from package to package.[17]

Among the 10 quantitative palliative care papers in my BMJ search that did report the software used, SPSS was the most commonly used package (three papers); it was probably used for several of the papers not reporting the software used. It is a relatively easy package to learn for non-statisticians, particularly with its point-and-click interface, and has an excellent Data Editor for data entry and browsing. It covers most types of analysis, but not the most up-to-date or advanced methods. For example, to estimate confidence intervals for proportions or percentages, you would have to download specially written command syntax,[18] or turn to other software such as StatsDirect. SPSS is not adequate for the analysis of data from cluster-randomized trials or survey designs involving stratification or clustering; you would have to turn to packages such as SAS or Stata for such complex analyses. Although both packages have a steep learning curve, they have made great strides recently in implementing point-and-click interfaces.

Important features to be considered when choosing software[3] (pp. 110–2) include the statistical methods available, the accuracy of their implementation and ease of use; you should try to use the same software for all analyses, if possible. The Association for Survey Computing maintains a software register.[19]

## Collecting data for the study

Once the design has been finalized, a statistician can advise on the way in which data are collected. He or she may make suggestions on the phrasing of questions or layout of questionnaires or pro formas, and how the data can be entered onto computer. You may need advice on getting started with your chosen statistical package, and practical tips on entering the data into the package.

Using a computer for data analysis involves coding the collected data into numbers, entering the numerical data into computer files and carefully checking them before analysis[20] (pp. 335–50). There is also some useful information online.[21] On the whole, however, published advice on collecting and entering data is rather scarce, and most researchers unfortunately have to learn by trial and error or rely on a friendly statistician's experience.

## Analysing data for the study

The statistical methods to be used for data analysis depend mainly on the *measurement levels* of the variables in the study (dichotomous, nominal, ordinal, interval or ratio) and the roles the variables play in analysis[1] (pp. 257–67). The statistical methods may also have underlying assumptions that need checking, and a statistician can help with appropriate choices of methods.

Among the 20 quantitative palliative care papers found at the BMJ website, nine used a combination of descriptive methods, confidence intervals or basic statistical hypothesis testing, while nine used more advanced statistical methods (Table 18.1). Analysis for roughly half of the studies could have been performed and reported by competent non-statisticians, but the other half would have required expert advice.

You should not run an analysis if you do not understand the rationale underlying the analysis, the meaning of the computer output or the underlying assumptions. If in doubt, talk with a statistician first to make sure you are using an appropriate approach, to learn what to look for in the output and to find out how to assess any underlying assumptions. Researchers often want to apply methods used in published papers to their own data, but this is only valid when the study design and the key variables are the same.

Some statistical textbooks give general guidelines on how to analyse data and report the results.[22] Others go through the common methods used in basic data analysis depending on the types of variables and the research problem[1] (pp. 257–67) or consider the appropriate methods for different research designs[4] (pp. 403–12). There are also several good introductions to statistics available on the web, including SurfStat,[23] The Little Handbook of Statistical Practice[24] and STATS.[6]

## Writing up the study

A statistician can provide advice on writing up the statistical sections of quantitative papers. If he or she has contributed to more than one stage of the work (design, data collection, data analysis, writing up) and is willing to defend the paper, then the statistician should be a co-author. As a statistical editor and reviewer, I can say that quantitative papers submitted to health care research journals generally fall down on basic statistical presentation. Study designs are usually sound, patient recruitment is usually well described, the correct statistical methods are usually applied, but the Results section is, frankly, often a mess. If a statistician is not going to read your paper before you send it off, it is well worth asking one for advice on correct statistical reporting.

Invaluable advice is available on how to structure and write a scientific paper, with illuminating comments on the editorial process.[25] Another source describes the growth of statistical reporting in medical research, looking at the statistical methods reported in practice and the types of errors in published papers, and gives advice on how to read and write a scientific paper[3] (pp. 477–504). Guidance to authors on statistical presentation in particular ranges from general advice[22] to highly detailed advice, from descriptive analyses through the more common multivariate techniques to meta-analysis.[17]

## How you can help the statistician

Time is precious for you, the statistician and, of course, for your patients. You can help all three by doing some research and background reading before any consultation. Try to think carefully about your research and data, and work out exactly what you want to know before the consultation. This will help you to ask intelligent questions, which in turn may allow the statistician to pick up extra clues. If you leave things until the last minute, and people usually do, the consultation may be too rushed or too late.

Discussing your research with a statistician will help you think more rigorously about your problem. You may have to grapple with new terminology and concepts, but you too may start to see things from a different point of view. In the short term, the statistician may suggest possible solutions that you can adopt immediately; in the long term, you should learn to help yourself by understanding the answers—you never know, you may be able to solve your own problems next time!

## Where to find a statistician

You should be able to find statisticians hiding in your local NHS Trust or Medical School, academic medical departments, or Mathematics/Statistics department—just follow the queue to their door! On the whole, statisticians try to be helpful and tend to be generous with their time. Good ones rapidly become rather overworked, so when you find a helpful statistician, check that you can continue to contact him or her in future.

Do not expect an immediate solution to your statistical problem, especially if you have a complicated question. Some questions may not have a simple answer, some may not have an answer at all, and the statistician, who tends to specialize in certain areas, may have to consult a colleague, textbook or a mailing list for further details.

## Conclusions

Good statistical advice is important at all stages of a quantitative study, from designing the study; estimating the required sample size; choosing software for data management and analysis; collecting data; analysing data; and writing up the study. It is important to get these stages right, so you should not be afraid to request advice or frightened by statistics itself. When you find a helpful statistician, check whether you can continue to consult him or her in future. You can help by preparing beforehand: think carefully about your problem, do some background reading or research, and work out exactly what you want to ask. Then make sure you can understand and apply the answers!

## References

1. Bland M (2000) *Introduction to Medical Statistics*, 3rd edn. Oxford: Oxford University Press.
2. McClelland G (1999) *Seeing Statistics*. Pacific Grove, CA: Duxbury Press. Also available at URL: http://www.seeingstatistics.com/
3. Altman DG (1991) *Practical Statistics for Medical Research*. London: Chapman & Hall/CRC.
4. Kirkwood B, Sterne JAC (2003) *Essential Medical Statistics*, 2nd edn. Oxford: Blackwell Science.

5. **Trochim WM.** The Research Methods Knowledge Base, 2nd edn. http://www.socialresearchmethods.net/kb/index.htm Accessed on 20 October 2006.

6. STATS—Steve's Attempts to Teach Statistics. http://www.childrensmercy.org/stats/index.asp Accessed on 20 October 2006.

7. **Bland JM, Butland BK, Peacock JL, Polonieki J, Reid F, Sedgwick P.** Statistics Guide for Research Grant Applications. http://www.sgul.ac.uk/depts/chs/chs-research/stat_guide/guide.cfm Accessed on 20 October 2006.

8. http://bmj.com/

9. **SPSS Inc.** (2004) SPSS® for Windows, Release 11.5.2.1, statistical software. Chicago, IL. URL: http://www.spss.com/

10. http://www.childrensmercy.org/stats/TopicList.asp#SamplesizeJustification Accessed on 20 October 2006.

11. **SAS Institute** (2004) SAS statistical software. Cary, NC. URL: http://www.sas.com/

12. **StataCorp** (2004) Stata statistical software. Stata Corporation, College Station, TX. URL: http://www.stata.com/

13. **StatsDirect** (2004) StatsDirect statistical software. Sale, Cheshire, UK. URL: http://www.statsdirect.com/

14. **Elashoff J** (2004) nQuery Advisor—software for sample size calculation, URL: http://www.statsol.ie/nquery/nquery.htm. Statistical Solutions, Cork, Eire.

15. http://home.clara.net/sisa/sampshlp.htm. Accessed on 20 October 2006.

16. **Moher D, Schulz KF, Altman D** (2001) The CONSORT statement: revised recommendations for improving the quality of reports of parallel-group randomized trials. *Journal of the American Medical Association* **285**: 1987–91. Also available at URL: http://www.consort-statement.org/

17. **Lang TA, Secic M** (1997) *How to Report Statistics in Medicine.* Philadelphia: American College of Physicians.

18. http://www.cardiff.ac.uk/medicine/epidemiology_statistics/research/statistics/newcombe/proportions/explanation.htm Accessed on 20 October 2006.

19. http://www.asc.org.uk/Register/index.htm Accessed on 20 October 2006.

20. **Bowling A** (2002) *Research Methods in Health*, 2nd edn. Maidenhead: Open University Press.

21. http://www.childrensmercy.org/stats/data.asp Accessed on 20 October 2006.

22. **Altman DG, Gore SM, Gardner MJ, Pocock SJ** (2000) Statistical guidelines for contributors to medical journals. In: Altman DG, Machin D, Bryant TN, Gardner MJ, (ed.) *Statistics with Confidence*, 2nd edn. London: BMJ Books.

23. Surfstat.australia: an online text in introductory statistics. http://www.anu.edu.au/nceph/surfstat/surfstat-home/surfstat.html Accessed on 20 October 2006.

24. **Dallal GE.** The Little Handbook of Statistical Practice. http://www.statisticalpractice.com Accessed on 20 October 2006.

25. **Hall GM,** (ed.) (1998) *How to Write a Paper*, 2nd edn. London: BMJ Books.

## Chapter 19

# How to write a paper

## Julia M. Addington-Hall

## How to write the paper

### Which journal?

Before you can start writing, you need to consider carefully which journal you intend to submit your paper to. Different journals have different requirements, depending on their academic discipline and 'house style'. In psychology journals, for example, it is usual for there to be a lengthy introduction which includes a full, critical review of all the relevant literature. In contrast, the same section in a medical journal is more likely to consist of one or two paragraphs, succinctly stating the background to the research question. The acceptable length of papers also varies widely, from 2000 words for some medical journals to 7000 words or more for some social science journals. If you start writing your paper without working out where you are aiming it at, you risk spending time later substantially revising it for content, length and 'house style'.

Deciding who your intended audience is will help you identify the appropriate journal. Often it will be clear to you that you are writing the paper for, for example, a palliative medicine audience or for a general academic nursing audience. On other occasions, there will be a number of options to consider with, perhaps, your findings having implications for family doctors, for specialist palliative care teams and also for sociological theory about end-of-life communication: in this case, thought needs to be given to whether there are sufficient substantive data to enable you to write separate papers for the different audiences (without, of course, committing publication fraud by writing a duplicate or redundant publication[1]) and, if not, who your priority audience is.

Other issues may come into play at this point. It may, for example, be important to you or to your fellow authors to aim at an academically prestigious journal; impact factors are often regarded as an important indicator of this,[2] but there is considerable debate about their value particularly in 'emerging' disciplines. Alternatively, you may want your paper read by large numbers of practitioners and feel that this would be better achieved by publishing in a professional journal. Another issue you may need to consider is the time taken by journals to review and publish papers, as these can vary considerably.

Once you and your co-authors have decided which journal to aim at, you next need to obtain, study and follow the journal's 'Instructions for Authors'. These are usually published in an edition of the journal each year and are available on the journal's website.

## Plan the content

You now need carefully to plan the paper's content. You need to keep an awareness of the ethics of publishing in mind while you do this: the data should not have already been published and care needs to be taken to avoid 'salami publishing', where the data are divided into small sections to increase the number of publications, resulting in potentially misleading papers.[1]

Research papers have to have a clear research question (or research questions), and they need a coherent structure within which that question is critically addressed. Everything in the paper has either to lead to or lead from the research question: the paper has to tell a clear 'story'. This will be refined as the paper is drafted and re-drafted. By the time the paper is finished, you should be able to write the paper's 'story' in one or two sentences. If you cannot do this, it suggests you have further refinement of your research questions and of the paper's story yet to do.

## The structure of papers

The basic format of papers is Abstract, Introduction, Methods, Results (or Findings), Discussion (which may be combined with Results in some journals taking qualitative research papers), Conclusions, Acknowledgements and References. Papers are often not written in this order, however. The Methods is often the most straightforward section and can be a useful one to start with, especially if writing is not proving easy. I usually write the Results section next as this clarifies exactly what the message of the paper is, and enables me to refine my plans for what to include in the Discussion, which I write next, and in the Introduction, which I then write. The Abstract is always the final thing I complete. You may prefer a different order, but you should not presume that you have to start at the beginning.

### Abstract

Once your paper is published, a few people will come across it because they subscribe to the journal: most people who become aware of it will do so following searches on bibliographic databases such as MEDLINE or CINAHL. They will read the abstract first, and then decide whether to obtain and read the whole paper. The abstract therefore needs to be both comprehensive and accurate. Some journals insist on a structured abstract.[3] Even where this is not necessary, following this structure when reporting quantitative research can greatly improve the quality of abstracts (it is also useful for qualitative work but needs some adjustment).

## Introduction

As described above, the Introduction's length varies considerably between disciplines. The basic content, however, does not. The current state of knowledge in relation to your research question needs to be described, the relevant literature critically reviewed, the need for your research made clear and its specific aims and objectives stated. It must all be related to the story you are trying to tell: a common mistake is to include interesting but irrelevant information. The ideal Introduction can be visualized as being funnel shaped, leading readers from the general area of your research down to your specific research question, and doing it so skilfully that it seems to the reader that your study was the obvious thing to do, given the state of knowledge in the field. It can be very helpful to read several 'Introductions' to papers in your chosen journal and to analyse critically how they have been constructed.

## Methods

You need to include sufficient detail in this section to enable another researcher to replicate your research, if they should do wish to do so. Journal requirements differ, but for a quantitative study you should expect to include information on your study design (including methods of randomization), the setting of the study, the participants (including eligibility criteria, and how they were recruited), issues relating to research ethics, data collection methods (including details of questionnaires, tests, investigations) and data analysis (what you did and why). If you are writing up a randomized controlled trial, you need to write this up in accordance with the CONSORT statement.[4] The same principles apply to a qualitative study, but the information needed by another researcher to repeat the study would both differ from that needed in quantitative research and differ between types of qualitative research[5] (Chapter 9). It would, however, be likely to include the theoretical basis of the study; how participants were sampled; method of data collection; how data were recorded; how they were analysed; and the steps taken to safeguard the trustworthiness of the analysis.

## Results

Whilst the Results and Discussion sections are often merged in qualitative papers, they are kept strictly separate in quantitative papers. Only those results relevant to the 'story' of the paper should be presented, but great care must be taken to ensure all relevant results are included to prevent misleading conclusions being drawn. Data should be presented in tables or graphically rather than in the text, and in sufficient detail to allow readers to draw their own conclusions. Detailed advice on the presentation of statistical data is available elsewhere[6] (Chapter 18), as are guidelines on writing up qualitative data.[5,7]

## Discussion

It can be useful to begin the Discussion section by succinctly re-stating the research question. This helps ensure you keep focused on the paper's story, and not get too distracted by interesting side issues which may make good papers in their own right, but are not the business of this paper. Next, state what you conclude from your findings. Be careful not to overinterpret these by failing to think of other interpretations or by overlooking conceptual or methodological limitations. However, do not ignore the good things about your research either: state clearly what your paper contributes to knowledge or practice. Some authors err on the side of overinterpreting their data and have to work hard at being sufficiently self-critical; others are so critical that they easily convince themselves, let alone their putative readers, that the work is useless. They need to be forced to begin their papers with a positive statement or two about the value of their findings (a particularly good response rate, perhaps, or the first study of its type). A well-written paper discusses the strengths and weaknesses of the research in a balanced way.

It is also describes and discusses the findings of other studies which support or refute the paper's findings. A common problem here is that authors rely on the literature review they did when they started the research, now sadly out of date, or they misinterpret other studies, perhaps because they cut corners and only read the abstracts of the papers (or, even worse, have only read what other authors have said about the papers).

Finally, it describes the practical and theoretical implications of the work, and makes suggestions for further research. Again, it is important to read some papers from your journal of choice as the emphasis and space allocated to theory as opposed to practical implications varies.

## Conclusion

To complete the paper, conclude by stating what you have found, what the implications are and what the next steps should be.

## Acknowledgements

Here, acknowledge the contribution of those who funded your research (most funding organizations will have a specific way in which they want to be acknowledged). You should also acknowledge the contribution of research participants, and of members of the research team whose contribution did not qualify them for authorship of the paper (see below). You may also want to acknowledge advice and support from other senior academics, members of your Advisory Committee, and so on.

### References

Make sure you know exactly what style your journal wants the referencing done in before you start writing the paper: this can save you considerable time and energy.

## Authorship

Who should—or should not—be an author of a paper can be a contentious issue. This is not surprising given on the one hand the importance of publishing for academics at every stage of the academic ladder and on the other the lack of clarity in the past about what justified authorship. There has been considerable debate on the topic over the past decade or so, with a number of organizations issuing guidelines appropriate to their disciplines.[1,8,9] Authorship issues are best discussed and resolved early in the life of a study, in the light of appropriate guidelines and institutional procedures. These discussions need to tackle not only who should be authors of which papers, but also the order of authorship—particularly who will be first author. Later revisions may be necessary, particularly if intended authors do not deliver papers on time. Care needs to be taken in all such discussions to ensure that those in more powerful positions do not overlook the rights of more junior team members, whilst at the same time ensuring that the contribution of more senior team members is not overlooked by those working on the study day by day. The discussion needs to be around who has made a significant intellectual contribution to the paper, and what that has been. The *British Medical Journal* and a number of other journals now ask authors to state what their contribution to the paper has been, which can help clarify the issue.[10] No-one should be an author without having read and commented on the intellectual content of the final paper.

## The submission process

### Submitting the paper

Make sure that you follow the journal's 'Instructions to Authors' precisely when you submit your paper. If you do not, you may well have your article returned to you unread. If you submit your paper by e-mail or in the post, do make sure you receive acknowledgement of the submission. Many journals have moved or are moving to online submissions which, although sometimes time consuming, does prevent papers getting lost is the post, which has happened!

## The review process

What happens once a paper reaches the journal varies. Some have an initial screening process, usually by the Editor or the Editor's Assistant. This eliminates papers which the journal feels would be better placed elsewhere, are clearly not of the necessary standard or are otherwise inappropriate. A rejection at this stage results in a rapid, if disappointing response. If the paper gets through this stage, it will be sent to one—or usually two—reviewers.

Journals without an initial screening process go directly to this stage. The Editorial Office decides on a number of peer reviewers, usually academics with relevant methodological or substantive expertise. They are then asked to critique the paper and to provide both a confidential recommendation for the Editor about whether the paper is suitable for publication and comments for the author. The reviewers' identity is not usually revealed to the authors, and many journals conceal the authors' identities too. An increasing number of journals are, however, now operating open reviewing, in which neither authors' identities nor the reviewer's are concealed. In most, but not all cases, the reviewer will suggest ways in which the paper could be improved if they think this is necessary. The Editor will then make the final decision, informed by the reviewers' comments, about whether to accept the paper as it is, to accept it if minor changes are made, to invite resubmission following more substantial revisions or to reject it. It is rare for papers to be published without any revisions. Most published papers will have been revised, often substantially, following receipt of the reviewers' comments. It is by no means uncommon for papers to be rejected by one journal, revised for another journal but rejected, revised and then finally accepted by a third (or a fourth ...). Novice authors presume they are the only people whose paper has been rejected and lose heart, whereas it is in fact a normal part of the academic process. The correct response is to revise the paper appropriately, and to send it off again.

It is not always appropriate to act on everything the reviewer suggests, however. The reviewers can often contradict each other, making this impossible. You may also feel that they misunderstood the study, or that they want you to write an entirely different paper (or do a different study) altogether. Sometimes their comments may seem completely unfair. If the Editor has asked for revisions, enclose a detailed letter when you resubmit the paper stating clearly what action you have taken in response to each of the reviewers' comments, and indicating why you disagree with the reviewer and have taken no action, if this is the case. If the Editor has rejected your paper, apparently on the basis of interpretations of your paper which seem incorrect or unfair, then it can on occasion be worth challenging her decision in a courteous and factual manner. This may change her mind. You do need to weigh the disadvantage of spending time appealing against her decision against the probability of her reconsidering, however, and only do this when you think you have a good case to answer.

## Your paper has been accepted

Well done! It has probably taken quite some time to get to this stage—3 months from submission at a minimum even if the first journal accepts it. You may be surprised to find there is probably still some time to wait before you see your work in print. This varies from journal to journal, and has eased recently as increasing numbers of journals make articles available as e-publications on the Internet before publication. In the meantime, you will be sent the proofs of the article to correct. Do not ignore these. They may well have been copy-edited in the house style in a way that has changed your original meaning, errors may have crept in at the typesetting stage, and so on. You need to read through it extremely carefully, checking it letter by letter against the original, including all the tables and references. If you can persuade a colleague to read out the original whilst you check the proofs, so much the better. The journal will give you instructions about how to mark up the proofs and you should follow these. Resist the temptation to rewrite the paper at this stage: the journal may charge you for all these changes. Make sure you return the proofs on time—there is usually a very short turnaround time.

## Your paper is out

At last—congratulations! Do not forget to send a copy to each of your co-authors, and to put one immediately in your personal reprint file (start one at once if this is your first paper—it will grow!).

# But I can't write

If you have read this article so far with sinking heart, because the problem for you is not knowing how to write a paper but writing itself, the following section is for you. Many of us find writing challenging. Although there are exceptions, paragons of virtue to whom writing seems to come as naturally as breathing and for whom no day is complete without a constructive spell at their word processor, most of us finding writing papers difficult.

## Is lack of time to blame?

I have carried out publishable research with a wide range of people: nurses, physiotherapists, social workers and doctors at senior and junior levels, some of whom undertook research as part of MSc and PhD programmes and others of whom initiated and carried out research as part of their clinical duties; as well as social science PhD students, post-doctoral fellows, lecturers, senior lecturers and professors. All of us without fail have cited work demands and lack of time as reasons why studies did not get written up, or have got written up slowly. As always with time management issues, there are notable exceptions: busy clinicians with demanding family lives who write up promptly and single PhD students who take up undemanding post-doctoral positions and still do not write the papers from their PhD. Time—or rather the lack of it— is, of course, a factor. However, it is not the only—or even the main—reason why writing papers can be difficult.

## Is lack of knowledge the problem?

Lack of 'how to ...' knowledge is another barrier to writing papers, especially for beginners. How should the paper be structured? How do I decide which journal to send my paper to? How do I know who else to include as authors? These are important barriers, and that is why I have addressed some of these issues above. However, again, they are often not the central reason, and they do not explain why even experienced authors can find writing hard.

## Fear of having others read your work

The main reason why we find paper writing so difficult is, I think, what has been described as 'the paralyzing fear of having others read your work'.[11] Writing down our research methods, our findings, our interpretations, our thoughts in black and white makes them accessible to other people, and thus exposes them, and by extension ourselves, to the possibility of negative criticism. Lively debate and critiquing of each other's work is an essential part of academic life, and of the advancement of knowledge. At the same time, we are often closely tied up in our research, so that criticism of it feels as if it is personal criticism. Also, as attendees of academic conferences will know, personal criticism dressed as professional criticism is not unknown in academia. Writing a paper can therefore face us with fears that others will think we are stupid to have reached the conclusion we have reached, that they will not be able to follow our argument and will dismiss us as lightweights, that—in short—we will be 'found out' as charlatans and exposed, or that the paper will be used as a vehicle for a more personal attack.

Some of the techniques we use which stop us writing also can be seen to stem from this 'paralyzing fear'. We may keep reading and making notes to ensure we cannot be criticized for missing some important literature, and to ensure our arguments, our conclusions are buttressed by as many authorities as possible. We may reanalyse the data, frantically check back to the original data, relisten to the tapes, to make sure—again—that our findings are correct and we are not going to be forced in 2 years' time to publish one of those embarrassing corrections. None of this is wrong: good researchers do read around and check out their theories, they do check and double-check their data—but they sit down and write the papers as well. We have to find a way (or even better—a number of ways) to overcome that 'paralyzing fear'.

## Motivations for writing

To balance the anxieties associated with writing papers, we need strong motivations for publishing. What finally motivates me to sit down and write is likely to differ from what will motivate you, and I have found different things particularly motivating at different stages of my career and for different writing projects. There are probably a number of motivating factors common to palliative care researchers, however.

### Responsibility to participants

The growth of user involvement in research in general is raising awareness of the extent to which research participants value knowing the outcomes of research, and that the results have been disseminated and used. In any research study, therefore, researchers have a responsibility to participants to ensure that findings are fully utilized. This can be a particularly strong motivating factor, I think, in palliative care research where the vast majority of our studies have involved palliative care patients, their families or the recently bereaved, all of who have participated in our studies at a particularly difficult time. I personally began to overcome my 'paralyzing fear' of writing whilst working on the Regional Study of Care of the Dying;[12] I felt strongly that I 'owed' it to the 3696 bereaved relatives who had often spent several hours painfully recounting the last months of a loved one's live to ensure that the findings were disseminated.

### Need to expand the knowledge base

Another important motivating factor for many palliative care researchers is an awareness of the importance of developing better knowledge about the problems experienced by palliative care patients, what interventions work and for whom. Doing good research studies is an essential part of building the much needed evidence base—but is of limited use if the study results sit locked in a filing cabinet drawer. This can lead to a waste of limited research resources when another researcher does the same, or a very similar study, not knowing that it has already been done. It can also lead to errors in our understanding of the effects of interventions, particularly as studies which fail to find statistically significant results are particularly likely not to be written up. It can be difficult, however, to persuade yourself that your study would add anything useful to the evidence base. Feedback following oral and poster presentations at conferences can be very helpful in developing a sense that there is interest in your findings, and in building your motivation to write it up.

## To encourage necessary changes

A colleague of mine reports that she has found it easiest to write, and has written her best papers, when she has felt angry at a particular clinical situation and thought that her research findings could make a difference both by bringing it to the attention of those with the power to instigate changes, and by suggesting what these changes should be (she was probably right—these papers have been widely cited). A sense of mission can be a dangerous thing if it is allowed to over-ride scientific judgement, but it can be an important motivator both for doing and for publishing research.

## Have to publish to get funding and/or build careers

Writing up your results because you consider that you owe it to your participants and/or because you want to add to the knowledge base of palliative care are, perhaps, rather altruistic motivations. A rather more pragmatic motivation is the knowledge that unless you write up and publish the research you have already done, you are unlikely to get the funding to do any more: most, if not all, research funding bodies will take into account your track record in completing previous studies and disseminating the findings when considering future funding requests. In addition, the number and quality of peer-reviewed publications are an essential part of the criteria by which academic researchers and clinicians are judged, making career progression and sustainability an important motivation for writing for many of us.

## Writing for writing's sake

Finally, in focusing on the difficulties of writing, it is important not to overlook how motivating writing itself can be. Some, perhaps many, people enjoy the process of writing itself once they get down to it: they enjoy shaping their ideas, finding a way of expressing them clearly, of searching for and then identifying just the right word. It can be very satisfying to complete a paper—or even just a difficult section. It is particularly satisfying to see the final paper in print with your name above it. It is not always easy to keep that final product in mind during the writing process or to believe that that will be the outcome, particularly if you are a novice writer, but it is worth hanging on to it as it can be a strong motivating factor!

What motivates you to get writing and, importantly given the often lengthy process of revisions, to keep writing will probably be different from what motivates me, and will vary from time to time. At some points you may find internal factors sufficient, such as the satisfaction of getting your ideas down on paper coherently and of knowing that you are keeping your side of the bargain with your research participants. At other times, you may be more motivated by external factors; awareness that you need more papers to get a research fellowship, or that your Professor is getting rather cross about the overdue paper (perhaps you can remind her about the one she said she would write …). What is important is that you find what motivates you to start—and keep—writing.

## Conclusion

In conclusion, this chapter has provided some of the information needed to publish a research paper in palliative care. It has also addressed some of the reasons why many of us find writing papers challenging, and considered some of the motivating factors which can help us start writing and then keep going through the often lengthy process of writing and rewriting, submitting and resubmitting. Many of us begin this process with some reluctance, are easily distracted from the word processor, and become down-hearted when our co-authors are critical or we receive another rejection letter. However, this is just one side of the coin. On the other side is the satisfaction of seeing the research we have done contributing to debates in palliative and end-of-life care, and to improvements in patient care. Research findings sitting in filing cabinets and on the computer can never do that—they have to be disseminated. Writing papers is an essential part of making a difference as a palliative care researcher. I hope this chapter has encouraged you to get (and keep) writing.

## References

1. **International Committee of Medical Journal Editors.** Uniform Requirements for Manuscripts Submitted to Biomedical Journals: Writing and Editing for Biomedical Publications. Updated February 2006. http://www.icmje.org Accessed 30 September 2006.

2. **Thomson Scientific.** The ISI Impact Factor. http://www.scientific.thomson.com/free/essays/journalcitationreports/impactfactor Accessed 30 September 2006.

3. http://bmj.bmjjournals.com/advice/sections.shtml Accessed 30 September 2006.

4. http://www.consort-statement.org/ Accessed 30 September 2006.

5. *Journal of Advanced Nursing.* Basic criteria for acceptability—qualitative research. http://www.journalofadvancednursing.com/default.asp?file=qualitative Accessed 30 September 2006.

6. **Peacock J, Kelly S** (2006) *Presenting Medical Statistics from Proposal to Publication: A Step-by-step Guide.* Oxford: Oxford University Press.

7. **Wolcott HF** (2001) *Writing up Qualitative Research*, 2nd edn. Thousand Oaks, CA: Sage Publications.

8. British Psychological Society. Principles of Publishing. http://www.bps.org.uk/publications/journal/principles-of-publishing.cfm

9. British Sociological Association. Authorship Guidelines for Academic Papers. 1 October 2006. http://www.britsoc.co.uk/library.authorship-01.doc

10. Smith R (1997) Authorship is dying: long live contributorship (editorial). *British Medical Journal* **315**: 696.

11. Becker HS (1986) *Writing for Social Scientists: How to Start and Finish Your Thesis, Book or Article.* Chicago: The University of Chicago Press.

12. Addington-Hall JM, McCarthy M (1995) The Regional Study of Care for the Dying: methods and sample characteristics. *Palliative Medicine* **9**: 27–35.

# Index